Respiratory Physiology

Look for these other *Mosby Physiology Monograph Series* titles:

Blankenship: **NEUROPHYSIOLOGY** (978-0-323-01899-9)

Blaustein et al: **CELLULAR PHYSIOLOGY** (978-0-323-01341-3)

Johnson: **GASTROINTESTINAL PHYSIOLOGY, 7th Edition** (978-0-323-03391-6)

Koeppen & Stanton: **RENAL PHYSIOLOGY, 4th Edition** (978-0-323-03447-0)

Levy & Pappano: **CARDIOVASCULAR PHYSIOLOGY, 9th Edition** (978-0-323-03446-3)

Porterfield & White: **ENDOCRINE PHYSIOLOGY, 3rd Edition** (978-0-323-03666-5)

Respiratory Physiology

■ ■ ■ ■ ■ ■ ■ ■ ■ ■ ■ ■ ■

MICHELLE M. CLOUTIER, MD

Professor of Pediatrics
University of Connecticut Health Center
Farmington, Connecticut
Director, Asthma Center
Connecticut Children's Medical Center
Hartford, Connecticut

MOSBY

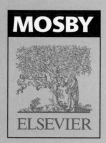

ELSEVIER

1600 John F. Kennedy Blvd.
Ste 1800
Philadelphia, PA 19103-2899

RESPIRATORY PHYSIOLOGY

ISBN-13: 978-0-323-03628-3

ISBN-10: 0-323-03628-7

Notice

Knowledge and best practice in this field are constantly changing. As new research and experience broaden our knowledge, changes in practice, treatment and drug therapy may become necessary or appropriate. Readers are advised to check the most current information provided (i) on procedures featured or (ii) by the manufacturer of each product to be administered, to verify the recommended dose or formula, the method and duration of administration, and contraindications. It is the responsibility of the practitioner, relying on their own experience and knowledge of the patient, to make diagnoses, to determine dosages and the best treatment for each individual patient, and to take all appropriate safety precautions. To the fullest extent of the law, neither the Publisher nor the Author assumes any liability for any injury and/or damage to persons or property arising out or related to any use of the material contained in this book.

The Publisher

Library of Congress Cataloging-in-Publication Data

Cloutier, Michelle M.
  Respiratory physiology / Michelle M. Cloutier.
    p. cm.
  ISBN 0-323-03628-7
    1. Respiration. I. Title.

  QP121.C56 2007
  612.21--dc22

2006046153

Acquisitions Editor: William Schmitt
Developmental Editor: Kevin Kochanski
Publishing Services Manager: Linda Van Pelt
Project Manager: Priscilla Crater
Design Direction: Lou Forgione

Printed in China
Last digit is the print number: 9 8 7 6 5 4 3 2 1

To
my parents and brother who have been my greatest fans
and to
my students who have been my best teachers.

PREFACE

My goal in writing this book is to provide students of respiratory physiology with a solid foundation that they will be able to use to understand how to approach pulmonary disease. My approach is to establish a firm base in physiology and to use that knowledge to understand mechanisms of pulmonary disease. Material is presented concisely in a manner in keeping with the limited time allotted to pulmonary physiology in medical school.

This book is written for all those individuals who have struggled to understand respiratory physiology. I was certainly one of them. While I knew that an understanding of respiratory physiology would be important in my future life as a physician, as a medical student, I couldn't grasp the concepts while I struggled with this new vocabulary. A wonderful teacher who subsequently became a good friend, Dr. Marvin Birnbaum of the University of Wisconsin, would ask me the same questions day after day and when I would confuse the answers, he would patiently re-explain the overarching themes and concepts. I did not know at the time, that during my residency, I would change the focus of my career and become a pulmonary specialist.

Each of the chapters stands alone but together they weave a story of the magnificence of the respiratory system, a system that is perfectly designed for its major function. I hope the reader will be amazed at the immense surface area for gas exchange in the lung that is contained within a small box called the thoracic cavity. It is an engineering marvel. At the same time, since the basic principles and concepts are directly related to the important functions of the lung and to states of disease in the lung, I hope the reader will find the information practical and not simply physiology for physiology's sake.

Having taught respiratory physiology to medical students for the past several years, I have been amazed at the ability of the student to ask some incredibly penetrating questions. I have tried to incorporate those questions frequently raised by students in this book and I have tried to use explanations that have been useful in explaining particularly difficult concepts. I look to their feedback to improve my teaching and the usefulness of this book. Hopefully, the material in this book will be useful not only to medical students but to graduate, allied health, and nursing students. This book is also intended for residents and fellows in all subspecialties who wish to review physiologic concepts in their approach to patients with pulmonary disease.

I am grateful to the many individuals at Elsevier who helped me in preparing this book and to Ms. Krissy Larrow who early on helped to format the chapters and get the figures in order. I hope you will enjoy reading this book as much as I enjoyed preparing it.

Michelle M. Cloutier

CONTENTS

CHAPTER 7

VENTILATION (V̇), PERFUSION (Q̇) & RELATIONSHIPS   101

CHAPTER 8

OXYGEN AND CARBON DIOXIDE TRANSPORT 113

CHAPTER 9

PULMONARY ASPECTS OF ACID-BASE BALANCE AND ARTERIAL BLOOD GAS INTERPRETATION 133

CHAPTER 10

CONTROL OF RESPIRATION . . 145

CHAPTER 11

NONRESPIRATORY FUNCTIONS OF THE LUNG 163

CHAPTER **12**

THE LUNG UNDER SPECIAL CIRCUMSTANCES 183

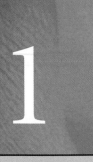

1

OVERVIEW OF THE RESPIRATORY SYSTEM: FUNCTION AND STRUCTURE

OBJECTIVES

1. Introduce the rules that govern gases in gaseous and aqueous phases.
2. Outline and briefly describe the components of respiration including:
   - The alveolar capillary unit
   - The alveolar surface
   - The pulmonary circulation

   - The conducting airways
   - The cells of the airway
   - The muscles of respiration
   - The central nervous system and neural pathways regulating respiration
3. Relate lung structure to lung function.

Breathing is essential to life. Without breathing and a fresh supply of oxygen, the cells in the body will die in approximately 5 minutes. In addition to supplying oxygen to the cells and tissues, carbon dioxide, a by-product of aerobic metabolism, must be eliminated. Thus, in order for tissues to function normally, a continuous supply of oxygen and a system for removing carbon dioxide are needed. *The principal function of the respiratory system is to bring oxygen from the external environment to the tissues in the body and to remove from the body the carbon dioxide produced by cell metabolism.* Other functions of the lung include acid-base balance (see Chapter 9), and host defense, metabolism, and handling of bioactive materials (see Chapter 11).

Respiratory physiology is the study of how oxygen is brought into the lungs and delivered to the tissues and how carbon dioxide is removed. It includes breathing and the circulation of blood to and from tissue capillaries. The **respiratory system** is composed of the lungs, the upper and lower airways including the nose,

the chest wall including the muscles of respiration (diaphragm, intercostal muscles, and abdominal muscles) and the rib cage, and those parts of the central nervous system that regulate respiration. The important components of gas exchange include the gases being inhaled, the characteristics of the conducting airways, the gas-exchanging unit, the pulmonary circulation that regulates blood flow through the gas-exchanging unit, and the muscles that move gas in and out of the lung.

Breathing is automatic, rhythmic, and under the control of the central nervous system. Gas exchange begins with inspiration, which is initiated by the contraction of the **diaphragm**, the major muscle of respiration. Upon contraction, the diaphragm moves into the abdominal cavity; this movement creates a negative pressure inside the chest. The upper airway (**glottis**) opens, creating an opening from the outside world to the inside of the lung. Because gases always flow from areas of higher pressure to areas of lower pressure and because the pressure inside the lung and airways during inspiration is less than atmospheric pressure, air moves into the lung in the same way that a vacuum cleaner sucks air into the canister. The volume of air inside the lung increases and gas moves into the **alveoli**, the gas-exchanging units of the body, where oxygen (O_2) is taken up and carbon dioxide (CO_2) is eliminated. During exhalation, the diaphragm and the other muscles of respiration relax, the pressure inside the chest and airways increases and becomes greater than atmospheric pressure, the glottis opens, and gas flows passively out of the lungs.

MOVEMENT OF GASES

An understanding of the rules that govern gases and the movement of gases from gaseous to liquid phases and familiarity with their terminology are essential to understanding respiratory physiology.

Air is composed of a mixture of gases that exert a pressure. Each individual gas exerts its own pressure, known as its **partial pressure**. The partial pressure of the individual gases is the product of the total gas pressure and the proportion of total gas composition made up by the specific gas of interest (see Chapter 5). For example, at sea level the total ambient pressure, also known as the **barometric pressure**, is 760 mm Hg. Air is composed of approximately 21% oxygen. Thus, at sea level the partial pressure of oxygen is 0.21×760 mm Hg = 160 mm Hg.

Of the various laws that govern gases, the most important in regard to the respiratory system is **Dalton's law**. Dalton's law states that the sum of the partial pressure of the gases in a gas mixture must be equal to the total pressure. That is, each individual gas in a gas mixture exerts its own partial pressure, and the sum of all of the partial pressures is equal to the total pressure. Because the total pressure is fixed, as the pressure exerted by one specific gas increases, the pressure exerted by another must decrease. As described later in Chapter 5, when carbon dioxide in the alveolus increases, the partial pressure of oxygen in the alveolus must decrease.

HOW A PRESSURE GRADIENT IS GENERATED

The second important property of gases, including air, is that gases move from regions of higher pressure to regions of lower pressure. The movement of air in and out of the lungs requires the creation of a pressure gradient from the inside of the alveoli to the outside world. Pressure changes within the airways are, by convention, referenced to barometric pressure. Since the absolute barometric pressure is different at different altitudes, again by convention, the pressure surrounding the chest wall (the barometric pressure) is considered to be zero when pressure gradients are being measured. Inspiration occurs when negative pressure is generated inside the alveoli; that is to say, when alveolar pressure is made lower than atmospheric pressure.

Alveoli are not capable of expanding on their own. They will expand only when there is an increase in the distending pressure across their walls. The distending pressure across the alveolar wall is called the **transmural** (mural, meaning any wall) or **transpulmonary** (across the lung; that is, from the alveolus to the pleura) pressure gradient and it is generated by the muscles of inspiration. Before airflow begins, the pressure inside the alveoli is the same as atmospheric pressure, which by convention, as described previously, is equal to 0 cm H_2O. An important principle of respiration is that pressures at the pleural surface generated by the muscles of respiration are transmitted through the alveolar walls to the more centrally located alveoli and small airways. Thus, alveolar units are structurally interdependent.

During inspiration, as the muscles of inspiration contract, the pressure inside the airways decreases relative to barometric pressure (that is, it becomes less than atmospheric pressure or "negative" relative to the "zero" atmospheric pressure) according to **Boyle's law**. Boyle's law states that in a closed container at a constant temperature, pressure multiplied by volume is constant. Thus, if the pressure in the alveoli decreases, the volume in the alveoli must increase. For example, during inspiration the pressure inside the airways is −5 cm H_2O. That is, it is 5 cm H_2O less than atmospheric pressure (zero), but the actual pressure, assuming that you are at sea level, would be 760 mm Hg −5 cm H_2O (note the different units). During exhalation, the process is reversed, and the pressure inside the airways becomes greater than atmospheric pressure. The important principle to remember is that gases always flow from an area of higher pressure to an area of lower pressure.

In the respiratory system, we must also consider the partial pressure of a gas in a liquid phase—namely, the blood. When a liquid is in contact with a gas mixture, the partial pressure of the particular gas in the liquid is the same as its partial pressure in the gas mixture, assuming that full equilibration has occurred. Therefore, the partial pressure of the gas acts as the "driving force" for the gas to be carried in the liquid phase.

However, the quantity of a gas that can be carried by the liquid medium (e.g., blood) depends on the "capacity" of the liquid for that particular gas. For example, if a gas is very soluble in the liquid, more of that particular gas will be carried in a given pressure compared to a less soluble gas. In addition, and most important for the respiratory system, if the liquid is able to bind or carry more of the gas, more of the gas will be transported at a particular partial pressure. The interaction of hemoglobin in the red blood cells and oxygen allows more oxygen to be transported at any partial pressure and is the major transport system in the body for oxygen (see Chapter 8).

STRUCTURE OF THE RESPIRATORY SYSTEM

Gas flows into the lung through either the nasopharynx or the oropharynx into the larynx, the trachea (windpipe) and then a series of branching tubes (Fig. 1-1). The trachea divides at the carina, or "keel" (so named because it looks like the keel of a boat), into the right and left main-stem bronchi that penetrate the lung **parenchyma** (tissue of the lung). Main-stem bronchi

branch into lobar bronchi (three on the right and two on the left) that in turn branch into segmental bronchi and an extensive system of subsegmental and smaller bronchi. Airway branching is dichotomous—that is, it is asymmetric. As a result, while in general there are between 15 and 20 generations of airways from the trachea to the level of the terminal bronchioles, there can be as few as 10 or as many as 20 generations (Fig. 1-2).

We now describe each of the important components of respiration. Many of these components are described in greater detail in subsequent chapters.

Alveolar-capillary Unit

Gas exchange occurs in the alveoli through a dense mesh-like network of capillaries and alveoli called the **alveolar-capillary network** (Fig. 1-3). The alveolar-capillary unit consists of the respiratory bronchioles, the alveolar ducts, the alveoli, and the pulmonary capillary bed. It is the basic **physiologic unit of the lung**. It is characterized by a large surface area and a blood supply that originates from the pulmonary arteries. In the adult, there are approximately 300 million alveoli, which are 250 microns in size and are entirely surrounded by capillaries. In addition, there are 280 billion capillaries in the lung or almost 1000 capillaries for each alveolus. The result of this incredible number of alveoli and capillaries is that there is a large surface area for gas exchange—approximately 50 to 100 m^2. This occurs in a space that is only 5 mm in length and is one of the most remarkable engineering feats in the body.

The barrier between the gas in the alveoli and the red blood cells is only 1 to 2 μ in thickness and consists of type I alveolar epithelial cells, capillary endothelial cells, and their respective basement membranes (Fig. 1-4). O_2 and CO_2 passively diffuse across this barrier into plasma and red blood cells. **Diffusion** is the passive thermodynamic flow of molecules between regions with different partial pressures. O_2 and CO_2 diffusion must occur between alveolar gas and blood in the pulmonary capillaries and between blood in the systemic capillary circulation and the cells in the tissue. Red blood cells pass through the pulmonary network in less than one second, which is sufficient time for CO_2 and O_2 gas exchange to occur.

In some regions of the alveolar wall, there is nothing between the airway epithelial cells and the capillary

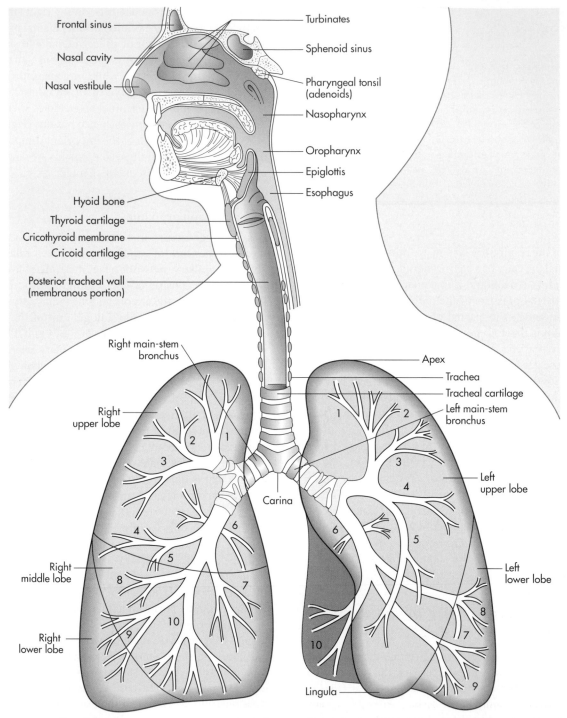

FIGURE 1-1 ■ Schematic diagram of the respiratory system including the bronchopulmonary segments; anterior view. Numbers refer to bronchopulmonary segments: 1, apical; 2, posterior; 3, anterior; 4, lateral (superior on the left); 5, medial (inferior on the left); 6, superior; 7, medial basal; 8, anterior basal; 9, lateral basal; 10, posterior basal.

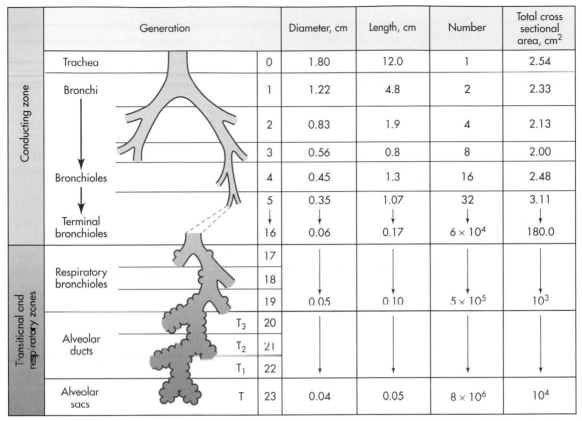

	Generation			Diameter, cm	Length, cm	Number	Total cross sectional area, cm^2
Conducting zone	Trachea		0	1.80	12.0	1	2.54
	Bronchi		1	1.22	4.8	2	2.33
			2	0.83	1.9	4	2.13
			3	0.56	0.8	8	2.00
	Bronchioles		4	0.45	1.3	16	2.48
			5 ↓ 16	0.35 ↓ 0.06	1.07 ↓ 0.17	32 ↓ 6×10^4	3.11 ↓ 180.0
	Terminal bronchioles						
Transitional and respiratory zones	Respiratory bronchioles		17				
			18				
			19	0.05	0.10	5×10^5	10^3
	Alveolar ducts	T$_3$	20				
		T$_2$	21				
		T$_1$	22				
	Alveolar sacs	T	23	0.04	0.05	8×10^6	10^4

FIGURE 1-2 ■ Airway generations and approximate dimensions in the human lung. In the adult, alveoli can be found as early as the 10th airway generation and as late as the 23rd generation. *(Redrawn from Weibel Er: Morphometry of the Human Lung. Springer Verlag, Berlin, 1963. Data from Bouhuys A: The Physiology of Breathing. Grune & Stratton, New York, 1977.)*

endothelial cells other than their basement membranes that are fused to form a single basement membrane. In other regions, there is a space between the epithelial and endothelial cells called the **interstitial space** or **interstitium** (see Fig. 1-4). The interstitium is composed of collagen, elastin, proteoglycans, a variety of macromolecules involved with cell-cell and cell-matrix interactions, some nerve endings, and some fibroblast-like cells. There are also small numbers of lymphocytes that have migrated out of the circulation in the interstitium.

Alveolar Surface

The alveolar epithelium is a continuous layer of tissue composed primarily of **type I cells** or squamous pneumocytes. These cells have broad, thin extensions that cover approximately 93% of the alveolar

surface (Fig. 1-5). They are highly differentiated cells that do not divide, which makes them particularly susceptible to injury from inhaled or aspirated toxins. The thin cytoplasm of the type I cell is ideal for optimal gas diffusion.

Type II cells, or granular pneumocytes, are more numerous than type I cells; however, because of their cuboidal shape, they occupy only approximately 7% of the alveolar surface and are located in the corners of the alveolus (see Fig. 1-5). The hallmarks of the type II cell are their microvilli and their osmiophilic lamellar inclusion bodies that contain **surfactant**, a compound with a high lipid content that acts as a detergent to reduce the surface tension of the alveoli (Fig. 1-6; also see Chapter 2). The type II cell is the progenitor cell of the alveolar epithelium. When there is injury to

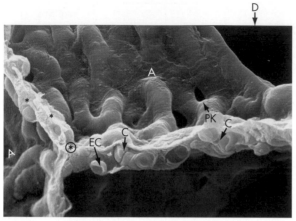

FIGURE 1-3 ■ Scanning electron micrograph of an alveolar surface demonstrating the alveolar septum. Capillaries (C) are seen in cross section in the foreground with erythrocytes (EC) in their lumen. At the *circled asteri*sk, three septae come together. The septae are held together by connective tissue fibers *(uncircled asterisks)*. A, alveolus; D, alveolar duct; PK, pores of Kohn. *(Micrograph Courtesy of Weibel ER, Institute of Anatomy, University of Berne, Switzerland.)*

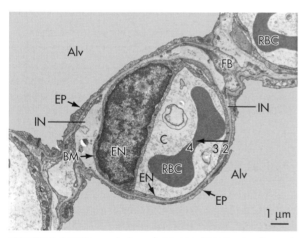

FIGURE 1-4 ■ Transmission electron micrograph of a pulmonary capillary in cross section. Alveoli (Alv) are on either side of the capillary that is shown with a red blood cell (RBC). The diffusion pathway for oxygen and carbon dioxide *(arrow)* consists of the areas numbered 2, 3, and 4, which are the alveolar-capillary barrier, plasma, and erythrocyte, respectively. BM, basement membrane; C, capillary; EN, capillary endothelial cell (note its very large nucleus); EP, alveolar epithelial cell; FB, fibroblast process; IN, interstitial space. *(Reproduced with permission from Weibel ER: Morphometric Estimation of Pulmonary diffusion capacity, I. Model & Method. Respir physiol 11:54, 1970.)*

the type I cell, the type II cell multiplies and eventually differentiates into a type I cell. In a group of diseases that result in pulmonary fibrosis, the type I cell is injured and the alveolar epithelium is now lined entirely by type II cells, a condition that is not conducive to optimal gas exchange. This repair system is an example of **phylogeny recapitulating ontogeny** because the epithelium of the alveolus is composed entirely of type II cells until very late in gestation.

The lumen of the alveolus is covered by a thin layer of fluid composed of a water phase immediately adjacent to the alveolar epithelial cell and covered by surfactant. Within the alveolar epithelium there are also a small number of **macrophages**, a type of phagocytic cell that patrols the alveolar surface and ingests (phagocytizes) bacteria and inhaled particles (see Chapter 11).

Pulmonary Circulation

The lung has two separate blood supplies (see Chapter 6). The **pulmonary circulation** brings deoxygenated blood from the right ventricle to the gas-exchanging units (alveoli). **Pulmonary perfusion** (Q) refers to pulmonary blood flow, which equals the heart rate multiplied by the right ventricular stroke volume. The lungs receive the entire right ventricular cardiac output and are the only organ in the body that functions in this manner. The **bronchial** (or lesser) **circulation** arises from the aorta and provides nourishment to the lung parenchyma. The dual circulation to the lung is another of the unique features of the lung.

The pulmonary capillary bed is the largest vascular bed in the body, with a surface area of 70 to 80 m^2. It is best viewed as a sheet of blood interrupted by small vertical supporting posts (Fig. 1-7). When the capillaries are filled with blood, about 75% of the surface area of the alveoli overlies the red blood cells. The capillaries allow red blood cells to flow through in single file only; this greatly facilitates gas exchange between the alveoli and the red blood cells. Once gas exchange is complete, the oxygenated blood returns to the left side of the heart through pulmonary venules and veins and is ready for pumping to the systemic circulation. At rest, the pulmonary capillaries contain about 70 mL of blood. This volume can almost triple (200 mL) during physical activity. The increase in

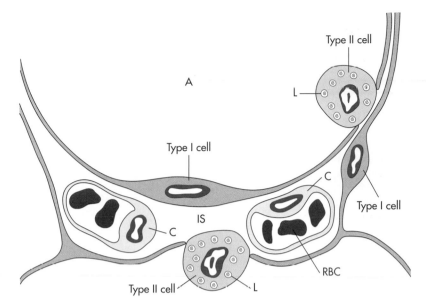

FIGURE 1-5 ■ Structure of the normal alveolus. The type I cell, with its long thin cytoplasmic processes, lines most of the alveolar surface, whereas the cuboidal type II cell, which is more numerous, occupies only about 7% of the alveolar surface. Capillaries (C) with red blood cells (RBC) are also shown. A, alveolar surface; IS, interstitial space; L, lamellar body, source of surfactant. *(Modified from Weinberger S: Principles of Pulmonary Medicine, 4th ed. Philadelphia, WB Saunders, 2003.)*

blood volume in the lung that occurs as a result of the increase in cardiac output during exercise is accomplished largely by the opening of capillary segments that are normally closed or compressed at rest. The capillaries are also capable of distending with increased flow. In contrast to the systemic circulation, the pulmonary circulation is a highly distensible, low-pressure system capable of accommodating large volumes of blood at low pressure. This is another unique feature of the lung.

The Conducting Airways

The conducting airways consist of those airways and their branches that bring (conduct) gas to the gas-exchanging units but do not actually participate in gas exchange. The conducting airways begin at the nose and end at the start of the alveoli. Thus, included in the conducting airways are the nasal cavity, the posterior pharynx, the glottis and vocal cords, the trachea, and all the divisions of the tracheobronchial tree to the end of the terminal bronchioles where the alveoli begin. The tracheobronchial tree includes the conducting airways and the airways that terminate in alveoli. The **upper airway** consists of all structures from the nose to the vocal cords, whereas the **lower airway** consists of the trachea and the bronchial structures to the alveolus.

The tracheobronchial system (also called the tracheobronchial *tree*, because if you turn the lung upside down and view the trachea as the trunk, the airways look like branches of a tree) begins with the trachea and consists of a series of branching tubes that become narrower, shorter, and more numerous as they penetrate deeper into the lung substance (parenchyma) (Fig. 1-8). The trachea is supported by C-shaped cartilage anteriorly and laterally and by smooth muscle posteriorly. Like the trachea, cartilage in large bronchi is also semicircular, but as the bronchi enter the lung, the cartilage rings disappear and are replaced by plates of cartilage. As the airways further divide, these plates of cartilage decrease in size and eventually disappear. The airways can thus be divided into two types: cartilaginous airways, or bronchi, and non-cartilaginous airways, or bronchioles (Table 1-1). Bronchi contain cartilage and are the conductors of air between the external environment and the distal sites of gas exchange. Bronchioles do not contain cartilage and can be further subdivided depending upon their function. Non-respiratory bronchioles include terminal bronchioles, which serve as conductors of the gas stream, whereas respiratory bronchioles function as sites of

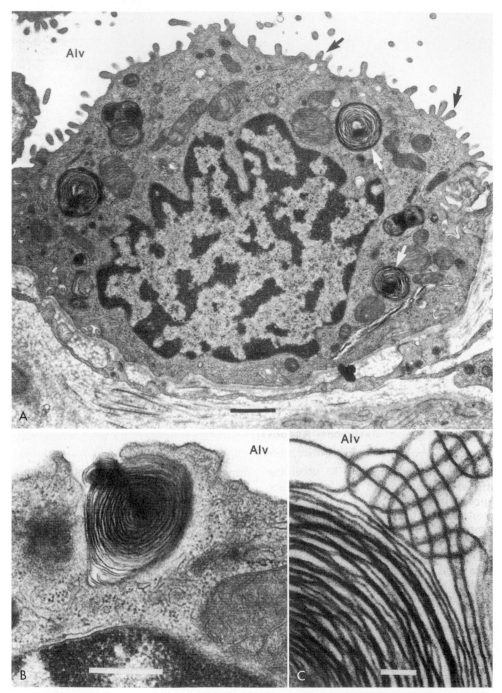

FIGURE 1-6 ■ Surfactant release by type II epithelial cells. Alv, alveolus. **A,** Type II epithelial cell from a human lung showing characteristic lamellar inclusion bodies *(white arrows)* within the cell and microvilli *(black arrows)* projecting into the alveolus. Bar = 0.5 μm. **B,** Early exocytosis of lamellar body into the alveolar space in a human lung. Bar = 0.5 μm. **C,** Secreted lamellar body and newly formed tubular myelin in alveolar liquid in a fetal rat lung. Membrane continuities between outer lamellae and adjacent tubular myelin provide evidence of intra-alveolar tubular myelin formation. Bar = 0.1 μm. *(Courtesy Dr. Mary C. Williams.)*

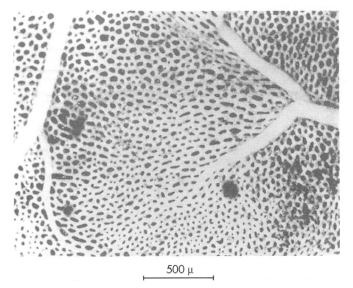

FIGURE 1-7 ■ Pulmonary capillary surface of the lung. View of alveolar wall (in a frog) demonstrating the dense network of capillaries. A small artery *(left)* and vein *(right)* can also be seen. The individual capillary segments are so short that the blood forms an almost continuous sheet. *(From Maloney JE, Castle BL: Respir Physiol 7:150, 1969.)*

500 μ

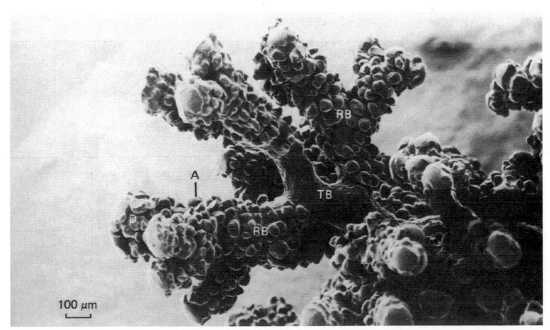

FIGURE 1-8 ■ Transition of terminal bronchiole. Scanning electron micrograph of airway branches peripheral to terminal bronchiole in a silicon-rubber cast of cat lung. A, alveolus; RB, respiratory bronchiole; TB, terminal bronchiole. Note absence of alveoli in terminal bronchiole. *(From Berne RM, Levy ML, Koeppen BM, Stanton BA (eds): Physiology, 5th ed. St. Louis, Mosby, 2004.)*

100 μm

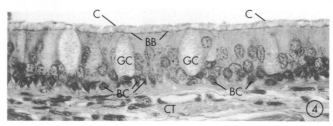

FIGURE 1-9 ■ Scanning electron micrograph of airway, showing the ciliated, pseudostratified, columnar epithelium of a bronchus. Each cilium is connected to a basal body (BB), which collectively appears at the base of the cilia (C) as a dark band. Goblet cells (GC) and basal cells (BC), the potential precursors of the ciliated cells, are shown. CT, connective tissue. *(From Berne RM, Levy ML, Koeppen BM, Stanton BA (eds): Physiology, 5th ed. St. Louis, Mosby, 2004.)*

gas exchange. The portion of the lung supplied by primary respiratory bronchioles is called an **acinus**. Because the conducting airways contain no alveoli and therefore take no part in gas exchange, they constitute the **anatomic dead space** (see Chapter 5). In normal individuals, the first 16 generations of airway branchings, with a volume of 150 mL, constitute the anatomic dead space.

Cells of the Airways

The respiratory tract (with the exception of the pharynx, the anterior one third of the nose, and the area distal to the terminal bronchioles) is lined by a pseudostratified, ciliated, columnar epithelium interspersed with mucus-secreting goblet cells and other secretory cells (Fig. 1-9; also see Chapter 11). In the distal airways, the columnar epithelium gives way to a more cuboidal epithelium. The airway epithelial cells are responsible for maintaining a thin, aqueous layer of fluid adjacent to the cells (**periciliary fluid**) in which the cilia can function. The depth of this periciliary fluid is maintained by the movement of ions across the epithelium.

Interspersed among the epithelial cells are **surface secretory cells,** which are also known as goblet cells. In general, there is one goblet cell per 5 to 6 ciliated cells. Goblet cells decrease in number between the 5th and 12th lung generation and in normal individuals disappear beyond the 12th tracheobronchial generation. In the bronchioles, goblet cells are replaced by **Clara cells**, another type of secretory cell.

Submucosal tracheobronchial glands are present wherever there is cartilage in the tracheobronchial tree. These glands empty to the surface epithelium through a ciliated duct and are lined by mucous and serous cells. Submucosal tracheobronchial glands increase in number and size in **chronic bronchitis**, a chronic lung disease primarily occurring in smokers, and extend down to the bronchioles in disease.

The ciliated epithelium, goblet cell, Clara cell, and tracheobronchial glands are important in host defense and are discussed in Chapter 11.

The Muscles of Respiration

The lung sits within the chest wall. Both the chest wall and the lung are in intimate contact, and normally the

TABLE 1-1						
Anatomic Characteristics of Bronchi and Bronchioles						
	CARTILAGE PRESENT	SIZE	EPITHELIUM	BLOOD SUPPLY	ALVEOLI	VOLUME
Bronchi	Yes	>1 mm	Psuedostratified columnar	Bronchial	No	~675 mL
Terminal bronchioles	No	<1 mm	Cuboidal	Bronchial	No	>150 mL
Respiratory bronchioles	No	<1 mm	Cuboidal	Pulmonary	Yes	2500 mL

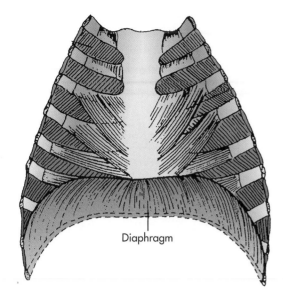

FIGURE 1-10 ■ The diaphragm. View from the inside of the thorax illustrates the position of the diaphragm in the thorax. *(From Fishman AP: Pulmonary Diseases and Disorders, vol 1, 2nd ed. New York, McGraw-Hill, 1988.)*

two structures move together. The lungs do not self-inflate. The force for lung inflation is supplied by the muscles of respiration, which are skeletal muscles. Like all skeletal muscles, their force of contraction increases when they are stretched and decreases when they are shortened. Thus, the force of contraction of the respiratory muscles increases with increasing lung volume.

Dividing the thoracic cavity from the abdominal cavity is the **diaphragm**, the major muscle of respiration (Fig. 1-10). The diaphragm is a thin, musculotendinous, dome-shaped sheet of muscle that is inserted into the lower ribs and separates the thoracic from the abdominal cavity. It is supplied by the phrenic nerve that arises from the second cervical vertebra. When it contracts, the abdominal contents are forced downward and forward and the vertical dimension of the chest cavity is increased. In addition, the rib margins are lifted and moved out, causing an increase in the transverse diameter of the thorax. In adults, the diaphragm is capable of generating airway pressures of 150 to 200 cm H_2O during a maximal

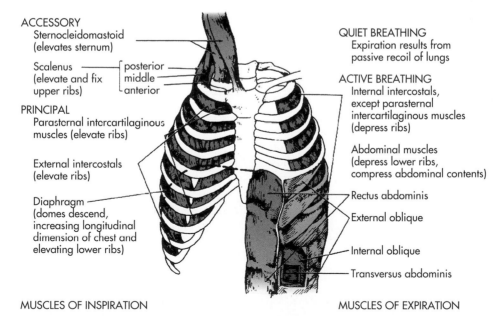

ACCESSORY
  Sternocleidomastoid
  (elevates sternum)

Scalenus ─────┌ posterior
(elevate and fix │ middle
upper ribs)   └ anterior

PRINCIPAL
  Parasternal intercartilaginous
  muscles (elevate ribs)

External intercostals
(elevate ribs)

Diaphragm
(domes descend,
increasing longitudinal
dimension of chest and
elevating lower ribs)

QUIET BREATHING
  Expiration results from
  passive recoil of lungs

ACTIVE BREATHING
  Internal intercostals,
  except parasternal
  intercartilaginous muscles
  (depress ribs)

  Abdominal muscles
  (depress lower ribs,
  compress abdominal contents)

Rectus abdominis

External oblique

Internal oblique

Transversus abdominis

MUSCLES OF INSPIRATION   MUSCLES OF EXPIRATION

FIGURE 1-11 ■ Muscles of respiration. Diagram of the anatomy of the major respiratory muscles. *Left side,* inspiratory muscles; *right side,* expiratory muscles. *(From Garrity ER, Sharp JT: Pulmonary and Critical Care Update, vol 2. Park Ridge, Ill, American College of Chest Physicians, 1986.)*

inspiratory effort. During quiet breathing (known as **tidal volume breathing**), the diaphragm moves approximately 1 cm, but during large-volume breathing, the diaphragm can move as much as 10 cm. If the diaphragm is paralyzed, it moves higher up in the thoracic cavity during inspiration because of the fall in intrathoracic pressure. This **paradoxical movement of the diaphragm** can be demonstrated using the radiographic technique called **fluoroscopy**.

Dyspnea is a feeling of shortness of breath or difficulty breathing and is often related to inspiratory muscle fatigue.

The other significant muscles of inspiration are the external intercostal muscles that pull the ribs upward and forward during inspiration, causing an increase in both the side-to-side and front-to-back diameters of the thorax (Fig. 1-11). Innervation of these muscles originates from intercostal nerves that originate off of the spinal cord at the same level. Paralysis of these muscles has no significant effect on respiration because of the dominance of the diaphragm as the major muscle of respiration. Accessory muscles of inspiration (scalene muscles, which elevate the sternocleidomastoid; the alae nasi, which cause nasal flaring; and small muscles in the neck and head) are quiet during quiet breathing but contract vigorously during exercise and with significant airway obstruction.

The upper airway must remain patent during inspiration; therefore, the pharyngeal wall muscles, the genioglossus and the arytenoid muscles are also considered muscles of inspiration.

Exhalation during quiet breathing is passive but becomes active during exercise and hyperventilation. The most important muscles of exhalation are those of the abdominal wall (rectus abdominis, internal and external oblique, and transversus abdominis) and the internal intercostal muscles that oppose the activity of the external intercostal muscles (i.e., pull the ribs downward and inward).

The Central Nervous System and Neural Pathways

The central nervous system (CNS), and in particular the brainstem, functions as the main control center for respiration (see Chapter 10). Breathing is both

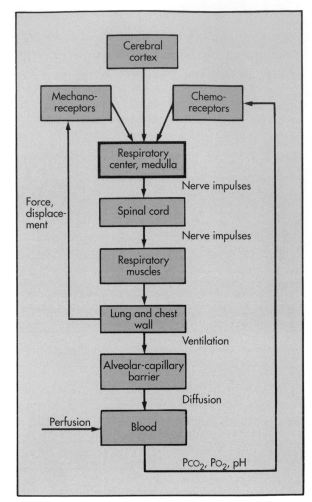

FIGURE 1-12 ■ Central control. Block diagram of the respiratory control system. Ventilation and perfusion come together near the bottom, and their output sets arterial and alveolar carbon dioxide and oxygen partial pressures (P_{CO_2} and P_{O_2}, respectively), and in part arterial hydrogen ion concentration (pH). These outputs feed back to the controllers via chemoreceptors located in strategic places. *(From Berne RM, Levy ML, Koeppen BM, Stanton BA (eds): Physiology, 5th ed. St. Louis, Mosby, 2004.)*

voluntary and automatic. Each breath begins in the brain, where the signal to breathe is carried to the respiratory muscles through the spinal cord and the nerves that innervate the respiratory muscles. It is remarkable that despite widely varying demands for O_2 uptake and CO_2 removal, the arterial levels of O_2 and CO_2 are normally kept within tight limits. Regulation of respiration requires three components:

1. Generation and maintenance of a respiratory rhythm (**central pattern generator**)
2. Modulation of the respiratory rhythm by sensory feedback loops and reflexes that allow adaptation to various situations and minimize energy costs
3. Recruitment of respiratory muscles that can contract appropriately for effective gas

exchange (Fig. 1-12). Unlike the heart, which begins beating at approximately 6 weeks' gestation, rhythmic respirations do not begin until birth.

The central pattern generator (CPG) is composed of several groups of cells that are located in the brainstem and that have the property of a pacemaker. Inspiration is the active phase of breathing and is initiated by impulses from the CPG. The CPG integrates both peripheral input from stretch receptors (**mechanoreceptors**) in the lung and oxygen receptors

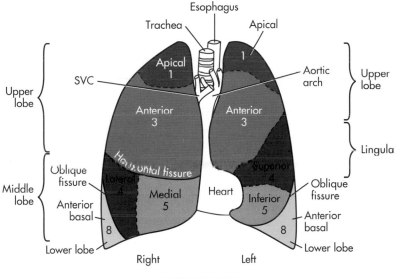

ANTERIOR VIEW

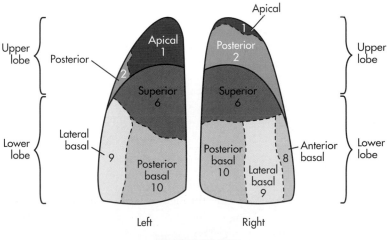

POSTERIOR VIEW

FIGURE 1-13 ■ Topography of the lung demonstrating the lobes, segments, and fissures. Numbers refer to specific bronchopulmonary segments that are also shown in Figure 1-1. SVC, Superior vena cava. *(From Berne RM, Levy ML, Koeppen BM, Stanton BA (eds): Physiology, 5th ed. St. Louis, Mosby, 2004.)*

(**chemoreceptors**) from the carotid body and CNS input from the hypothalamus and amygdala. This input may be excitatory or inhibitory in nature. In addition, because phrenic nerve output is absent between inspiratory efforts, there is an inspiratory on-off switch in the system with a feedback system that inhibits the CPG during exhalation.

ANATOMIC AND PHYSIOLOGIC CORRELATES

Lung structure is closely correlated with lung function in health and disease. Because lung disease is described in anatomic terms (e.g., right middle lobe pneumonia), a knowledge of lung anatomy is essential. The **bronchopulmonary segment** is the region of the lung supplied by a segmental bronchus. It is the **functional anatomic unit of the lung**, so named because disease usually involves one segment at a time and because surgical resection follows along segments. When using a stethoscope (auscultation), all of the bronchopulmonary segments can be examined with one

exception—namely the hilar segments of the lower lobes (Fig. 1-13). The **hilum** is the area of the lung where the main-stem bronchi and pulmonary arteries and veins enter and leave the right and left lung. These segments face inward and have no topographic relationship to the chest.

The various lobes of the lung (three on the right and two on the left) are subdivided by **fissures**. The division into the lobes, however, is incomplete, which allows for collateral ventilation. **Collateral ventilation** is an accessory pathway that connects airspaces supplied by other airways. There are two types of accessory pathways in the lung: (1) **canals of Lambert**, which connect respiratory bronchioles and terminal bronchioles to airspaces supplied by other airways, and (2) **pores of Kohn**, which are openings in the alveolar walls that connect adjacent alveoli. These accessory pathways help to prevent collapse of terminal respiratory units when their supplying airway becomes obstructed (atelectasis) and are particularly important in individuals with lung diseases such as **emphysema**.

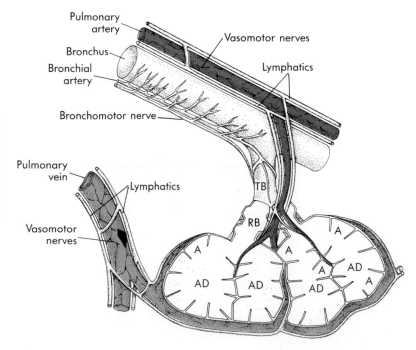

FIGURE 1-14 ■ The anatomic relation between the pulmonary artery, the bronchial artery, the airways, and the lymphatics. A, alveoli; AD, alveolar ducts; RB, respiratory bronchioles; TB, terminal bronchioles. *(From Berne RM, Levy ML, Koeppen BM, Stanton BA (eds): Physiology, 5th ed. St. Louis, Mosby, 2004.)*

Physiologically, the lung demonstrates functional unity; that is, every alveolar unit has the same structure and the same function as every other alveolar unit. This is in contrast to the heart, in which the various chambers have both a different structure and a different function. The significance of functional unity is that a large portion of the lung can be removed without significantly compromising overall lung function (i.e., gas exchange).

Both the right and the left lung are covered by two pleural membranes—the **visceral pleura** and the **parietal pleura**. The visceral pleural membrane completely envelops the lung except at the hilum where the bronchus, pulmonary vessels and nerves enter the lung parenchyma. The parietal pleural membrane lines the inner surface of the chest wall, mediastinum, and diaphragm and becomes continuous with the visceral pleura at the hilum. Under normal conditions, the space between the two pleuras contains a small amount of clear, serous fluid that facilitates smooth gliding of the lung as it expands in the chest. It also creates a potential space that can be involved in disease. Air can enter this potential space between the visceral and parietal pleuras because of trauma, rupture of a weakened area at the surface of the lung, or surgery producing a **pneumothorax**. Fluid can also enter this space, creating a **pleural effusion**. Because the pleuras of the right and left lung are separate, a pneumothorax involves only the right or the left hemithorax.

Pulmonary arteries that contain deoxygenated blood follow the bronchi, whereas pulmonary veins cross segments on their way to the left atrium (Fig. 1-14). Bronchial arteries also follow the bronchi and divide with them. In contrast, one third of the blood from the bronchial veins (deoxygenated blood) drains into the right atrium, and the remainder drains into pulmonary veins that drain into the left atrium. Thus, a small amount of deoxygenated blood that has nourished the lung parenchyma mixes with oxygenated blood in the left atrium.

SUMMARY

1. The principal function of the respiratory system is gas exchange. Other functions include acid-base balance, host defense and metabolism, and the handling of bioactive materials.
2. Respiratory gases obey the gas laws. Gases in a gas mixture exert a partial pressure; the sum of the partial pressures of individual gases is equal to the total pressure (Dalton's law). Gases move from areas of higher pressure to areas of lower pressure. Pressure gradients in the lung are referenced to atmospheric pressure, which by convention is considered to be zero.
3. The partial pressure of a gas acts as the driving force for the gas to be carried in the liquid or blood phase. The capacity of the liquid (blood) for the gas depends on the solubility of the gas and the ability of the liquid to bind or carry more of the gas than would be normally transported at a particular partial pressure.
4. Gas exchange occurs in the alveolar capillary unit, the basic physiologic unit of the lung.
5. The bronchopulmonary segment is the segment of the lung supplied by a segmental bronchus. It is the functional anatomic unit of the lung.
6. The alveolar surface is lined by type I and type II cells. The thin cytoplasm of the type I cell is ideal for optimal gas diffusion, whereas the type II cell is important for the production of surfactant, which decreases the surface tension of the alveolus.
7. The lung has two separate circulations. The pulmonary circulation brings deoxygenated blood from the right ventricle to the gas-exchanging units. The bronchial circulation arises from the aorta and nourishes the lung parenchyma.
8. The circulation to the lung is unique in its dual circulation and in its ability to accommodate large volumes of blood at low pressure.
9. The anatomic deadspace is composed of all of the airways that do not participate in gas exchange— that is, the airways to the level of the respiratory bronchioles.
10. The cells of the conducting airways include the pseudostratified, ciliated, columnar epithelial cells, surface secretory cells, Clara cells, and submucosal tracheobronchial gland cells.

11. The diaphragm is the major muscle of respiration.
12. Breathing is both voluntary and automatic.
13. The lung demonstrates both anatomic and physiologic unity—that is, each unit is structurally identical and functions just like every other unit.

KEY WORDS

- Alveolar macrophage
- Alveolus
- Anatomic deadspace
- Atelectasis
- Boyle's law
- Bronchopulmonary segment
- Bronchus
- Canals of Lambert
- Central pattern generator
- Chemoreceptor
- Clara cell
- Collateral ventilation
- Dalton's law
- Diaphragm
- Diffusion
- Dyspnea
- Emphysema
- Fissure
- Functional unity
- Glottis
- Hilum
- Interstitium/interstitial space
- Mechanoreceptor
- Parietal pleura
- Partial pressure
- Periciliary fluid
- Pneumothorax
- Pores of Kohn
- Surface secretory cells (goblet cells)
- Surfactant
- Torr
- Tracheobronchial glands
- Type I cell
- Type II cell
- Visceral pleura

SELF-STUDY PROBLEMS

1. What are the principal muscles of inspiration?
2. What are the principal muscles of exhalation?
3. If the pulmonary artery that supplies the left lung was occluded for a short period of time, and the cardiac output remained unchanged (that is, all of the blood from the right ventricle now goes to the right lung), would the pressure inside the right pulmonary artery approximately double?
4. What are the components of the blood-gas barrier?
5. What are the anatomic features that make the lung ideally suited for its principal function?

REFERENCES

Baile EM: The anatomy and physiology of the bronchial circulation. J Aerosol Med 9:1-6, 1996.

Boggs DS, Kinasewitz GT: Review: Pathophysiology of the pleural space, Am J Med 309:53-59, 1995.

Fehrenbach H: Alveolar epithelial type II cell: Defender of the alveolus revisited. Respir Res 2:33-46, 2001.

Fishman AP (ed): Pulmonary Diseases and Disorders, 3rd ed. New York, McGraw-Hill, 1998.

Gandevia SC, Allen GM, Butler J, et al: Human respiratory muscles: Sensations, reflexes and fatigability. Clin Exp Pharm Physiol 25:757-763, 1998.

Horsfield K, Cumming G: Morphology of the bronchial tree in man. J Appl Physiol 24:373-383, 1968.

Leff AR, Schumacker PT: Respiratory Physiology: Basics and Applications. Philadelphia, WB Saunders, 1993.

Massaro D, Massaro GD: Invited review: Pulmonary alveoli: Formation, the "call for oxygen," and other regulators. Am J Physiol Lung Cell Mol Physiol 282:L345-L358, 2002.

Murray JF, Nadel JA, Mason RJ, et al (eds): Textbook of Respiratory Medicine, 3rd ed. Philadelphia, WB Saunders, 2000.

Nettesheim P, Koo JS, Gray T: Regulation of differentiation of the tracheobronchial epithelium. J Aerosol Med 13:207-218, 2000.

Poole DC, Sexton WL, Farkas GA: Diaphragm structure and function in health and disease. Med Sci Sports Exerc 29:738-754, 1997.

Rogers DE: Airway goblet cells: Responsive and adaptable frontline defenders. Eur Respir J 7:1690-1706, 1994.

Weibel ER: The Pathway for Oxygen: Structure and Function of the Mammalian Respiratory System. Cambridge, MA, Harvard University Press, 1984.

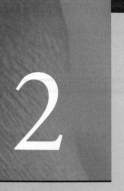

MECHANICAL PROPERTIES OF THE LUNG AND CHEST WALL

OBJECTIVES

1. Describe static lung mechanics and the measurement of lung volumes.
2. Define lung compliance and its measurement.
3. Relate lung and chest wall compliance to lung volumes.
4. Characterize lung and chest wall interactions in terms of pressure gradients and pressure volume relationships.
5. Describe surfactant and its role in altering surface tension.

STATIC LUNG MECHANICS

Before examining further how air moves in and out of the lung, it is important to begin to describe several properties of the lung and chest wall. **Lung mechanics** is the study of the mechanical properties of the lung and chest wall. Two different mechanical properties are used to characterize the lung and chest wall. **Static lung mechanics,** which is the study of the mechanical properties of the lung and chest wall whose volume is not changing with time, is discussed in this chapter. In contrast, **dynamic lung mechanics,** which is the study of the lung and chest wall in motion (i.e., changing volume), is discussed in Chapter 3.

The study of static and dynamic lung mechanics can be further separated into two components. The first is the lung itself, which is composed of the airways, lung parenchyma, interstitial matrix (composed of fibrin, collagen, and a few cells), alveolar surface, and pulmonary circulation. Each of these components contributes to the overall mechanical properties that are referred to as the **mechanical properties of the lung.** The second component is the **chest wall and its mechanical properties.** *Chest wall* is a term commonly used in lung mechanics to describe the properties of all of the structures outside of the lungs that move during breathing, including the rib cage, diaphragm, abdominal cavity, and anterior abdominal muscles. The interaction between the lung and the chest wall determines lung volumes, and static lung volumes play a major role in gas exchange and in the work of breathing.

LUNG VOLUMES

The static volumes of the lungs are shown in Figure 2-1. All lung volumes are subdivisions of the total lung capacity (TLC) and are measured in liters. They are reported either as volumes (e.g., residual volume) or capacities (e.g., vital capacity). A **capacity** is composed of two or more volumes.

The total volume of air that is contained in the lung is called the **total lung capacity** (TLC). It is composed of the volume of air that an individual can exhale from a maximum inspiration to a maximum exhalation, known as the **vital capacity** (VC), and the volume of

17

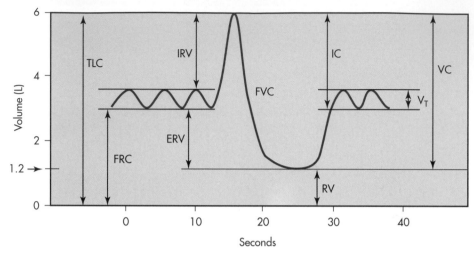

FIGURE 2-1 ■ The various lung volumes and capacities. ERV, expiratory reserve volume; FRC, functional residual capacity; FVC, forced vital capacity; IC, inspiratory capacity; IRV, inspiratory reserve volume; RV, residual volume; TLC, total lung capacity; VC, vital capacity; V_T, tidal volume. *(From Berne RM, Levy ML, Koeppen BM, Stanton BA (eds): Physiology, 5th ed. St. Louis, Mosby, 2004.)*

air that is left in the lung after a maximal exhalation, known as the **residual volume** (**RV**). Two other lung volumes of importance are the **tidal volume** (**TV, or V_T**) and the **functional residual capacity** (**FRC**). The TV is the volume of air that is breathed into and out of the lung during quiet breathing. The FRC is the volume of air contained in the lung after a normal exhalation. It is composed of the residual volume and the volume of air that can be exhaled from the end of a normal exhalation to residual volume. This latter volume is called the expiratory reserve volume (ERV); clinically, it is not a volume that is often reported, but physiologically it is important. The FRC is an important capacity because it represents the resting volume of the respiratory system, in which the forces of the chest wall to increase in size and the forces of the lung to decrease in size are equal but opposite.

To get a sense of the importance of lung volumes in respiration, breathe quietly close to your TLC (take a deep breath in, and breathe at this high lung volume for a few minutes). Now breathe out until you can't force any more air out and try breathing at this volume that is close to your residual volume. Both of these maneuvers should be uncomfortable; both breathing at a high lung volume and breathing at a low lung volume are present with pulmonary disease and occur as a result of a change in lung mechanics associated with disease. The measurement of lung volumes is used to detect and follow the progression of lung disease and is discussed in Chapter 4.

USING AND INTERPRETING RESULTS OF LUNG VOLUME MEASUREMENTS

Two major types of pathophysiologic abnormalities involving the lung and chest wall can be described using lung volumes. One group of diseases is called **obstructive pulmonary disease** (OPD). In OPD, during exhalation the airways close (*premature airway closure,* the hallmark of OPD) trapping air behind them (see Chapter 3). This results in an increase in TLC, RV, and FRC. In contrast, in **restrictive pulmonary disease**, the other major pathophysiologic abnormality involving the lung and chest wall, lung volumes are reduced.

One of the most useful tests for distinguishing obstructive and restrictive types of lung disease is the measurement of the **RV/TLC ratio**. In normal individuals, the RV/TLC ratio is less than 0.25. An elevated

RV/TLC ratio, characterized by an increase in RV out of proportion to any increase in TLC, is due to air trapping secondary to airway obstruction and is seen in individuals with OPD. An elevated RV/TLC ratio due to a *decrease* in TLC out of proportion to any change in RV is seen in individuals with restrictive types of pulmonary disease.

LUNG COMPLIANCE

Lung compliance (CL) is a measure of the elastic properties of the lung and is a reflection of lung distensibility. These distensibility properties of the lung are seen in the **pressure volume relaxation curve** for the lung that is called the *compliance curve of the lung*. Compliance of the lungs is defined as the change in lung volume resulting from a change in the distending pressure of the lung equal to 1 cm H_2O. The units of compliance are mL (or L)/cm H_2O. A lung with high lung compliance refers to a lung that is easily distended. A lung with low compliance or a "stiff" lung is a lung that is not easily distended. Thus, the compliance of the lung (CL) is:

$$CL = \frac{\Delta V}{\Delta P}$$

where ΔV is the change in volume and ΔP is the change in pressure.

The compliance of the isolated lung is measured in animals by removing the lung and measuring the changes in volume that occur with each change in transpulmonary pressure. As transpulmonary pressure increases, lung volume increases (Fig. 2-2A). The line that is generated however, is curvilinear, not linear. That is, at low lung volumes the lung distends easily, but at high lung volumes large increases in transpulmonary pressure produce only small changes in lung volume. This is because at high lung volumes all of the alveolar units and airways have been maximally stretched.

Lungs that are highly complaint will have a steeper slope than lungs with a low compliance. Looking at this relationship, it should be apparent that lung compliance or distensibility is the inverse of elasticity or **lung elastic recoil** (PEL). Compliance is the ease with which something is stretched, whereas elastic recoil is the tendency to resist or oppose stretching.

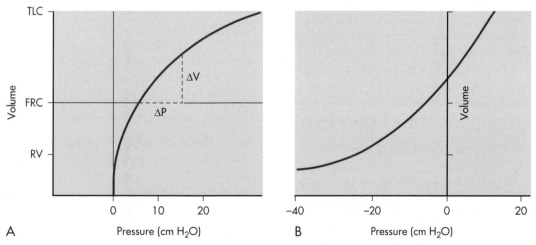

FIGURE 2-2 ■ Deflation pressure volume (PV) curve of the lung (**A**) and chest wall (**B**). **A,** The compliance of the lung at any point along the curve is the change in volume (ΔV) per the change in pressure (ΔP). From the curve, it is apparent that the compliance of the lung changes with lung volume. By convention, the deflation pressure volume curve is used, and lung compliance is the change in pressure when going from functional residual capacity (FRC) to FRC + 1 L. RV, residual volume; TLC, total lung capacity. **B,** PV curve of the chest wall demonstrating a change in compliance with change in lung volume. Note that at volumes greater than 60% of the TLC, the pressure needed to expand the chest wall is positive (inward recoil), whereas at lower lung volumes, the chest wall pressure is negative (outward recoil).

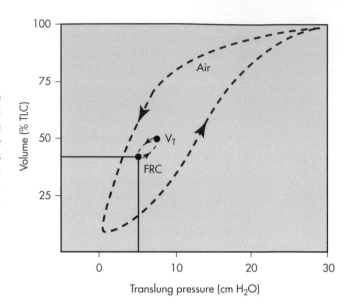

FIGURE 2-3 ■ Inflation: deflation pressure-volume curve of the lung. The direction of inspiration and exhalation is shown by the *arrows*. The difference between the inflation and deflation pressure-volume curves is due to surface tension variation with changes in lung volume. FRC, functional residual capacity; TLC, total lung capacity; V_T, tidal volume. *(From Berne RM, Levy ML, Koeppen BM, Stanton BA (eds): Physiology, 5th ed. St. Louis, Mosby, 2004.)*

By convention, the compliance of the lung is the slope of the line between any two points on the **deflation limb** of the pressure volume loop. The compliance of the lung is greater when measured from TLC to RV (deflation) than from RV to TLC (inflation) (Fig. 2-3). This is due in large part to the changes in surface tension with changing lung volume and is discussed later in this chapter. This difference between the inflation and exhalation curve is called *hysteresis*. As we will see later in this chapter, one of the important reasons for hysteresis is surfactant.

COMPLIANCE OF THE CHEST WALL

When the lungs are removed, the chest wall has a spring-like character with a relatively high resting volume. In much the same way as the lung, the compliance curve of the chest wall relates the volume of gas enclosed by the chest wall to the pressure across the chest wall. The curve (Fig. 2-2B) is relatively flat at low volumes; that is, the chest wall is stiff with the shortened respiratory muscles maximally contracted. The curve is also flat at high lung volumes in which the respiratory muscles are maximally stretched. At both high and low lung volumes, large changes in pressure across the chest wall result in small changes in the volume enclosed by the chest wall.

COMPLIANCE OF THE RESPIRATORY SYSTEM

Like the lungs and chest wall, the respiratory system also has its own compliance curve (Fig. 2-4). Because the lungs and chest wall function as a unit, the compliance of the respiratory system is a combination of the individual compliance curves of the lungs and chest wall. The compliances of the lung and the chest wall are physically in series with each other, and therefore their individual compliances add as reciprocals; that is,

1/compliance of the respiratory system =
1/compliance of the lung + 1/compliance of the chest wall

In contrast, compliances in parallel add directly. For example, the compliance of the lungs in the two hemithoraces is the sum of the compliances of the lung in each hemithorax.

CLINICAL USES OF COMPLIANCE

The compliance of the lung and chest wall is affected by a number of respiratory disorders. In *emphysema*, the lung is more compliant; that is, for every increase of 1 cm of H_2O pressure, there is a larger increase in volume than in the normal lung (Fig. 2-5). In contrast, a proliferation of connective tissue in the lung called

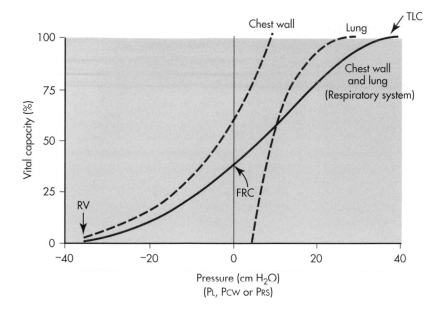

FIGURE 2-4 ■ The relaxation pressure-volume curve of the lung, chest wall, and respiratory system. The curve for the respiratory system is the sum of the individual curves. The curve for the lung is the same as in Figure 2-2A, and the curve for the chest wall is the same as in Figure 2-2B. FRC, functional residual capacity; Pcw, chest wall pressure; PL, transpulmonary pressure; Prs, respiratory system pressure; TLC, total lung capacity. *(From Berne RM, Levy ML, Koeppen BM, Stanton BA (eds): Physiology, 5th ed. St. Louis, Mosby, 2004.)*

pulmonary fibrosis can be seen in lung diseases such as interstitial pneumonitis and sarcoidosis or in association with chemical or thermal lung injury. The lungs in these diseases are "stiff," or non-compliant; that is, for every change of 1 cm H_2O pressure, there

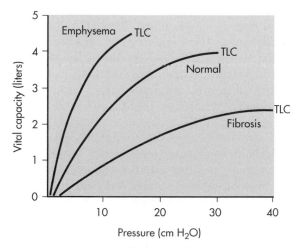

FIGURE 2-5 ■ Fibrosis/emphysema pressure-volume curve. TLC, total lung capacity. *(From Berne RM, Levy ML, Koeppen BM, Stanton BA (eds): Physiology, 5th ed. St. Louis, Mosby, 2004.)*

is a smaller change in volume. Similarly, in diseases associated with increased fluid in the interstitial spaces such as *pulmonary edema* or in diseases associated with fluid, blood, or infection in the intrapleural space (*pleural effusion, hemothorax,* or *empyema,* respectively), lung compliance is reduced.

The compliance of the chest wall is decreased in individuals with obesity in whom adipose tissue results in an additional load on the chest wall muscles and the diaphragm. Individuals with decreased mobility of the rib cage such as in *kyphoscoliosis* or other types of musculoskeletal diseases that affect chest wall movement also have decreased chest wall compliance.

Individuals with decreased compliance must generate greater transpulmonary pressures to produce changes in lung volume than individuals with normal compliance. This results in increased work associated with breathing (see Chapter 3).

As noted previously, lung compliance varies with lung volume (see Fig. 2-2). It is greater at lower lung volumes than at higher lung volumes. For this reason, **specific compliance**, or compliance divided by lung volume (usually FRC), is used (Fig. 2-6). As an example, consider the individual with chronic bronchitis in whom FRC is increased. As a result, pulmonary compliance, which is now being measured at this higher

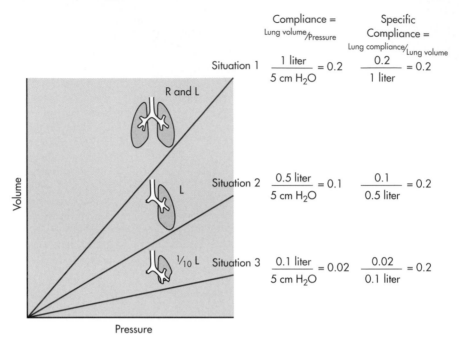

FIGURE 2-6 ■ Relationship between compliance and lung volume. Imagine a lung in which a change in pressure of 5 cm H_2O results in a change in volume of 1 liter. If half of the lung is removed (Situation 2), the compliance will decrease, but when corrected for the volume of the lung there is no change (specific compliance). Even when the lung is reduced by 90% (Situation 3), the specific compliance is unchanged. R, right lung; L, left lung. *(From Berne RM, Levy ML, Koeppen BM, Stanton BA (eds): Physiology, 5th ed. St. Louis, Mosby, 2004.)*

lung volume, would also be increased. However, when corrected for the FRC (specific compliance), the compliance is normal. In individuals with normal FRC, the compliance of the lung is about 0.2 L/cm H_2O, of the chest wall is 0.2 L/cm H_2O, and of the respiratory system is 0.1 L/cm H_2O.

DETERMINANTS OF LUNG VOLUME

Why can't we inspire above TLC or exhale beyond RV? The answers lie in the properties of the lung parenchyma and in the interaction between the lungs and the chest wall. Both the lungs and the chest wall have elastic properties. Both have a resting volume (or size) that they would assume if there were no external forces or pressures exerted on them. Both expand when stresses are applied and recoil passively when stresses are released. If the lungs were removed from

the chest and no external forces were applied, they would become almost airless. To expand these lungs would require either the exertion of a positive pressure on the alveoli and airways or the application of a negative pressure from outside the lungs. Either would result in a positive transpulmonary pressure. Both situations are analogous to the balloon and the vacuum canister. A balloon is airless unless positive pressure is exerted at the opening to distend the balloon walls (positive-pressure "ventilation"). In the case of the vacuum, negative external pressure is applied and results in sucking materials (air) into the canister (negative-pressure "ventilation").

The lungs are enclosed by the chest wall, which expands during inspiration. The lungs and chest wall always move together in healthy individuals. Lung volumes are determined by the balance between the lung's elastic recoil properties and the properties of the muscles of the chest wall. TLC occurs when the forces of inspiration decrease because of chest wall muscle lengthening and are insufficient to overcome the increasing force required to distend the lung and chest wall (Fig. 2-4).

At RV, a significant amount of gas remains within the lung. As RV is approached, the chest wall becomes so stiff that additional effort by the expiratory chest wall muscles is unable to further reduce the volume. Thus, RV occurs when the expiratory muscle force is insufficient to cause a further reduction in chest wall volume (see Fig. 2-4). As the chest wall is squeezed by the expiratory muscles, the recoil pressure of the chest wall (the chest wall wanting to increase in size) increases. The expiratory muscles shorten and their capacity to generate force decreases; the point at which the force generated by the expiratory muscles is insufficient to overcome the outward recoil of the chest wall determines the RV. This simple model of RV applies to (young) individuals with normal lungs. In older individuals and in individuals with lung disease, premature airway closure, a property of the lung (see Chapter 3), becomes the major determinant of RV rather than outward chest wall recoil.

The FRC is the volume of the lung at the end of a normal exhalation and is determined by the balance between the elastic recoil pressure generated by the lung parenchyma to become smaller and the pressure generated by the chest wall to become larger (see Fig. 2-4). In the presence of chest wall weakness, the FRC decreases (lung elastic recoil is greater than chest wall muscle force). In the presence of airway obstruction, the FRC increases because of premature airway closure that traps air in the lung. Always, however, the FRC will be that lung volume at which the outward recoil of the chest wall is equal to the inward recoil of the lung.

LUNG–CHEST WALL INTERACTIONS

The lung and chest wall move together in healthy people. The pleural space that separates the lung and the chest wall is best thought of as a "potential" space because of its small volume. Because the lung and chest wall move together, changes in their respective volumes are the same. The pressure changes across the lung and across the chest wall are defined as the **transmural pressures**. For the lung, this transmural

pressure is called the **transpulmonary pressure** (P_L) (also called the *translung pressure*) and is defined as the pressure difference between the airspaces (alveolar pressure [P_A]) and the pressure surrounding the lung (pleural pressure [P_{PL}]); that is,

$$P_L = P_A - P_{PL}$$

The lung requires a positive P_L in order to increase its volume and lung volume increases with increasing P_L. The lung assumes its smallest size when the transpulmonary pressure is zero. The lung, however, is not airless when the P_L is zero because of the surface tension–lowering properties of surfactant (discussed later).

The **transmural pressure across the chest wall** (P_W) is the difference between the pleural pressure and the pressure surrounding the chest wall, which is the barometric pressure (P_B) or body surface pressure. That is,

$$P_W = P_{PL} - P_B$$

During the inspiratory phase of quiet breathing, the chest wall expands to a larger volume. Because the pleural pressure is negative relative to atmospheric pressure during quiet breathing, the transmural pressure across the chest wall is negative.

The pressure then across the respiratory system (P_{rs}) is the sum of the pressure across the lung and the pressure across the chest wall; that is,

$$P_{rs} = P_L + P_W$$
$$= (P_A - P_{PL}) + (P_{PL} - P_B)$$
$$= P_A - P_B$$

The important relationship between the lung and chest wall is illustrated in the static pressure volume curves for the lung and the chest wall (see Fig. 2-4). These curves are obtained by asking participants to breathe into a spirometer (see Chapter 4) to measure lung volumes. An esophageal balloon is placed in the distal one third of the esophagus to measure intrapleural pressure. In addition, pressure at the mouth is measured. Participants then inspire to a specific lung volume; a stopcock in the spirometer tubing near the mouth is closed, and the participant is instructed to relax the respiratory muscles. The pressure at the mouth is equal to alveolar pressure because there is no airflow, and this is equal to the recoil pressure of the lungs (P_L) and the chest wall (P_W). This is the

pressure of the respiratory system ($Prs = P_L + P_W$). Because the intrapleural pressure is known, the individual recoil pressure of the lungs and the chest wall can be calculated.

A number of important observations can be made by examining the pressure volume curves of the lung, chest wall, and respiratory system. First, the lung volume at which the pressure across the respiratory system is 0 is the FRC. The resting volume of the chest wall is approximately 60% of the VC. Thus, in the absence of the lungs, the resting volume of the chest wall would be approximately 60% of the VC. Below 60% of the VC, the chest wall has outward elastic recoil. At lung volumes greater than 60% of the VC, the chest wall, like the lung, has inward elastic recoil.

The transmural distending pressure for the lung alone flattens at pressures greater than 20 cm H_2O because the elastic limits of the lung have been reached. Thus, further increases in transmural pressure produce no change in volume, and compliance is low. Further distention is limited by the connective tissue of the lung (collagen, elastin). If further pressure is applied, the alveoli close to the lung surface can rupture and air can escape into the pleural space. This is called a *pneumothorax*.

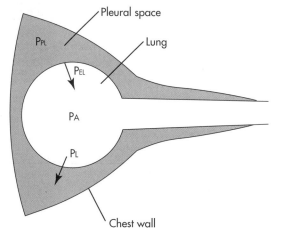

FIGURE 2-7 ■ The relationship between transpulmonary pressure (P_L) (the pressure across the lung) and the pleural (P_{PL}), alveolar (P_A), and elastic recoil (P_{EL}) pressures in the lung. The alveolar pressure is the sum of the pleural and the elastic recoil pressures; that is, $P_A = P_{PL} + P_{EL}$. *(From Berne RM, Levy ML, Koeppen BM, Stanton BA (eds): Physiology, 5th ed. St. Louis, Mosby, 2004.)*

As lung volume increases above FRC, the pressure across the respiratory system becomes positive because of two factors: the increased elastic recoil of the lung and the decreased outward elastic recoil of the chest wall. Below FRC, the relaxation pressure at the mouth is negative because the outward recoil of the chest wall is now greater than the reduced inward recoil of the lungs.

This relationship between pleural, alveolar, and elastic recoil pressure is shown in Figure 2-7. The alveolar pressure is the sum of the elastic recoil pressure P_{EL} and the pleural pressure of the lung:

$$P_A = P_{EL} + P_{PL}$$

Because

$$P_L = P_A - P_{PL}$$

Then

$$P_L = (P_{EL} + P_{PL}) - P_{PL}$$

Therefore,

$$P_L = P_{EL}$$

In general, P_L is the pressure distending the lung and P_{EL} is the pressure tending to collapse the lung. As we will show later, P_{EL} is the driving pressure for expiratory gas flow.

If the seal between the chest wall and the lung is broken, such as by a penetrating knife injury, the inward elastic recoil of the lung is no longer opposed by the outward recoil of the chest wall and their interdependence ceases. As a result, lung volume will decrease and airways and alveoli will collapse. At the same time, the chest wall will expand because its outward recoil is no longer opposed by the inward recoil of the lung. When the chest is opened, as during thoracic surgery, the lung recoils until the transpulmonary pressure is zero and the chest wall increases in size (to approximately 60% of the VC). The lungs do not, however, become totally airless but retain approximately 10% of their total lung capacity.

What happens in the supine position? The supine position has no effect on lung elastic recoil. However, when an individual is supine, the position of the diaphragm is changed due to gravitational effects, and the result is that the recoil pressures for the chest wall, and as a consequence for the respiratory system, are shifted to the right. Upright, the diaphragm is pulled down by gravity; supine, the abdominal contents push inward against the relaxed diaphragm. The displacement of the diaphragm into the chest decreases the overall outward recoil of the chest wall and displaces the chest wall elastic recoil pressure to the right. This change from the upright to the supine position results in a decrease in FRC.

PRESSURE/VOLUME RELATIONSHIPS

Based on what we have described so far, it is now possible to describe the volume changes in the lung associated with changes in pressure. Prior to the start of inspiration, the pressure in the pleural space in normal individuals is slightly negative (approximately –5 cm H_2O). That is, pleural pressure is less than atmospheric pressure. This negative pressure is created by the elastic recoil pressure of the lung, which acts to pull the lung away from the chest wall. Alveolar pressure at this point is zero because there is no airflow and at points of no airflow, alveolar and atmospheric pressures must be equal. As inspiration begins, the diaphragm contracts and moves into the abdominal cavity and the rib cage moves out and upward. The volume of the thoracic cavity increases and because of Boyle's law (see Chapter 1) the pressure inside the alveoli decreases.

As alveolar pressure decreases below atmospheric pressure, the glottis opens and air rushes into the airways. The decrease in alveolar pressure is small during tidal volume breathing in normal individuals (1-3 cm H_2O), but is much larger in individuals with airway obstruction who must generate larger inspiratory pressures to overcome the obstructed airways.

As alveolar pressure falls during inspiration, intrapleural pressure also falls. The decrease in intrapleural pressure is equal to the sum of the elastic recoil pressure, which increases as the lung inflates and the pressure drops along the airways as gas flows into the lung from higher (atmospheric or 0 pressure) to lower pressure (alveolar, subatmospheric pressure). Airflow stops when alveolar pressure and atmospheric pressure become equal.

On exhalation, the diaphragm moves back into the chest, intrapleural pressure increases (i.e., becomes less negative), alveolar pressure rises, the glottis opens, and gas again flows from higher to lower pressure. In the alveoli, the driving pressure for expiratory gas flow is the sum of the elastic recoil of the lung and the intrapleural pressure. The pressure volume events that occur during inspiration and exhalation are shown in Figure 2-8; Figure 2-9 shows the relationship between transpulmonary, intrapleural, and elastic recoil at end exhalation and during inspiration.

SURFACE TENSION

The elastic properties of the lung, including elastin, collagen, and other constituents of the lung tissue, are responsible for some but not all of the elastic recoil of the lung. The other important factor that contributes to lung elastic recoil is the surface tension at the air-liquid interface in the alveoli. **Surface tension** is a measure of the attractive force of the surface molecules per unit length of the material to which they are attached. The units of surface tension are those of a force applied per unit length (dynes/cm).

The role of surface tension forces in lung elastic recoil can be illustrated by comparing the volume pressure curves of saline-filled and air-filled lungs (Fig. 2-10). Similar to Figure 2-3, in this experiment a pressure volume curve is generated using an excised lung. When the lung is inflated with air, an air-liquid interface is present in the lung and surface tension contributes to alveolar elastic recoil. After all the gas is removed, the lung is inflated again, but this time saline instead of air is used. In this situation, surface tension forces are absent because there is no air-liquid interface. The difference between the two curves is the recoil due to surface tension forces.

For a sphere such as an alveolus, the relationship between the pressure within the sphere (Ps) and the tension in the wall is described by **Laplace's law**:

$$Ps = \frac{2T}{r}$$

or

$$T = \frac{Ps \times r}{2}$$

where T is the wall tension (dynes/cm) and r is the radius of the sphere.

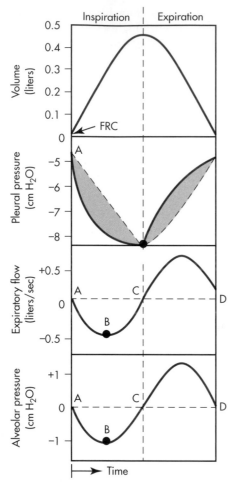

FIGURE 2-8 ■ Changes in alveolar and pleural pressure, expiratory flow, and lung volume during a tidal volume breath. Inspiration is to the left of the vertical dotted line, and exhalation is to the right. Positive (relative to atmosphere) pressures are above the horizontal dotted line, and negative pressures are below. At points of no airflow (A, C and D), alveolar pressure is zero. Point B represents the mid-point of inspiration. Intrapleural pressure has two different courses noted by the solid and the dotted lines. The *dotted line* represents the pleural pressure changes needed to overcome the elastic recoil of the alveoli; the *solid line* includes the additional pressure changes required to overcome tissue and airflow resistance. Thus, the *dotted line* is a more accurate representation of intrapleural pressure. FRC, functional residual capacity. *(From Berne RM, Levy ML, Koeppen BM, Stanton BA (eds): Physiology, 5th ed. St. Louis, Mosby, 2004.)*

Consider what would happen in the alveolus. Note here that the surface of most liquids (such as water) is constant and is not dependent on the area of the air-liquid interface. Imagine two alveoli of different sizes connected by a common airway (Fig. 2-11A). If the surface tension in both of these alveoli is equal, Laplace's law states that the pressure in the smaller alveolus must be greater than the pressure in the larger alveolus, and because gas always flows from higher to lower pressure, the smaller alveolus will empty into the larger alveolus.

Alveoli in the lung are of variable sizes. With a constant surface tension, these interconnected alveoli would be unstable—that is, the smaller alveoli would empty into the larger alveoli. The collapsed alveoli would have significant cohesive forces at their liquid-liquid interface and would, therefore, require a significant distending pressure to open. The result would be a marked increase in the distending pressures and in the work of breathing due to "stiff" alveoli. Two major factors cause the alveoli to be more stable than would be expected based on a constant surface tension. The first factor is pulmonary surfactant; the second is the structural interdependence of the alveoli.

SURFACTANT

Surfactant is a component of the alveolar surface fluid that lowers the elastic recoil due to surface tension even at high lung volumes. It increases the compliance of the lungs above that predicted by an air-water interface, and as a result, it decreases the work of breathing.

Surfactants are generally considered to be soaps or detergents. Pulmonary surfactant is a complex mixture of phospholipids, neutral lipids, fatty acids, and proteins. This substance constitutes a thin film that lines the surface of the alveoli. In addition to its surface tension–lowering properties, surfactant has "anti-stick" properties, and it acts as a barrier at the air-liquid interface.

Surfactant stabilizes the inflation of alveoli, because it allows the surface tension to increase as the alveoli become larger and to decrease as the alveoli become smaller (Fig. 2-11B). As a result, the transmural pressure required to keep an alveolus inflated increases as lung volume (and transpulmonary pressure) increases,

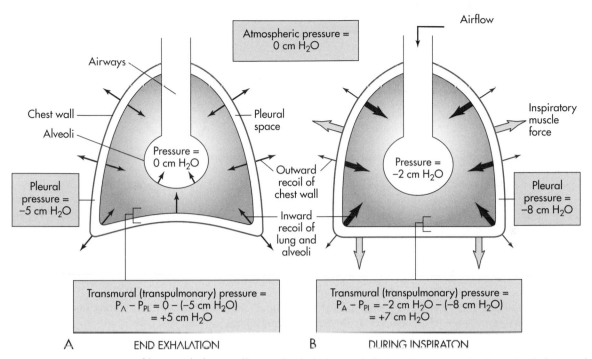

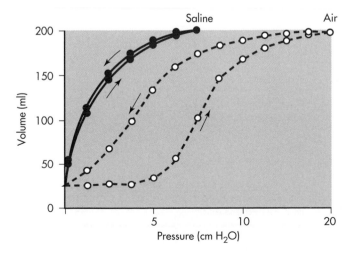

FIGURE 2-9 ■ Interaction of lung and chest wall at end exhalation and during inspiration. **A,** At end exhalation, the respiratory muscles are relaxed, the diaphragm sits high in the thoracic cavity, and there is no airflow because there is no difference between atmospheric and alveolar pressure. Lung elastic recoil pulls the lung inward, whereas chest wall elastic recoil pulls the chest wall outward. The tension created by the two opposing forces creates a negative pleural pressure. **B,** During inspiration, the diaphragm and other muscles of inspiration contract, resulting in a further decrease in pleural pressure. This negative pleural pressure is transmitted to the alveoli, causing a drop in alveolar pressure. Gas flows into the lung along the pressure gradient. Note that as lung volume increases, lung elastic recoil increases *(solid arrows)* and the outward recoil of the chest wall *(open arrows)* decreases.

FIGURE 2-10 ■ Volume-pressure curves of lungs filled with saline and with air. The *arrows* indicate whether the lung is being inflated or deflated; note that when using saline, hysteresis (i.e., the difference between inflation and deflation limbs of the curve) is virtually eliminated. *(From Clements JA, Tierney DF. In Fenn WO, Rahn H (eds): Handbook of Physiology, Section 3: Respiration, vol II. Washington, DC, American Physiological Society, 1964.)*

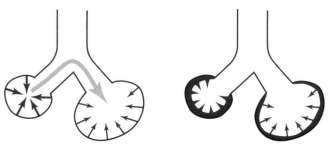

FIGURE 2-11 ■ Surface tension in a sphere. Surface forces in a sphere attempt to reduce the area of the surface and generate a pressure within the sphere. By Laplace's law, the pressure generated is inversely proportional to the radius of the sphere. **A,** Surface forces (Ps [surface pressure]) in the smaller sphere generate a higher pressure *(heavier arrows)* than the forces (PL [transpulmonary pressure]) in the larger sphere *(lighter arrows)*. As a result, air moves from the smaller sphere (higher pressure) to the larger sphere (lower pressure); see *large shaded arrow.* This causes the smaller sphere to collapse and the larger sphere to become over distended. **B,** Surfactant *(dark areas)* lowers surface tension, decreasing it more in the smaller sphere than in the larger sphere. The net result is that Ps is approximately equal to PL, and the spheres are stabilized. *(From Berne RM, Levy ML, Koeppen BM, Stanton BA (eds): Physiology, 5th ed. St. Louis, Mosby, 2004.)*

and it decreases as lung volume decreases. In the absence of surfactant, the surface tension at the air-liquid interface would remain constant and the transmural (transalveolar) pressure needed to keep it at that volume would be greater at lower lung (alveolar) volumes. Thus, it requires a greater transmural pressure to produce a given increase in alveolar volume at lower lung volumes than at higher lung volumes. Stated another way, in the absence of surfactant the transmural pressure necessary to keep an alveolus inflated would decrease as the transpulmonary pressure (i.e., lung volume) increases; conversely, the transmural pressure necessary to keep an alveolus inflated would increase as the transpulmonary pressure (i.e., lung volume) decreases. This would create instability of alveolar inflation and alveolar collapse.

As shown in Table 2-1, surfactant contains 85% to 90% lipids (of which 85% are phospholipids and 5% are neutral lipids) and 10% to 15% protein. The major phospholipid in surfactant is phosphatidylcholine, of which approximately 75% is present as dipalmitoyl phosphatidylcholine (DPPC). DPPC is the major active component in surfactant, and it readily decreases surface tension. The second most abundant phospholipid is phosphatidylglycerol (PG), which constitutes 7% to 10% of total surfactant. Both of these lipids are important in the formation of the liquid monolayer on the alveolar-air interface,

and PG is important in the spreading of surfactant over a large surface area.

Pulmonary surfactant is secreted from the small cuboidal type II cells, which occupy only about 2% to 7% of the surface area of the alveoli. The surfactant must then spread over the remaining surface area. This is accomplished with the aid of surfactant components such as PG, with spreading properties. Cholesterol and cholesterol esters account for the majority of the neutral lipids; their precise role is not yet determined, but they may aid in stabilizing the lipid structure.

TABLE 2-1	
Composition of Mature Surfactant	
COMPONENT	WEIGHT (%)
Total lipids	85-90
Protein	10-15
Specific lipids	
Phospholipids	85-90
Neutral lipids	5
Glycolipids	5-10
Specific phospholipids	
Phosphatidylcholine	70-80
Dipalmitoyl phosphatidylcholine	45-50
Phosphatidylglycerol	7-10
Phosphatidylethanolamine	3-5

Four important specific surfactant proteins (SPs) constitute a small part (2%-5%) of the weight of surfactant. SP-A, which is expressed in alveolar type II epithelial cells and in Clara cells in the lung, is the most studied surfactant protein. SP-A regulates surfactant turnover and is involved in the immune regulation within the lung and in the formation of **tubular myelin**. Tubular myelin is the term used to describe a precursor stage of surfactant as it is initially secreted from the type II cell and that has not yet spread (see Fig. 1-6C).

SP-B and SP-C are two hydrophobic surfactant-specific proteins. SP-B may be involved in the formation of tubular myelin. SP-B is involved in the surface activity of surfactant, and may increase the intermolecular and intramolecular order of the phospholipid bilayer and the lateral stability of the phospholipid layer. The 25 amino-terminal peptides of SP-B may further stabilize the phospholipid layer by increasing the collapse pressure of surfactant phospholipids. This action may prevent the squeezing out of the phospholipids from the monolayers at the alveolar air-liquid interface. A specific charge interaction between the cationic peptide and an anionic lipid, such as PG, may be responsible for this stabilization.

SP-C may be involved in the spreading ability and in the surface activity of surfactant. Another recently discovered surfactant-specific protein, SP-D, is a glycoprotein with an apparent molecular weight of 43 kDa. This substance contains an N-terminal collagenous domain and a carboxy-terminal, glycosylated domain similar to SP-A. The function of SP-D is unknown.

Pulmonary surfactant, synthesized in the alveolar type II epithelial cell, is stored as preformed units in lamellar bodies in the cytoplasm. These preformed lamellar bodies have distinctive swirling patterns that are readily observed by electron microscopy, and they are uniquely characteristic of type II epithelial cells (see Fig. 1-6). Secretion of surfactant into the airway occurs via exocytosis of the lamellar body by both constitutive and regulated mechanisms. Numerous agents, including β-adrenergic agonists, activators of protein kinase C, leukotrienes, and purinergic agonists, have been shown to stimulate the secretion of surfactant.

Pulmonary surfactant is cleared from the alveolus primarily through reuptake by type II cells, with minor contributions through absorption into lymphatics and clearance by alveolar macrophages. After being taken up by the type II cell, the phospholipids either are recycled for future secretion or are degraded and subsequently reutilized in the synthesis of new phospholipids. These processes are regulated developmentally in the fetal lung.

CLINICAL IMPORTANCE OF SURFACTANT

In 1959, Avery and Mead discovered that the lungs of premature infants who died of hyaline membrane disease (HMD) were deficient in surfactant. HMD, also know as respiratory distress syndrome (RDS), is characterized by increased work of breathing, progressive atelectasis (lung unit collapse), and respiratory failure in premature infants. It is a major cause of morbidity and mortality in the neonatal period. The major surfactant deficiency in premature infants is the lack of PG. In general, as the level of PG increases in amniotic fluid, the mortality rate decreases. This work culminated in successful attempts to treat HMD in premature infants with surfactant replacement therapy. Today, surfactant replacement therapy is the standard care for premature infants.

In summary, pulmonary surfactant reduces the work of breathing by reducing surface tension forces, prevents collapse and sticking of alveoli upon exhalation with anti-stick properties, and stabilizes alveoli, especially those that tend to deflate at low surface tension.

ALVEOLAR INTERDEPENDENCE

In addition to surfactant, another mechanism, namely interdependence, contributes to the stability of the alveoli (Fig. 2-12). Except for alveoli on the pleural surface, all alveoli are surrounded by other alveoli. The collapse of one alveolus is opposed by the traction exerted by the surrounding alveoli. Thus, the collapse of a single alveolus stretches and distorts the surrounding alveoli, which in turn are connected to other alveoli. The pores of Kohn and the canals of Lambert provide collateral ventilation and also prevent alveolar collapse (atelectasis).

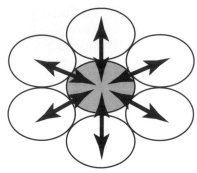

FIGURE 2-12 ■ Interdependence. The tendency of one alveolus to collapse *(shaded area)* is countered by opposing traction from the surrounding alveoli. *(From Berne RM, Levy ML, Koeppen BM, Stanton BA (eds): Physiology, 5th ed. St. Louis, Mosby, 2004.)*

SUMMARY

1. Lung volumes play a major role in gas exchange and work of breathing. Lung volumes are determined by the balance between the lung's elastic recoil properties and the properties of the muscles of the chest wall.

2. The vital capacity (VC) is the maximum amount of air that an individual can either inspire or exhale.

3. The functional residual capacity (FRC) is the resting volume of the lung. It is determined by the balance between the lung elastic recoil pressure operating to decrease lung volume and the pressure generated by the chest wall to become larger. At FRC, the pressure across the respiratory system is zero.

4. Limits to expiratory muscle lengthening and shortening are important determinants of TLC and RV, respectively, in young individuals.

5. The pressure across the lung (transpulmonary pressure [P_L]) is the difference between alveolar pressure and pleural pressure ($P_L = P_A - P_{PL}$). The pressure across the chest wall is the difference between pleural and barometric pressure ($P_W = P_{PL} - P_B$). The pressure across the respiratory system is the sum of the recoil pressures of the lung and the chest wall.

6. Lung compliance is a measure of the elastic properties of the lung. A loss of elastic recoil is seen in patients with emphysema and is associated with an increase in lung compliance. In contrast, in diseases associated with pulmonary fibrosis, lung compliance is decreased.

7. A positive transpulmonary pressure is needed to increase lung volume. The pressure across the respiratory system is zero at points of no airflow (end inspiration and end exhalation).

8. Surfactant in the alveolus changes the surface tension of the air-liquid interface as lung volume changes. The transmural pressure required to keep an alveolus inflated increases as lung volume (and transpulmonary pressure) increases and decreases as lung volume decreases.

9. Alveolar interdependence, the pores of Kohn, and the canals of Lambert help to prevent alveolar collapse (atelectasis).

KEY WORDS

- Alveolar interdependence
- Boyle's law
- Chest wall
- Chest wall mechanics
- Dynamic lung mechanics
- Functional residual capacity (FRC)
- Lamellar bodies
- Laplace's law
- Lung compliance
- Phosphatidylcholine
- Pleural effusion
- Pulmonary edema
- Residual volume (RV)

- Respiratory distress syndrome (RDS)
- Respiratory system
- Static lung mechanics
- Surface tension
- Surfactant
- Surfactant B (SP-B)
- Tidal volume (TV or V_T)
- Total lung capacity (TLC)
- Transmural pressure
- Transpulmonary pressure (P_L)
- Type I cell
- Type II cell
- Vital capacity (VC)

SELF-STUDY PROBLEMS

1. What factors determine total lung capacity?
2. What factors determine residual volume?
3. Describe the lung volume changes in an individual with acute hypersensitivity pneumonitis (a condition associated with interstitial pneumonia and the presence of proteinaceous fluid with increased numbers of alveolar macrophages in the alveoli).

REFERENCES

Brown RH, Mitzner W: Effects of lung inflation and airway muscle tone on airway diameter in vivo. J Appl Physiol 80: 1581-1588, 1996.

Cheung D, Schot R, Zwindermann AH, et al: Relationship between loss in parenchymal recoil pressure and maximal airway narrowing in subjects with alpha-1-antitrypsin deficiency. Am J Respir Crit Care Med 155:135-140, 1997.

D'Angelo E, Robatto FM, Calderini E, et al: Pulmonary and chest wall mechanics in anesthetized paralyzed humans. J Appl Physiol 70:2602-2610, 1991.

George RB, Light RW, Matthay MA, Matthay RA (eds): Chest Medicine: Essentials of Pulmonary and Critical Care Medicine, 3rd ed. Baltimore, Williams and Wilkins, 1995.

Lai-Fook SJ, Rodarte JR: Pleural pressure distribution and its relationship to lung volume and interstitial pressure. J Appl Physiol 70:967-978, 1991.

Zapletal A, Desmond KJ, Demizio D, et al: Lung recoil and the determination of airflow limitation in cystic fibrosis and asthma. Pediatr Pulmonol 15:13-18, 1993.

3

DYNAMIC LUNG MECHANICS

■ ■ ■ ■ ■ ■ ■ ■ ■ ■ ■ ■ ■

OBJECTIVES

1. Understand the principles of laminar and turbulent airflow.

2. Define airway resistance and its measurement.

3. Discuss three factors that contribute to or regulate airway resistance in health and disease.

4. Describe the concepts of flow limitation, the equal pressure point, and dynamic airway compression.

5. Define work of breathing and the factors that contribute to work of breathing.

D ynamic lung mechanics is that aspect of mechanics that studies the lung in motion. To cause air to move from the outside of the body into the distal airways, three opposing forces must be overcome: (1) the elastic recoil of the lungs and chest wall, (2) the frictional resistances of the airways and of the tissues of the lung and chest wall, and (3) the inertance or impedance of acceleration of the respiratory system. The elastic forces of the lung and chest wall depend on lung volume and are not affected by motion. Inertance depends on the rate of airflow but is negligible during quiet breathing. Thus, the major force that must be overcome to achieve airflow is frictional resistance. Frictional resistance is determined by flow and not by a change in lung volume.

AIRFLOW IN AIRWAYS

Air or liquid flows through a tube or a set of tubes when there is a pressure difference from one end of the tube to the other. The same is true in the airways, in which air flows when a pressure difference exists from one point in the airways to another. Thus, during inspiration, with contraction of the diaphragm the pressure in the pleural space (also called **intrathoracic pressure**) becomes more negative relative to atmospheric pressure. When the glottis then opens, gas flows into the airways (from higher to lower pressure) and lung volume increases. The speed or average velocity (in cm/sec) of flow is equal to the overall flow rate (in mL/sec) divided by the cross-sectional area of the tube (cm^2).

There are two major patterns of gas flow—**laminar** and **turbulent** (Fig. 3-1). Gas flow patterns in between laminar and turbulent also occur and are called transitional, or disturbed. The pattern of gas flow depends on the velocity and the characteristics of the airway. Laminar flow occurs when the stream of gas in a cylindrical tube is parallel to the walls of the tube. Laminar flow occurs at low flow rates. As the flow rate increases, and particularly as the airways divide, the flow stream becomes unsteady and small eddies occur; this is known as **transitional flow** or disturbed flow. At higher flow rates, there is disorganization of the flow stream with flow occurring both parallel and perpendicular to the overall flow axis and **turbulence** occurs.

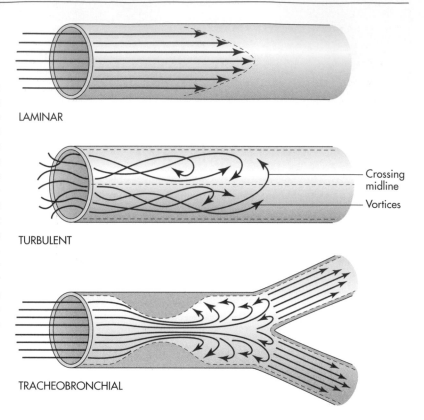

FIGURE 3-1 ■ Types of airflow. In laminar flow, air moves in the same direction parallel to the walls of the airways. The fluid in the center moves twice as fast as the fluid toward the edges while the fluid at the wall does not move. In turbulent flow, air moves irregularly in axial, radial, and circumferential directions and vortices are common. Gas density is important but viscosity is not. Turbulent flow requires higher pressures than laminar flow. Flow changes from laminar to turbulent when the Reynolds number exceeds 2000. Turbulent flow occurs in the large airways (tracheobronchial) and wherever there are irregularities in the airways (e.g., bifurcations, mucus).

In laminar flow, the gas traveling in the center of the tube moves most rapidly while the gas in direct contact with the wall of the tube remains stationary. In laminar flow, pressure (P) and flow ($\dot{V}$) are proportional (i.e., $P = k \times \dot{V}$). This telescope arrangement of multiple cylinders within the tube results in the cylinder closest to the vessel wall having the slowest velocity (due to frictional forces) and the center cylinder, where K is a constant, having the highest velocity. This changing velocity across the diameter of the tube is known as the **velocity profile** and occurs because fluid velocity decreases with the square of the radial distance away from the center of the tube. Thus, laminar flow has a parabolic velocity profile. In fact, when laminar flow is fully developed, the gas in the center of the tube moves exactly twice as fast as the average velocity.

In **turbulent flow**, gas movement occurs both parallel and perpendicular to the axis of the tube. Pressure is no longer proportional to the flow rate but to the flow rate squared (i.e., $P = k \times \dot{V}^2$). Viscosity of the gas becomes unimportant, but an increase in gas density increases the pressure drop for a given flow. Gas along the wall still remains stationary, but there is less variation in gas velocity as a function of position in the tube. Overall, gas velocity is blunted because energy is consumed in the process of generating the eddies and chaotic movement. As a consequence, all things being equal, a higher driving pressure is needed to support a given flow under turbulent conditions compared with laminar flow conditions. Stated another way, during laminar flow conditions, doubling the driving pressure (P) will double the flow rate. In contrast, during turbulent flow conditions, doubling the driving pressure will result in less than a doubling of the flow rate since some of the flow is perpendicular to the axis of the tube. Thus, there is a linear relationship between pressure and flow under laminar conditions and a nonlinear relationship under turbulent conditions (Fig. 3-2).

In transitional or disturbed flow, characteristics of both laminar and turbulent flow are seen. Flow through

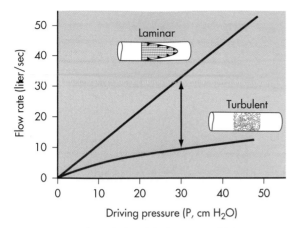

FIGURE 3-2 ■ The relationship between driving pressure and flow through a tube. Under laminar flow conditions, an increase in the driving pressure is associated with an increase in flow. In contrast, in turbulent flow, at any driving pressure, flow is less than under laminar conditions. The reason for this is that in turbulent flow some of the increase in driving pressure is expended by moving air in directions perpendicular to the airway axis. *(Redrawn from Leff A, Schumacker P. Respiratory Physiology: Basics and Applications. Philadelphia, WB Saunders, 1993.)*

much of the tube may be laminar but becomes more turbulent at sites where the tubes narrow or branch or where the walls of the tubes become irregular.

REYNOLDS NUMBER DETERMINES WHETHER FLOW IS LAMINAR OR TURBULENT

Whether flow through a tube is laminar or turbulent depends upon the Reynolds number (Re). Re is a dimensionless value that expresses the ratio of two dimensionally equivalent terms (kinematic/viscosity):

$$Re = \frac{2\ rvd}{n}$$

where r is the radius, v is the average velocity, d is the density, and n is the viscosity.

In straight tubes, turbulence occurs when the Reynolds number is greater than 2000. From this relationship, it can be seen that turbulence is most likely to occur when the average velocity of gas flow is high and the radius is large. In contrast, a low-density gas such as helium is less likely to cause turbulent flow

at any given flow rate. Airflow in the trachea during tidal volume (V_T) breathing is turbulent because the trachea has a large diameter (3 cm in the adult) and gas flow at the mouth during quiet breathing is approximately 1 L/sec, which results in an average velocity of 150 cm/sec. Thus, the Reynolds number for the trachea during quiet breathing is greater than 2000. For example,

$$Re = \frac{2 \times 1.5\ cm \times 150\ cm/sec \times 0.0012\ g/mL}{1.83 \times 10^{-4}\ g/sec \bullet cm} = 2951$$

where 0.0012 g/mL is the density of air and 1.83×10^{-4} g/sec • cm is the viscosity of air. Airflow becomes less turbulent as airway radius and flow decrease.

In such a complicated system as the bronchial tree, with its many branches, changes in caliber, and irregular wall surfaces, fully developed laminar flow probably only occurs in the very small airways, whereas flow is transitional in most of the bronchial tree.

Turbulence is also promoted by the glottis and vocal cords that produce some "irregularity" and obstruction in the tubes. As gas flows more distally, the total cross sectional area increases dramatically, and gas velocities decrease significantly. As a result, gas flow becomes more laminar in smaller airways even during maximal ventilation. The bottom line is that gas flow in the larger airways (nose, mouth, glottis, and bronchi) is turbulent, whereas gas flow in the smaller airways is laminar. Breath sounds heard with a stethoscope are due to turbulent airflow. Laminar flow is silent. As we describe later, this is one of the factors responsible for the difficulty in recognizing clinically small airway disease, which is said to be "silent."

RESISTANCE

The pressure flow characteristics of laminar flow were first described by the French physician Poiseuille. In straight circular tubes, the flow rate ($\dot{V}$; the dot above the letter V signifies a change in volume with respect to time—that is, a flow rate) is given by:

$$\dot{V} = \frac{P\pi r^4}{8nl}$$

where P is the driving pressure, r is the radius, n is the viscosity, and l is the length. Thus, it can be seen that the driving pressure (P) is proportional to the flow rate ($\dot{V}$); that is, $P = k \times \dot{V}$. The flow resistance, R, across a set of tubes is defined as the change in driving pressure (ΔP) divided by the flow rate, or

$$R = \frac{\Delta P}{\dot{V}} = \frac{8nl}{\Pi r^4}$$

The units of resistance are cm $H_2O/L \cdot$ sec. A number of important observations can be made based on this equation, including the role of the radius in determining resistance. If the radius of the tube is reduced in half, the resistance will increase 16-fold. If, however, the length is increased to twofold, the resistance will only increase twofold. Thus the radius of the tube primarily determines resistance. Stated another way, resistance is inversely proportional to the fourth power of the radius and directly proportional to the length of the tube and the gas viscosity. The radius is thus the main factor that affects resistance. The smaller the airway, the greater the resistance of that individual airway.

Resistance to airflow in the respiratory system is composed of three individual resistances; airway resistance, pulmonary (parenchyma or lung tissue) resistance, and chest wall resistance. **Airway resistance** is defined as the frictional resistance of the entire system of airways from the tip of the nose (for nasal breathing) or mouth (for mouth breathing) to the alveoli. **Pulmonary resistance** (or lung resistance) is defined as the frictional resistance afforded by the lungs and the airways combined. **Chest wall resistance** is the frictional resistance of the chest wall and abdominal structures. In turn, airway resistance is composed of the resistance of the upper airway (from nose to glottis) and the resistance of the lower airways (from glottis to alveoli).

Approximately 25% to 40% of the total resistance to airflow is located in the upper airways—namely the nose, nasal turbinates, oropharynx, nasopharynx, and larynx (Fig. 3-3). Respiratory system resistance is thus higher when you breathe through your nose than when you breathe through your mouth. During V_T breathing, the vocal cords open slightly during inspiration and close slightly during exhalation. During inspiration, airways inside the chest are surrounded by a negative intrathoracic (pleural) pressure, and airways outside the chest (extrathoracic airways) are surrounded by atmospheric pressure. As a result, the pressure

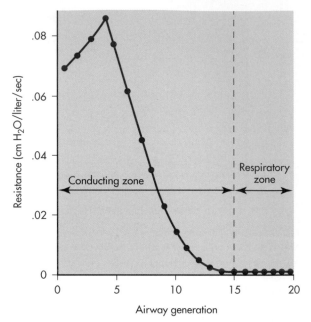

FIGURE 3-3 ■ Airway resistance as a function of the airway generation. As the airways branch from the trachea to main-stem bronchi to lobar bronchi, and so on, the daughter airways at each branch point are described as belonging to the next generation. In the normal lung, most of the resistance to airflow occurs in the first 8 generations. *(From Berne RM, Levy ML, Koeppen BM, Stanton BA (eds): Physiology, 5th ed. St. Louis, Mosby, 2004.)*

surrounding the extrathoracic airways is greater than the pressure inside the airways and these extrathoracic airways are pulled inward, resulting in partial or complete airway obstruction, especially during deep inspirations.

This inward pulling of extra thoracic airways during inspiration is most easily demonstrated in the nose. Making a rapid inspiratory effort while breathing through the nose results in collapse of the anterior portion of the nose (a "sniff"). Counteracting the collapse of the extrathoracic airways during inspiration are the muscles of the oropharynx that contract during inspiration. Reflex contraction of these pharyngeal dilator muscles dilates and stabilizes the upper airway. In the anterior nose, active contraction of the alae nasi minimizes the collapse associated with sniffing. Failure of these muscles to contract can occur, especially during sleep and can result in airway obstruction and obstructive sleep apnea (see Chapter 10).

Airflow resistance in the lower airways (Raw) can be divided between that in the large airways (>2 mm in diameter: first 8 airway generations), the medium-sized airways (subsegmental bronchi, ≥2 mm in diameter), and the small airways (bronchioles, <2 mm in diameter). Therefore, Raw is equal to the sum of each of these individual resistances; that is,

$$Raw = R_{large} + R_{medium} + R_{small}$$

From Poiseuille's equation, you might conclude that the major site of resistance in the airways is in the smallest airways. For many years, this was thought to be true. In fact, however, the major site of resistance along the bronchial tree is the large bronchi. The smallest airways contribute very little to the *overall* total resistance of the bronchial tree even though their *individual* resistance is high. The reason for this is twofold. First, airflow velocity becomes very low as the effective cross-sectional area increases (Fig. 3-4). Second, and most important, the airways exist in parallel rather than in series. The resistance to airflow in the lower airways is analogous to electrical resistance in that resistances in series are added together ($R_{TOT} = R_1 + R_2 ...$) and resistances in parallel are added as reciprocals ($1/R_{TOT} = 1/R_1 + 1/R_2 ...$). An *individual* small airway has a high resistance, but resistance of the small airways *in total*, because they exist in parallel, is the inverse of the sum of the individual resistances. Thus, the resistance of the small airways is very small. As an example, assume that there are three tubes each with a resistance of 3 cm $H_2O/L \cdot$ sec (Fig. 3-5). If the tubes are in series, the total resistance (R_{TOT}) is the sum of the individual resistances:

$$R_{TOT} = R_1 + R_2 + R_3 = 3 + 3 + 3 = 9 \text{ cm } H_2O/L \cdot sec$$

If the tubes are in parallel (as they are in small airways), the total resistance is the sum of the inverse of the individual resistances:

$$\frac{1}{R_{TOT}} = 1/R_1 + 1/R_2 + 1/R_3 =$$
$$1/3 + 1/3 + 1/3 = 1 \text{ cm } H_2O/L \cdot sec$$

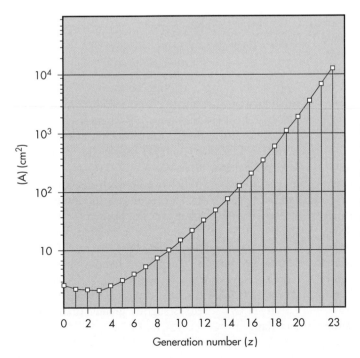

FIGURE 3-4 ■ Change in surface area (A) of the airways with increasing airway generation number. Although each individual airway gets smaller with each increase in generation number, (Z) the total cross-sectional area of each generation is greater than the total of area of the previous generation. *(From Weibel ER: Morphometry of the Human Lung. Heidelberg, Springer-Verlag, 1963.)*

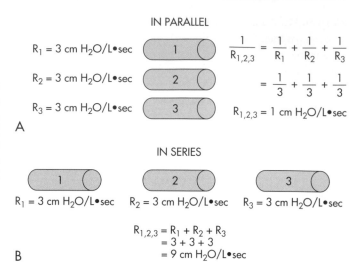

FIGURE 3-5 ■ Resistance in airways in parallel and in series. Resistance of airways in parallel (**A**) is always much less than the resistance in airways in series (**B**). This means that the total resistance of the small airways is less than the total resistance of the large airways even though the individual resistances of the small airways are much greater than the individual resistances of the large airways.

In the lung, the trachea divides into the main-stem bronchi, which in turn divide into the lobar, then segmental, and then subsegmental bronchi. In going from the trachea to the respiratory bronchioles, the number of airway branches increases as the size of each branch decreases. The smaller diameter increases the resistance offered by each individual airway, but the large increase in the number of parallel pathways reduces the resistance at each generation of branching (see Fig. 3-4). During normal breathing, approximately 80% of the resistance to airflow at functional residual capacity (FRC) occurs in airways with diameters greater than 2 mm. This is in contrast to the pulmonary blood vessels, in which most of the resistance is in the small vessels. Because the small airways contribute so little to total lung resistance, the measurement of airway resistance (see Chapter 4) is a poor test to detect small airway obstruction.

The partitioning of Raw between large and small airways can be further illustrated by the following example. If the resistance of the respiratory system (Raw) equals 2 cm $H_2O/L \cdot$ sec, and if the "large" airways (from the trachea to the segmental bronchi) contribute 80% to the total resistance, the subsegmental "medium-sized" airways (≥2 mm in diameter) contribute 15%, and the "small" airways (<2 mm in diameter) contribute

the remainder, then the individual resistances of the small, medium, and large airways can be determined as follows:

Large airways = 0.80 × 2 cm $H_2O/L \cdot$ sec =
1.6 cm $H_2O/$Lsec
Medium airways = 0.15 × 2 cm $H_2O/L \cdot$ sec =
0.30 cm $H_2O/$Lsec
Small airways = 0.05 × 2 cm $H_2O/L \cdot$ sec =
0.10 cm $H_2O/$Lsec

In this example, tripling of the resistance in the small airways due to obstruction would only increase Raw to 2.2 cm $H_2O/L \cdot$ sec, a 10% change. Thus, significant small airway disease can exist without a significant change in Raw. This is another reason why small airway disease is "silent."

There is also a difference between inspiratory and expiratory resistance. During quiet inspiration, the difference in pressure between the open mouth and the alveoli is 0.5 cm H_2O and the average airflow rate is 0.25 L/sec. Thus Raw = 0.5/0.25 = 2.0 cm $H_2O/L \cdot$ sec during inspiration. During exhalation, there is the same pressure difference, but the airflow rate is slightly slower at 0.2 L/sec. Thus, expiratory Raw (0.5/0.2 = 2.5 cm $H_2O/L \cdot$ sec) is slightly greater than inspiratory Raw.

FACTORS CONTRIBUTING TO RESISTANCE

Airway resistance is determined by a number of factors, including the number, length, and cross-sectional area of the conducting airways. The number of airways is established by the 16th week of gestation and is determined by the pattern of branching. Airway length varies from person to person and is dependent on age and body size and the phase of the respiratory cycle. Airways lengthen during inspiration as lung volume increases and shorten during exhalation. Of all the factors contributing to airway resistance, the cross-sectional area of the conducting airways is the most important because Raw varies inversely with the fourth power of the radius of the airway.

LUNG RESISTANCE

In healthy individuals, **lung resistance** is approximately 1 cm $H_2O/L \cdot$ sec. Lung resistance includes airway resistance and the resistance of the lung parenchyma to changing lung volume. Refer to the pleural pressure diagram shown in Figure 2-8. In this illustration, when the lung is inflated very slowly (known as a quasi-steady state), the dashed pleural pressure curve is generated. In contrast, during tidal volume breathing, the solid pleural pressure curve is generated. The difference between the two curves represents the additional pressure that is required to overcome the resistance encountered during changing lung volume. It is composed of the

resistance due to the acceleration of gas as it moves toward (or away from) the lung periphery as a result of the changing cross-sectional area and the viscous impedance encountered in changing lung volume.

The cross-sectional area of a conducting airway is determined by the balance of two opposing forces (Fig. 3-6). The elastic forces in the airways and the tension of airway smooth muscle surrounding the airways tend to contract the walls and decrease the cross-sectional area. Increasing the cross-sectional area is the outward traction either from a positive transpulmonary pressure or from the interdependence of alveoli and terminal bronchioles. The strength of these two opposing forces is largely determined by lung volume, elastic recoil, and the effect of neural and humoral agents on smooth muscle tone.

LUNG VOLUME AND AIRWAY RESISTANCE

Lung volume is one of the most important factors affecting airway resistance because the length and diameter of the airways increase with increasing lung volume and decrease with decreasing lung volume. As a result, resistance to airflow decreases with increasing lung volume and increases with decreasing lung volume. The relationship between Raw and lung volume is, however, curvilinear (Fig. 3-7). Specifically, Raw does not change significantly with changes in lung volume greater than FRC. Between FRC and residual volume

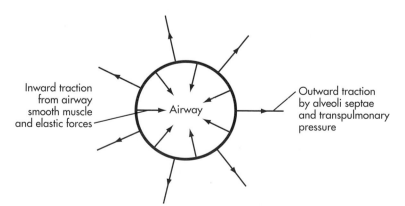

Inward traction from airway smooth muscle and elastic forces

Airway

Outward traction by alveoli septae and transpulmonary pressure

FIGURE 3-6 ■ Factors responsible for airway size. Airway smooth muscle and elastic forces in the airways tend to constrict the airways and decrease cross-sectional area. This tendency to constriction is opposed by the outward traction on the airways due to the interdependence of alveoli and terminal bronchioles or because of a positive transpulmonary pressure.

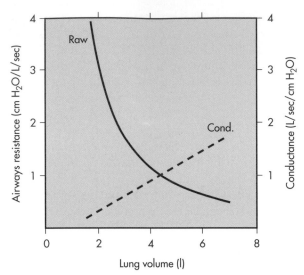

FIGURE 3-7 ■ Airway resistance (Raw) and conductance (Cond.) as a function of lung volume. *(From Berne RM, Levy ML, Koeppen BM, Stanton BA (eds): Physiology, 5th ed. St. Louis, Mosby, 2004.)*

(RV), however, Raw increases rapidly and approaches infinity (no airflow) at RV. The reciprocal of RAW is called the conductance (G = 1/Raw). When conductance is plotted against lung volume, the relationship becomes linear (see Fig. 3-7). As can be seen from the graph in Figure 3-7, conductance varies with lung volume. It also will vary in children compared with adults as a result of differences in body size. Specific airway conductance (SGAW) is airway conductance (GAW) divided by the lung volume at which it is measured. SGAW takes into account these variations in body size. From this relationship it can be seen that in the presence of increased airway resistance, breathing at a higher lung volume will reduce airway resistance. Individuals with increased airway resistance frequently breathe at higher than normal lung volumes. Although this will tend to normalize their GAW, their SGAW will remain abnormal. Factors known to increase resistance include airway mucus, edema, and contraction of bronchial smooth muscle, all of which decrease the caliber of the airways.

Applying Poiseuille's law, it can be seen that the density and viscosity of the inspired gas also affect resistance. When gas density increases, such as during a dive, airway resistance increases. When an oxygen-helium mixture is breathed instead of oxygen-nitrogen, the decrease in gas density results in a decrease in airway resistance. This decrease has been exploited in the treatment of *status asthmaticus*, a condition associated with increased airway resistance due to a combination of bronchospasm, edema, and mucus, in which breathing in an oxygen-helium gas admixture, results in decreased airway resistance.

ELASTIC RECOIL AND AIRWAY RESISTANCE

The elastic recoil of the lung also affects airway caliber through direct traction on small intrapulmonary airways and by effects on intrapleural pressure (see Fig. 3-6). Because of its effects on airway size in normal individuals, elastic recoil is the major determinant of intrathoracic airway resistance when individuals are breathing under quiet conditions in which flow is not limited.

As previously mentioned, the *airway* resistance at FRC in normal adults is 1 to 3 cm $H_2O/L \cdot$ sec. Resistance is higher in young children because their airways are smaller. As we shall see later, there is a strong negative correlation between resistance and maximal expiratory flow. A high resistance is associated with decreased expiratory flows.

NEUROHUMORAL REGULATION OF AIRWAY RESISTANCE

Airway resistance is also affected or regulated by neural and humoral agents through their effects on airway smooth muscle (Table 3-1). Airway smooth muscle from the trachea to the alveolar ducts is under the control of efferent fibers of the autonomic nervous system. These submucosal smooth muscle bands encircle the airways and can change the diameter of bronchi and bronchioles independent of lung volume or pleural pressure. Stimulation of cholinergic, parasympathetic postganglionic fibers, either directly or reflexively, leads to airway constriction (recall that the vagus nerve innervates airway smooth muscle) with an increase in airway resistance and a decrease in anatomic dead space. In contrast, stimulation of the sympathetic nerves and release of the postganglionic neurotransmitter norepinephrine inhibits airway constriction. Airway smooth muscle tone is mediated by β_2-adrenergic receptors that predominate in the airways. In general, parasympathetic tone in bronchial smooth muscle is

TABLE 3-1
Active Control of the Airways

CONSTRICT

Parasympathetic stimulation
Acetylcholine
Histamine
Leukotrienes
Thromboxane A_2
Serotonin
Alpha-adrenergic agonists
Decreased P_{CO_2} in small airways

DILATE

Sympathetic stimulation β_2 receptors
Circulating β_2 agonists
Nitric oxide
Increased P_{CO_2} in small airways
Decreased P_{CO_2} in small airways

greater than sympathetic tone, and thus even normal individuals can have a small decrease in airway resistance after inhalation of a bronchodilator.

Reflex stimulation of the vagus nerve due to smoke inhalation, dust, cold air, or other irritants can result in airway constriction and/or cough. Agents such as histamine, acetylcholine, thromboxane A_2, prostaglandin F_2, and leukotrienes (LTB4, C4, and D4) are released by various resident and recruited airway cells in response to various triggers and act directly on airway smooth muscle, causing constriction and an increase in airway resistance.

O_2 and CO_2 also affect airway caliber. Decreased CO_2 at bifurcations of the airways causes a local constriction of nearby airway smooth muscle while increased CO_2 or decreased O_2 causes dilation. O_2 and CO_2 responsiveness of airway smooth muscle may be an important homeostatic mechanism in balancing ventilation and perfusion when there is a pulmonary embolus.

The responsiveness of airway smooth muscle to humoral agents is used to determine whether an individual has heightened airway sensitivity. Measurement of pulmonary function after inhalation of methacholine, a histamine-like compound, is used in individuals suspected of having asthma in order to provoke airway constriction. Although all individuals will eventually respond to high concentrations of methacholine, individuals with asthma develop airway obstruction at low methacholine concentrations.

DYNAMIC COMPLIANCE

In Chapter 2, we examined compliance in terms of static changes—that is, compliance at discrete points. By way of review, the static compliance of the lungs is defined as the change in lung volume resulting from a change of 1 cm H_2O in the distending pressure. Breathing and the component of time create a set of dynamic mechanical properties that affect the pressure in the lung and chest wall. **Dynamic compliance** is the change in the volume of the lungs divided by the distending pressure during the course of a breath.

A dynamic pressure volume curve can be created by having an individual breathe over a normal lung volume range (usually from FRC to FRC + 1 L). The mean dynamic compliance of the lung (dyn CL) is calculated as the slope of the line that joins the end-inspiratory and end-expiratory points of no flow (Fig. 3-8).

Dynamic and static compliance are closely related in normal individuals. At a respiratory frequency of 15 breaths per minute or lower, dynamic compliance is

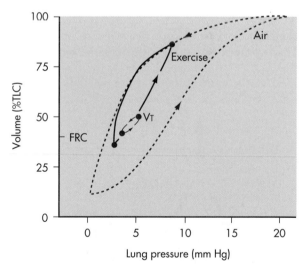

FIGURE 3-8 ■ Dynamic pressure-volume loops of the lung: resting tidal volume (VT) *(small loop)* and VT during exercise *(mid-sized loop)*. The maximum air-filled lung pressure-volume loop *(red loop)* from Figure 2-9 is also shown. The dynamic compliance of the tidal breath (slope of the line connecting end inspiration with end expiration) is less than that of the lung during exercise. FRC, functional residual capacity; TLC, total lung capacity; VT, tidal volume. *(Modified from Berne RM, Levy ML (eds): Principles of Physiology, 3rd ed. St. Louis, Mosby, 1999.)*

slightly less than static compliance. This is because during tidal volume breathing, there is a small change in alveolar surface area that is insufficient to bring additional surfactant molecules to the surface, and so the lung is less compliant. At higher respiratory frequencies, such as during exercise dynamic compliance is slightly greater than static compliance. This is because during exercise, there are big changes in tidal volume and more surfactant material is incorporated into the air-liquid interface, and thus the lung is more compliant. In individuals with increased airway resistance, the ratio of dynamic compliance to static compliance decreases significantly as respiratory rate increases. Thus, dynamic compliance is affected not only by changes in lung compliance but also by changes in airway resistance.

How does airway resistance contribute to the difference between static and dynamic compliance in individuals with obstructive pulmonary disease? Consider two alveoli supplied by the same airway (Fig. 3-9). If the resistance and compliance of the two units were equal, the two units would fill and empty with identical time courses. Imagine now that the resistance of the airways supplying each of the units was equal but the compliance of one of the units was decreased by half. The two units would fill with the same time course,

but the unit with the decrease in compliance would receive only half of the volume of air of the other unit. Now imagine a situation where the compliance of the two lung units is the same but the resistance of one unit is twice the resistance of the other unit. The unit with the elevated resistance would fill more slowly than the other lung unit although, given sufficient time, both units would fill to the same volume.

As the respiratory rate increases, the unit with the lower resistance will accommodate a larger volume of air per breath. In addition, there will be a redistribution of air at the end of inspiration because one alveolus will have more air than the other. As a result, because the compliance characteristics are the same, the more distended alveolus will have a higher elastic recoil pressure, and air will follow the pressure gradient and move to the other alveolus.

Alveoli supplied by airways with increased resistance (e.g., small airway obstruction/disease) are referred to as having long **time constants**. As respiratory frequency increases in individuals with small airway obstruction, these alveoli with long time constants will have insufficient time to fill and will not contribute to the dynamic compliance. Dynamic compliance will decrease as the respiratory rate increases, and more and more of these alveoli with long time constants will drop out.

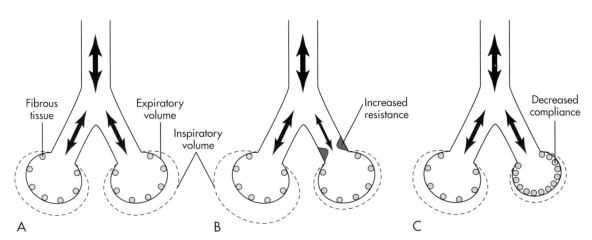

FIGURE 3-9 ■ Relationship between compliance and resistance. **A,** Two respiratory units with equal resistance and compliance will fill and empty with identical time courses. **B,** If the resistance of one airway is increased, the unit with the higher resistance will fill more slowly (note *smaller arrow*) and more of the ventilation will be distributed to the other unit (note larger inspiratory volume). **C,** If the compliance of one unit is decreased, the two units will fill with the same time course, but the volume of the unit with the decreased compliance will be less than the volume of the other unit. *(Modified from Berne RM, Levy ML (eds): Principles of Physiology, 3rd ed. St. Louis, Mosby, 1999.)*

Sighing and yawning increase dynamic compliance by increasing tidal volume via restoring the normal surfactant layer. Both of these activities are important to maintaining normal compliance. In contrast to the lung, the **dynamic compliance of the chest wall** is not significantly different from its static compliance.

DYNAMIC AIRWAY COMPRESSION AND FLOW LIMITATION

Take a deep breath in and blow the air out while feeling the force of air movement against your hand. Note that as lung volume decreases, the flow rate felt by your hand decreases. Try now to increase that flow rate at low lung volumes by exerting greater expiratory effort. No matter how hard you try, expiratory flow rates decrease as lung volume decreases, and the maximum expiratory flow rate occurs at a relatively modest level of effort. This is called **expiratory flow limitation**. What is the mechanism for expiratory flow limitation? Flow limitation occurs when the airways, which are intrinsically floppy, distensible tubes, become compressed (**dynamic airway compression**). Airways become compressed when the pressure outside the airway is greater than the pressure inside the airway.

Consider the events that occur during expiratory flow at two different lung volumes (Fig. 3-10). The collective airways and alveoli are shown surrounded by

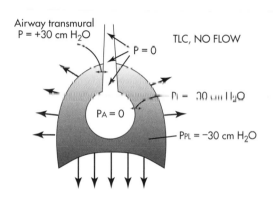

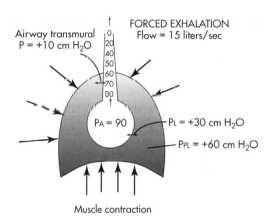

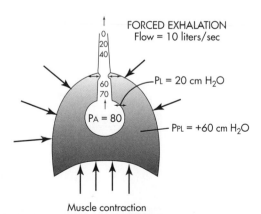

FIGURE 3-10 ■ Flow limitation. End inspiration, before the start of exhalation (**A**) and at the start of a forced exhalation (**B**). **C,** Expiratory flow limitation later, in a forced exhalation. Expiratory flow limitation occurs at locations where airway diameter is narrowed as a result of a negative transmural pressure. See text for further explanation. *(From Berne RM, Levy ML, Koeppen BM, Stanton BA (eds): Physiology, 5th ed. St. Louis, Mosby, 2004.)*

the pleural space and the chest wall. In Figure 3-10, the airways are shown as tapered tubes because the total or collective airway cross-sectional area decreases from the alveoli to the trachea. At the start of exhalation, but before any gas flow occurs, the alveolar pressure (PA) is zero (no airflow) and the pleural pressure (PPL) in this example is −30 cm H_2O. The transpulmonary pressure (PL) is thus +30 cm H_2O (PL = PA − PPL). Since there is no flow, the pressure inside the airways is zero and the pressure across the airways (PTA, transairway pressure) is also +30 cm H_2O (PTA = P_{airway} − PPL = 0 − [−30 cm H_2O]). This positive transpulmonary and transairway pressure holds the alveoli and the airways open.

Exhalation now begins, and with relaxation of the diaphragm the pleural pressure rises to +60 cm H_2O. Alveolar pressure also rises; in part, this is due to the increase in pleural pressure (60 cm H_2O) (recall that at zero flow, pleural pressure and alveolar pressure are equal), and in part this is due to the elastic recoil pressure (PEL) of the lung at that lung volume. The alveolar pressure is thus the sum of the pleural pressure and the elastic recoil pressure (which in this case is +30 cm H_2O). This is the driving pressure for expiratory gas flow. Because alveolar pressure (PA = PEL + PPL = 30 cm H_2O + 60 cm H_2O = 90 cm H_2O in this example) is greater than atmospheric pressure, gas begins to flow from the alveolus to the mouth when the glottis opens. As gas flows out of the alveoli, the transmural pressure across the airways decreases (i.e., the pressure head for expiratory gas flow dissipates). This occurs for two reasons: first, there is a resistive pressure drop caused by the frictional pressure loss associated with flow (expiratory airflow resistance). The second reason is that as the cross-sectional area of the airways decreases toward the trachea, the gas velocity increases. This acceleration of gas flow further decreases the pressure due to the **Bernoulli principle** effect (Fig. 3-11).

Thus, as air moves out of the lung, the driving pressure for expiratory gas flow decreases. In addition, the mechanical tethering (traction) that helps to hold the airways open at high lung volumes becomes less as lung volume decreases. There is a point between the alveoli and the mouth at which the pressure inside the

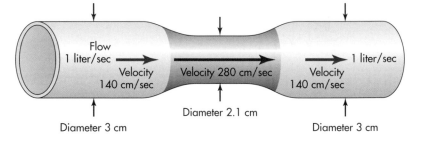

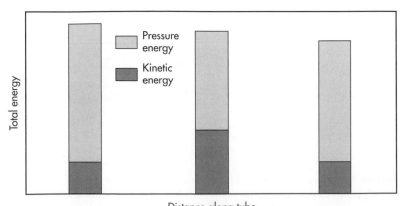

FIGURE 3-11 ■ The Bernoulli principle. As fluid moves through a tube at a constant flow rate, the total energy (kinetic plus potential energy) decreases as a result of frictional resistance (converting some of the energy into heat). At points of narrowing, fluid velocity increases, causing an increase in kinetic energy at the expense of potential energy. When the tube then widens, the fluid decelerates and the kinetic energy is converted into pressure energy. Thus, as air moves from the larger to the smaller airways, rates of airflow decrease. Similarly, during exhalation, as small airways empty into large airways, rates of airflow increase. (*Redrawn from Leff A, Schumacker P: Respiratory Physiology: Basics and Applications. Philadelphia, WB Saunders, 1993.*)

airways is equal to the pressure surrounding the airways. This point is called the **equal pressure point**. Airways toward the mouth become compressed because the pressure outside is greater than the pressure inside (dynamic airway compression). As a consequence, the transairway pressure now becomes negative ($P_{TA} = P_{airway} - P_{PL} = 58 - [+60] = -2$ cm H_2O just beyond the equal pressure point), and no amount of greater effort will increase the flow further because the higher pleural pressure will tend to collapse the airway at the equal pressure point just as much as it tends to increase the driving gradient for expiratory gas flow. Under these conditions, airflow is independent of the total driving pressure. This is why effort independent expiratory flow limitation occurs. It is also why airway resistance is higher during exhalation than inspiration.

In normal individuals, dynamic airway compression does not occur during a passive exhalation (Fig. 3-12). Consider a lung inflated to the same lung volume as before with the same elastic recoil. In the absence of forceful contraction of the muscles of exhalation, pleural pressure is slightly negative. The driving pressure for expiratory gas flow is the sum of the pleural pressure (−5 cm H_2O in this example) and elastic recoil pressure (+30 cm H_2O in this case) or 25 cm H_2O.

Gas flows out of the lung when the glottis opens, and the pressure head is dissipated as lung volume decreases secondary to frictional resistance. However, at every point in which there is gas flow (alveolar pressure − atmospheric pressure > 0), the transmural pressure across the airway is positive, tending to hold the airway open. Thus, during quiet breathing in normal individuals there is no flow limitation and no dynamic airway compression.

In contrast, coughing is the best example of dynamic compression in normal individuals. At the start of a cough, the individual takes a deep breath (usually $1\frac{1}{2}$ times tidal volume), increasing elastic recoil; the glottis closes and the chest wall muscles contract, increasing pleural pressure. The glottis then opens and gas is forcefully expelled. During the cough, the posterior membranous portion of the trachea is compressed and the tracheal diameter is narrowed (Fig. 3-13). Airflow at the site of compression is turbulent and makes the sound that we call a cough.

The measurement of expiratory flow rates is discussed in Chapter 4.

In the absence of lung disease, the equal pressure point occurs in airways that contain cartilage and thus resist deformation. The equal pressure point, however,

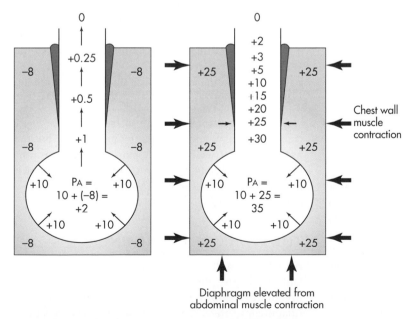

PASSIVE EXHALATION   FORCED EXHALATION

Diaphragm elevated from abdominal muscle contraction

Chest wall muscle contraction

FIGURE 3-12 ■ Dynamic airway compression. **A,** During passive exhalation intra-airway pressure remains positive and greater than pleural pressure; no dynamic compression occurs. **B,** With a forced exhalation, the driving pressure for expiratory gas flow is still the sum of the elastic recoil pressure (+10) and the pleural pressure (+25). As gas moves out of the alveoli, the pressure head is dissipated due to frictional resistance. At some point in the airways, the intra-airway pressure is equal to the pleural pressure (equal pressure point; *red arrows*). Beyond this point the pleural (outside) pressure is greater than airway (inside) pressure and airways are compressed. P_A, alveolar pressure.

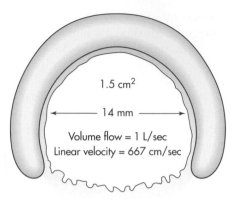

TRACHEA DURING NORMAL BREATHING

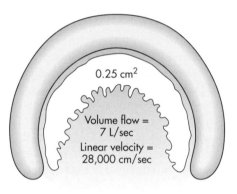

TRACHEA DURING COUGH

FIGURE 3-13 ■ Tracheal dimensions and air velocity during cough. With coughing, the noncartilaginous posterior membrane of the trachea is inverted, decreasing the size of the tracheal lumen to one-sixth of normal. With an increase in flow rate of 7-fold during a cough, the linear velocity of air increases 42-fold. *(Redrawn from Comroe JH: Physiology of Respiration. Chicago, Year Book Medical Publishers, 1965.)*

is not static. As lung volume decreases and the elastic recoil pressure decreases, the equal pressure point moves closer to the alveoli. What happens in individuals with lung disease? Picture an individual with airway obstruction secondary to a combination of mucus and airway inflammation. At the start of exhalation, the driving pressure for expiratory gas flow is the same as in a normal individual—that is, it is the sum of the elastic recoil pressure and the pleural pressure. As exhalation proceeds, however, there is a greater

resistive drop in the pressure head due to the decrease in airway radius secondary to mucus and inflammation. As a result, the point at which the pressure inside the airway is equal to the pressure outside now occurs in smaller airways without cartilage. These airways become compressed and readily collapse as the equal pressure point moves even closer to the alveolus. **Premature airway closure** occurs, resulting in air trapping and an increase in lung volume. The increase in lung volume initially helps to offset the increase in airway resistance due to the mucus and inflammation by increasing airway caliber and increasing elastic recoil. As inflammation progresses or mucus increases, flow limitation occurs and maximal expiratory flow rates decrease. Premature airway closure is the mechanism responsible for the appearance of crackles on auscultation in individuals with lung disease. It can be due to mucus, airway inflammation, fluid in the airways, or any mechanism responsible for airway narrowing or compression and can also be due to loss of elastic recoil (emphysema). In fact, acute and chronic lung diseases can alter the expiratory flow volume relationship as a result of any of the following:

- Changes in static lung recoil pressures
- Changes in airway resistance and the distribution of resistance along the airways
- Loss of mechanical tethering of intraparenchymal airways
- Changes in stiffness or mechanical properties of the airways
- Differences in the severity of the above changes among lung regions

Airway closure can be demonstrated only at especially low lung volumes in healthy individuals, but the lung volume at which airway closure occurs in individuals with obstructive pulmonary diseases is much higher. The measurement of this closing volume is discussed in Chapter 4.

THE WORK OF BREATHING

Before leaving the area of lung mechanics it is important to discuss the concept of work of breathing. Breathing requires the use of respiratory muscles (diaphragm, intercostals, etc.) that expend energy; thus, work is involved in inspiration and (to a lesser extent) in exhalation. Work is required to overcome the inherent mechanical properties of the lung (i.e., elastic and flow resistive forces) to move both the lungs and the chest wall. In the respiratory system, the work of breathing is the change in volume multiplied by the pressure exerted across the respiratory system. The pressure change is the change in transpulmonary pressure that is required to overcome the elastic work of breathing and the resistance work of breathing. The volume change is the volume of air that is moving in and out of the lung (e.g., the tidal volume at rest; that is,

$$\text{Work of breathing (W)} = \text{pressure (P)} \times \text{change in volume } (\Delta V)$$

The elastic component of the work of breathing is composed of the work associated with overcoming the elastic recoil of the chest wall and lung parenchyma and the work associated with overcoming the surface tension of the alveoli. The resistive component of the work of breathing is the work associated with overcoming the tissue (lung) and airway resistance.

Although methods are not available to measure the total amount of work involved in breathing, one can estimate the mechanical work necessary by measuring volume and pressure changes during a respiratory cycle. Work of breathing can be illustrated by analysis of the pressure-volume curves shown in Figure 3-14. Panel A is representative of a respiratory cycle of a normal lung. The static inflation-deflation curve is represented by line ABC. The total mechanical workload is represented by the trapezoidal area 0AECD. A breakdown of the trapezoidal areas in Panel A enables one to appreciate individual aspects of the mechanical work load, which includes the following areas:

0ABCD—work necessary to overcome elastic resistance
AECF—work necessary to overcome non-elastic resistance
AECB—work necessary to overcome non-elastic resistance during inspiration
ABCF—work necessary to overcome non-elastic resistance during exhalation (represents stored elastic energy from inspiration)

In restrictive lung diseases such as pulmonary fibrosis in which lung compliance is decreased or in obese individuals who have increased inward chest elastic recoil pressure, the elastic work of breathing is increased,

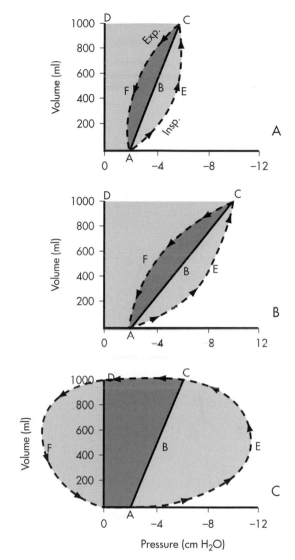

FIGURE 3-14 ■ The mechanical work done during a respiratory cycle in a normal lung (**A**), a lung with reduced compliance (**B**), and a lung with increased airway resistance (**C**). Exp., expiratory; F, flow; Insp., inspiratory. *(From Berne RM, Levy ML, Koeppen BM, Stanton BA (eds): Physiology, 5th ed. St. Louis, Mosby, 2004.)*

the pressure-volume curve is shifted to the right. and thus the work of breathing is increased significantly (Panel B in Fig. 3-14), as seen by the increase in the trapezoidal area 0AECD. In obstructive lung diseases such as asthma and chronic bronchitis, in which airway resistance is elevated, or in diseases associated with increased tissue resistance such as sarcoidosis, greater negative pleural pressures are needed to maintain proper inspiratory flow rates. In addition to the increase in total inspiratory work (area 0AECD), these individuals have an increase in positive pleural pressure during exhalation due to the increase in resistance and also an increased expiratory workload visualized as area DF0. This is because the stored elastic energy in area ABCF in Panel A is not sufficient, and additional energy is needed for exhalation. For these individuals, the resistive work of breathing can be extremely high during a forced exhalation associated with dynamic compression. Respiratory muscles are capable of performing increased work over long periods of time, but like other skeletal muscles, they can fatigue. Respiratory muscle fatigue is a major problem in individuals with lung disease and can result in respiratory failure.

In addition to the diseases just mentioned, work of breathing is influenced by breathing patterns. Work of breathing is increased when deeper breaths are taken (increase in tidal volume requires more elastic work to overcome) or when there is an increase in the respiratory rate (increase in minute ventilation requires more flow-resistance forces to overcome) (Fig. 3-15). As would be anticipated, individuals with normal lungs and individuals with lung disease adopt the respiratory patterns at which the work of breathing is the lowest. Individuals with pulmonary fibrosis (high elastic work) breathe more shallowly and rapidly, whereas individuals with obstructive lung disease (nonelastic work, high resistive work) breathe more slowly and deeply.

In normal individuals, the oxygen cost of quiet breathing is less than 5% of the total body

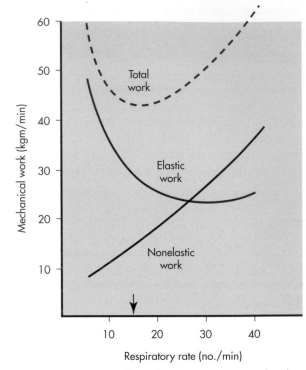

FIGURE 3-15 ■ The effect of respiratory rate on the elastic, nonelastic, and total mechanical work of breathing at a given level of alveolar ventilation. Subjects tend to adopt the respiratory rate at which the total of work of breathing (the sum of the elastic work and the nonelastic work) is minimal *(arrow). (From Berne RM, Levy ML, Koeppen BM, Stanton BA (eds): Physiology, 5th ed. St. Louis, Mosby, 2004.)*

oxygen uptake. This oxygen cost can increase to 30% during maximal exercise. In individuals with obstructive pulmonary disease, the work of breathing is high and can become the limiting factor in exercise.

SUMMARY

1. Resistance is the change in pressure per unit of flow. Airway resistance is determined by airway caliber and length as well as gas velocity and density.
2. Airway resistance is highly sensitive to changes in airway radius and varies with the inverse of the fourth power of the radius. Resistance is higher in turbulent than in laminar flow.
3. The Reynolds number determines whether flow is laminar or turbulent. Only flow in small airways is laminar; laminar flow is "silent."

4. The first 8 airway generations are the major site of airway resistance. Small airways contribute little to overall airway resistance.

5. Airway resistance decreases with increases in lung volume and with increases in elastic recoil.

6. Neural and humoral agents regulate or affect airway resistance through their effects on airway smooth muscle.

7. Dynamic and static compliance are closely related in normal individuals, but dynamic compliance is much lower in individuals with obstructive pulmonary disease.

8. Airway resistance contributes to the long time constants present in individuals with obstructive pulmonary disease.

9. Flow limitation occurs when dynamic airway compression is present.

10. The equal pressure point is the point at which the pressure inside and the pressure surrounding the airway are the same. As lung volume and elastic recoil decrease during exhalation, the equal pressure point moves toward the alveolus in normal individuals resulting in dynamic compression and expiratory flow limitation. In individuals with chronic obstructive pulmonary disease (COPD), at any lung volume the equal pressure point is closer to the alveolus, resulting in greater expiratory flow limitation and decreased expiratory flow rates.

11. Work of breathing is the change in volume times the pressure exerted across the respiratory system and is composed of elastic and nonelastic (resistive) components. Work of breathing is elevated in individuals with obstructive pulmonary diseases. All individuals breathe at a respiratory frequency that minimizes the work of breathing.

KEY WORDS

- Airway resistance (Raw)
- Alveolar interdependence
- Bernoulli principle
- Dynamic airway compression
- Dynamic compliance
- Equal pressure point
- Flow limitation
- Laminar flow
- Oxygen cost (of breathing)
- Poiseuille's law
- Reynolds number
- Transitional flow
- Turbulent flow
- Velocity profile
- Work of breathing

SELF-STUDY PROBLEMS

1. What is the effect of lung volume on airway resistance?
2. What are the factors that control the cross-sectional area of an airway?
3. What is the effect of a reduction in elastic recoil pressure on the location of the equal pressure point?
4. Why are large airways the major contributors to the resistance of the respiratory system as compared with small airways?

REFERENCES

Brown RH, Mitzner W: Effects of lung inflation and airway muscle tone on airway diameter in vivo. J Appl Physiol 80:1581-1588, 1996.

Cheung D, Schot R, Zwindermann AH, et al: Relationship between loss in parenchymal recoil pressure and maximal airway narrowing in subjects with alpha-1-antitrypsin deficiency. Am J Respir Crit Care Med 155:135-140, 1997.

D'Angelo E, Robatto FM, Calderini E, et al. Pulmonary and chest wall mechanics in anesthetized paralyzed humans. J Appl Physiol 70:2602-2610, 1991.

George RB, Light RW, Matthay MA, Matthay RA (eds): Chest Medicine: Essentials of Pulmonary and Critical Care Medicine, 3rd ed. Baltimore, Williams and Wilkins, 1995.

Lai-Fook SJ, Rodarte JR: Pleural pressure distribution and its relationship to lung volume and interstitial pressure. J Appl Physiol 70:967-978, 1991.

Zapletal A, Desmond KJ, Demizio D, et al: Lung recoil and the determination of airflow limitation in cystic fibrosis and asthma. Pediatr Pulmonol 15:13-18, 1993.

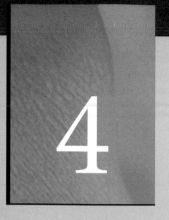

TESTS OF LUNG FUNCTION

OBJECTIVES

1. Describe lung volumes and their measurement using three different methods.
2. Discuss the uses of spirometry in clinical practice.
3. Define the effort-dependent and effort-independent portions of the flow volume curve.
4. Outline an approach to the interpretation of lung volumes, spirometry, and flow volume curves.
5. Describe the physiology behind the diffusion capacity for carbon monoxide and list three diseases associated with abnormal results.
6. Briefly outline the measurement of resistance and compliance.

A discussion of lung mechanics would be incomplete without a discussion of pulmonary function tests. Pulmonary function tests are designed to identify and quantify abnormalities in lung function. With the exception of exercise-induced asthma, pulmonary function tests do not make a clinical diagnosis. Rather, they can describe pathophysiologic processes and can help to distinguish between cardiac and pulmonary disease. The two major groups of pathophysiologic processes that can be distinguished using pulmonary function tests are **obstructive pulmonary disease (OPD)** and **restrictive pulmonary disease.** Pulmonary function test results are used as an additional, albeit important, element of the history, physical examination, and laboratory data that aid the clinician in making a diagnosis and in assessing response to therapy and disease progression. In this chapter, we describe the measurement and interpretation of a variety of pulmonary function tests that are used clinically.

LUNG VOLUMES

Before examining how to measure lung volumes, the reader should review the definition of the important lung volumes (see Chapter 2).

As a general rule, all lung volumes are measured in liters. The **vital capacity** (**VC**) is the total volume of air that an individual is able to exhale from a full and maximal inspiration to a maximal exhalation and is one of the most important pulmonary function tests. When measured as a rapid exhalation, it is called the **forced vital capacity** (**FVC**). The FVC varies with age, height, gender, and ethnicity but is approximately 4 liters in a healthy adult male.

The VC can also be measured as a slow exhalation (called the **slow vital capacity** [**SVC**]). In individuals with normal lung function, the FVC and the SVC are the same. In the presence of premature airway closure, however, the SVC is greater than the FVC because air trapping occurs during a forced maneuver secondary to dynamic airway closure. The difference between the

SVC and the FVC is thus a measure of dynamic airway closure. It is, however, of greater interest to physiologists than to clinicians.

The **residual volume** (**RV**) is the air remaining in the lung after a complete exhalation. This volume is established with the first several breaths of extrauterine life and disappears with the last breath.

The **total lung capacity** (**TLC**) is the sum of the VC and the RV. TLC occurs when the forces of inspiration (because of muscle fiber lengthening) are insufficient to overcome the increasing force required to distend the lung and chest wall.

The **functional residual capacity** (**FRC**) is the resting volume of the lung and is composed of the RV and the **expiratory reserve volume** (**ERV**) (the volume of air that can be exhaled from FRC to RV). The FRC is the volume of air in the lung at the end of a normal exhalation and is determined by the balance between the pressure generated by the lung parenchyma to become smaller (lung recoil pressure) and the pressure generated by the chest wall to become larger. In the presence of chest wall muscle weakness, the chest wall outward recoil pressure is decreased, the lung recoil pressure is less opposed, and the FRC decreases. In contrast, in the presence of air trapping, the FRC increases.

The relationship between RV and TLC is called the RV/TLC ratio and is often used to help distinguish between restrictive pulmonary disease and OPD (Table 4-1). In normal individuals, the RV/TLC ratio is less than 25%. An elevated RV/TLC ratio due to an increase in RV is caused by air trapping secondary to airway obstruction. An elevated RV/TLC ratio due

TABLE 4-1

Lung Volume Abnormalities in Obstructive and Restrictive Pulmonary Diseases

	OBSTRUCTIVE LUNG DISEASE	RESTRICTIVE LUNG DISEASE
TLC	N → ↑	↓
RV	↑	↓ → N
FRC	↑	↓
RV/TLC (%)	↑	N → ↑

FRC, functional residual capacity; RV, residual volume; TLC, total lung capacity; N, normal; ↑, increased; ↓, decreased.

to a decrease in TLC is seen in individuals with restrictive lung disease.

MEASUREMENT OF LUNG VOLUMES

There are three commonly used methods to measure lung volumes: inert gas dilution, plethysmography, and nitrogen washout.

Inert Gas Dilution Technique

In the inert gas dilution technique (Fig. 4-1), a known concentration of an inert gas such as helium, argon, or neon (this example uses helium) is added to a spirometer system that has a known volume. At FRC, the subject is connected to the system and breathes in the closed system until the helium concentration reaches a plateau, indicating equal concentrations of helium

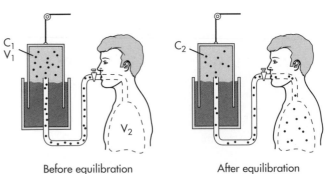

FIGURE 4-1 ■ Measurement of lung volume by helium dilution. C, concentration of helium; V, volume. *(From Berne RM, Levy ML, Koeppen BM, Stanton BA (eds): Physiology, 5th ed. St. Louis, Mosby, 2004.)*

Before equilibration   After equilibration

$$C_1 \times V_1 = C_2 \times (V_1 + V_2)$$

in the spirometer system and in the subject's lung. Because helium is inert, the new helium concentration after equilibrium in the subject's lung has occurred can be used to determine the subject's FRC by solving for V_2 using the mass balance equation:

$$C_1V_1 = C_2(V_1+V_2)$$

where C_1 is the initial concentration of helium in the spirometer system, V_1 is the volume of the spirometer system, C_2 is the new concentration of helium at equilibrium in the subject's lung and spirometer, and V_2 is the subject's FRC. By measuring the FRC, other lung volumes such as RV and TLC can be determined by subtracting the ERV from the FRC to get RV and by adding the RV to the FVC to get TLC.

Plethysmography

Plethysmography can also measure lung volumes and is the preferred method. The principle of plethysmography is based upon Boyle's law, which states that the product of pressure (P) times volume (V) (i.e., PV) of a gas is constant when temperature is constant (isothermal). The gas in the lungs is isothermal because of its intimate contact with capillary blood.

A plethysmograph (also known as a body box) is an airtight box with pressure transducers for measuring the pressure inside the box and at the mouth (Fig. 4-2). Recall that pressure measured at the mouth with an open glottis and no airflow reflects alveolar pressure. The change in pressure inside the box is related to volume by introducing a small volume of gas into the box and measuring the change in pressure. The subject sits inside the airtight box and breathes through a mouthpiece connected to the outside. With temperature constant, the shutter on the mouthpiece closes and the individual gently and slowly pants against the closed mouthpiece (Fig. 4-3). The change in pressure in the mouthpiece reflects alveolar pressure (recall there is essentially no airflow). Pressure changes inside the box reflect changes in pulmonary gas volume as gas within the chest is alternately compressed and decompressed by the action of the respiratory muscles. If the valve at the mouth closes while the subject is making an expiratory effort, alveolar pressure increases by an amount that is measured by the mouth pressure sensor, lung volume decreases as a result of

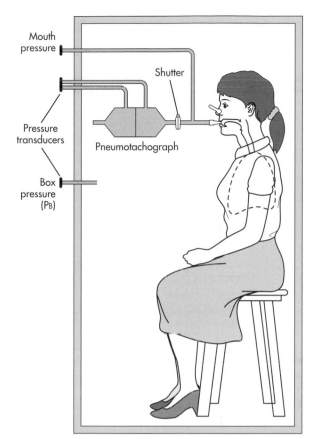

FIGURE 4-2 ■ Body plethysmograph. *(From Berne RM, Levy ML, Koeppen BM, Stanton BA (eds): Physiology, 5th ed. St. Louis, Mosby, 2004.)*

gas compression, and, with no airflow, the pressure inside the plethysmograph decreases. This pressure change is related back to a change in volume, and all the elements of Boyle's law are now present to solve for lung volume at FRC.

In individuals with normal lungs, FRC measured by helium dilution and by plethysmography is the same. The inert gas technique, however, can markedly underestimate FRC in individuals with OPD because equilibration of the helium in markedly obstructed airways may not have occurred during the test (these areas have very long time constants). In contrast, plethysmography measures all gas in the lung at FRC, including trapped gas. Because of this, the difference

FIGURE 4-3 ■ Measurement of functional residual capacity by body plethysmography. See text for details. *(Modified from Hyatt RE, Scanlon PD, Nakamura M: Interpretation of Pulmonary Function Tests: A Practical Guide. Philadelphia, Lippincott Williams & Wilkins, 1997.)*

Boyle's law:
$$PV = P_1V_1$$

$P = P_B$ (Barometric pressure)
V_{UN} = Unknown vol (FRC)

Closed shutter
$P_1 = P_B + \Delta P$
where ΔP is the increase in alveolar pressure measured at the mouth

$V_1 = V_{UN} - \Delta V$
where ΔV is the decrease in volume due to compression

Therefore
$$P_B V_{UN} = (P_B + \Delta P)(V_{UN} - \Delta V)$$

$$V_{UN} = \frac{\Delta V}{\Delta P}(P_B + \Delta P*)$$

$$\text{or } V_{UN} = \frac{\Delta V}{\Delta P}(P_B)$$

*ΔP is negligible compared to P_B.

Nitrogen Washout Technique

The nitrogen washout technique is similar in many ways to the inert gas technique. The subject is connected to the system at end exhalation and breathes nitrogen-free air (Fig. 4-4). At the start of the test, the lung contains 80% nitrogen that is evenly distributed. The volume of exhaled gas is collected into a bag and the nitrogen concentration is measured. Using the simple mass balance equation ($C_1V_1 = C_2V_2$), the concentration of nitrogen at the start (C_1) (i.e., in the lung) and at the end (C_2) (i.e., in the bag) is known, and the volume in the bag is known (V_2). The equation is then solved for the volume in the lung (V_1). The nitrogen washout technique is used infrequently because, like the inert gas technique, it underestimates FRC in individuals with airway obstruction; it can also

in FRC measured by plethysmography and FRC measured by helium dilution has been used (primarily by physiologists) as a measure of trapped gas.

be uncomfortable for subjects, and it requires a nitrogen analyzer and bags to collect expiratory gas.

SPIROMETRY

The rapidity with which air can flow out of the lung (known as the expiratory flow rate) can be measured using spirometry, an important clinical tool for diagnosing and monitoring the course of many respiratory diseases. Spirometry measures the rate at which the lung changes volume during a forced breathing maneuver (Fig. 4-5). When performed from TLC, spirometry measures the FVC, and this is the single most important pulmonary function test. In this test, known as the **"FVC maneuver,"** the subject breathes in and out of a mouthpiece that is connected to a spirometer. The subject is then instructed to inhale maximally and then exhale as rapidly, as forcibly and as completely as possible until he is unable to exhale further.

The FVC maneuver can be displayed in two different ways: as a **spirogram** and as a **flow volume loop.**

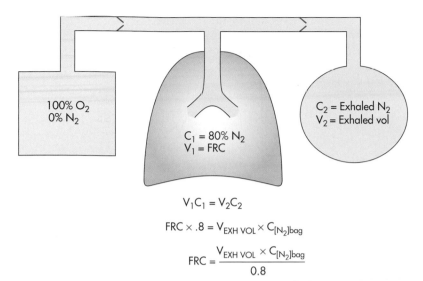

$$V_1 C_1 = V_2 C_2$$

$$FRC \times .8 = V_{EXH\ VOL} \times C_{[N_2]bag}$$

$$FRC = \frac{V_{EXH\ VOL} \times C_{[N_2]bag}}{0.8}$$

FIGURE 4-4 ■ Measurement of functional residual capacity (FRC) by the nitrogen washout method. See text for details. $V_{EXH\ VOL}$, Volume of the bag in which the exhaled gas is collected, or the exhaled volume of gas. (Modified from Hyatt RE, Scanlon PD, Nakamura M: Interpretation of Pulmonary Function Tests: A Practical Guide. Philadelphia, Lippincott Williams & Wilkins, 1997.)

Spirogram Display

In a spirogram (or volume/time curve), the volume of gas exhaled is plotted against time, as shown in Figure 4-6A. The spirogram reports four major test results:

1. The forced vital capacity (FVC)
2. The forced expiratory volume in 1 second (FEV_1)
3. The ratio of the FEV_1 to the FVC (FEV_1/FVC)
4. The average mid-maximal expiratory flow (MMEF) or, as more commonly called, the FEF_{25-75}).

The FVC is measured directly from the spirogram tracing and is the total volume of air that is exhaled during a forced exhalation; it is usually reported in liters. The volume of air that is exhaled in the first second during the maneuver is called the FEV_1, and it too is measured directly from the spirogram tracing and is reported in liters. In normal individuals, at least 72% of the FVC can be exhaled in the first second. Thus, the **FEV_1/FVC ratio** in individuals with normal lungs should be greater than 72%. A ratio less than 72% suggests obstruction to expiratory gas flow and is a hallmark of OPD. The fourth test that can be measured

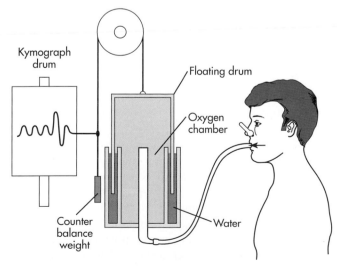

FIGURE 4-5 ■ Simple water-seal spirometer. (From Berne RM, Levy ML, Koeppen BM, Stanton BA (eds): Physiology, 5th ed. St. Louis, Mosby, 2004.)

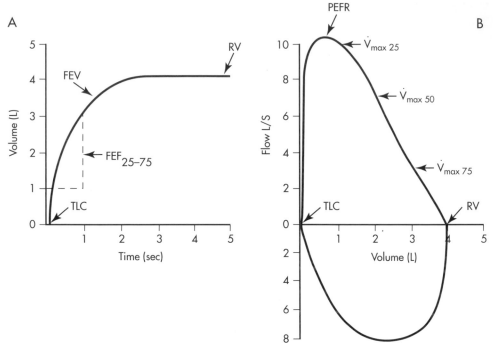

FIGURE 4-6 ■ The clinical spirogram (**A**) and expiratory flow volume curve (**B**). The subject takes a maximal inspiration and then exhales as rapidly, forcefully, and maximally as possible. The volume exhaled is plotted as a function of time. In the spirogram that is reported in clinical settings, exhaled volume increases from the bottom of the trace to the top (A). This is in contrast to the physiologist's view of the same maneuver (see Fig. 2-2) in which the exhaled volume increases from the top to the bottom of the trace. Note the locations of TLC and RV on both tracings. FEF, forced expiratory flow; FEV, forced expiratory volume; PEFR, peak expiratory flow rate; RV, residual volume; TLC, total lung capacity; $\dot{V}_{max}$, maximal expiratory flow rate. *(From Berne RM, Levy ML, Koeppen BM, Stanton BA (eds): Physiology, 5th ed. St. Louis, Mosby, 2004.)*

from the spirogram is the average flow rate over the middle section of the VC. This test has several names, including MMEF (mid-maximal expiratory flow) and FEF_{25-75} (forced expiratory flow from 25% to 75% of the VC). It can be calculated from the spirogram tracing by dividing the VC into quarters, dropping a line from the first (25%) and third (75%) quartiles and then connecting the lines and measuring the slope (see Fig. 4-6A). Volume/time is a flow rate and thus the slope of this line is an expiratory flow rate, the only flow rate that can readily be obtained from the spirogram. Although the maximum or **peak expiratory flow rate** (PEFR) can also be obtained from the spirogram by measuring the maximum slope, this is rarely done, as there are easier and more accurate ways of making this measurement. Occasionally, other measures are obtained using the spirogram, including FEV_3 and FEV_6, forced expiratory volume exhaled at

3 seconds and 6 seconds, respectively. The value of these additional measurements compared to FEV_1 and FVC is not clear.

Flow Volume Loop Display

The FVC maneuver can also be displayed as a **flow volume loop** in which the instantaneous flow rate is plotted against volume. The flow volume loop can record instantaneous flow both during exhalation (expiratory flow volume curve) and during inspiration (inspiratory flow volume curve) (see Fig. 4-6B). It is created in the same way as the spirogram. The subject puts his mouth around a mouthpiece and breathes normally (tidal volume [VT]). The subject is then asked to take a maximal inspiration to TLC and to breathe out as fast, as forcefully, and as rapidly as he can until he can exhale no further (a maximal exhalation to RV) at which time he takes a rapid and maximal inspiration back to TLC. Flow rates above the horizontal line are expiratory, whereas flow rates below the horizontal line are inspiratory. The point on the flow volume loop at which maximal inspiration has occurred is the TLC, and the point at which maximal exhalation has occurred is the RV.

Expiratory Flow Volume Curve

The expiratory flow volume curve gives results for four main pulmonary function tests. Again, the total amount of air that can be exhaled is the FVC. The greatest flow rate achieved during the maneuver is the **PEFR**. The expiratory flow volume curve can also be divided into quarters. The instantaneous flow rate at which 50% of the VC remains to be exhaled is called the **FEF_{50}** (also known as the $\dot{V}_{max50}$). The flow rate at which 75% of the VC has been exhaled is called the $\dot{V}_{max75}$, and the flow rate at which 25% of the VC has been exhaled is called the $\dot{V}_{max25}$.*

DETERMINANTS OF MAXIMAL FLOW

Upon closer inspection of the flow volume loop, it can be seen that in general, the maximum inspiratory flow rate is the same or slightly greater than the maximal expiratory flow rate. Three major factors are responsible for the maximum inspiratory flow rate. The first factor is the force generated by the inspiratory muscles that is greatest at RV and then decreases as lung volume increases above RV; the second factor is the increase of the static recoil pressure of the lung as the lung volume increases above RV and as lung elastic fibers are stretched. This opposes the force generated by the inspiratory muscles and tends to reduce maximum inspiratory flow rates. The third factor is the airway resistance that decreases with increasing lung volume as airway

caliber increases. The combination of the inspiratory muscle force, the static recoil of the lung, and the changes in airway resistance causes maximal inspiratory flow to occur about halfway between TLC and RV.

During exhalation, maximal flow occurs early (in the first 20%) in the maneuver, and flow rates decrease progressively as lung volume decreases. Even with increasing effort, maximal flow will decrease as RV is approached ("expiratory flow limitation"; see later for an explanation of why this occurs). Expiratory flow limitation can be demonstrated by asking an individual to perform three forced expiratory maneuvers with increasing effort. Figure 4-7 shows the superimposed results of these maneuvers. As effort increases, peak expiratory flow increases. However, the flow rates at lower lung volumes converge, indicating that with modest efforts maximal expiratory flow is achieved. No amount of effort will increase these flow rates at lower lung volumes. For this reason, expiratory flow rates at lower lung volumes are said to be **effort-independent**, because maximal flow is achieved with modest effort. In this range, the expiratory flow rate is flow limited by the lung and no amount of additional effort can increase the flow rate beyond this limit. In contrast, events early in the expiratory maneuver are said to be **effort-dependent**. That is, increasing effort generates increasing flow rates. In general, the first 20% of the flow in the expiratory flow volume loop is effort-dependent.

INTERPRETING THE VITAL CAPACITY MANEUVER

Two important principles are useful in interpreting the VC maneuver: (1) events that occur early in the maneuver reflect large airway function, and (2) different patterns of abnormalities are found in obstructive and restrictive lung disease, the two broad categories of pulmonary disease. It is important to not only look at the values reported for the various tests but also to examine carefully the shape of the spirogram or flow volume curve.

In general, OPD is categorized by premature airway closure, which is manifested in pulmonary function tests, by decreases in expiratory flow rates secondary to airway obstruction, and by increases in lung volumes due to air trapping. In OPD, the usual sequence of abnormalities in pulmonary function is an increase in

---

*In the pediatric literature, the flow rate at which 75% of the FVC has been exhaled is called the V_{max25} (25% of the FVC remained to be exhaled), and the flow rate at which 25% of the VC has been exhaled is called the V_{max75} (75% of the FVC remained to be exhaled). To distinguish which nomenclature system is being used, you must look at the lowest of the V_{max} flow rates. This will be the flow rate closest to residual volume.

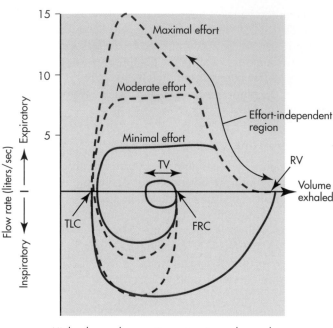

FIGURE 4-7 ■ Isovolume curves. Three superimposed expiratory flow maneuvers are made with increasing effort. Note that peak inspiratory and expiratory flow rates are effort-dependent, whereas expiratory flow rates later in expiration are effort-independent. FRC, functional residual capacity; RV, residual volume; TLC, total lung capacity; TV, tidal volume. *(From Berne RM, Levy ML, Koeppen BM, Stanton BA (eds): Physiology, 5th Ed. St. Louis, Mosby, 2004.)*

RV and in the RV/TLC ratio, followed by a decrease in expiratory flow rates, then by a decrease in FEV_1, and finally by a decrease in FVC; that is, air trapping and decreases in expiratory flow rates are seen with early airway obstruction or mild disease. Decreases in FEV_1 (in addition to greater decreases in expiratory flow rates) occur with moderate airway obstruction and decreases in FVC (in conjunction with a marked decrease in FEV_1 and in expiratory flow rates) occur with more advanced airway obstructive disease.

In OPD, the FEV_1 is decreased out of proportion to any change in FVC. Thus, the hallmark of OPD is a decrease in the FEV_1/FVC ratio due to a decrease in FEV_1 out of proportion to any change in FVC. This latter distinction is important, as we will see later, because the FEV_1 is also decreased in restrictive pulmonary disease (Table 4-2).

Early events, such as the PEFR, reflect large airway function, whereas events that occur late (the last 80%) reflect small airway obstruction. For example, in someone with small airway obstruction, the only abnormality on spirometry might be a decrease in the $Vmax_{75}$. In contrast, in someone with large airway obstruction such as paralysis of a vocal cord, the only abnormality might be a decrease in PEFR.

The shapes of the spirogram and flow volume curve can also help in determining the presence of airway obstruction. In OPD, the slope of the rise in volume with time is reduced; these changes are reflected both in the FEF_{25-75} and in the FEV_1. On the flow volume curve, the shape of the downward slope changes and becomes concave or sags. As disease progresses, these changes become more severe. A flattening of the

TABLE 4-2		
Patterns of Abnormalities in Pulmonary Function Tests		
PULMONARY FUNCTION MEASUREMENT	**OPD**	**RPD**
FVC (L)	↓	↓
FEV_1 (L)	↓	↓
FEV_1/FVC	↓	N
FEF_{25-75} (L/sec)	↓	N
PEFR (L/sec)	↓	N
FEF_{50} (L/sec)	↓	N
FEF_{75} (L/sec)	↓	N
Slope of FVC curve	↓	N to ↑

OPD, obstructive pulmonary disease; FEV, forced expiratory volume; FVC, forced vital capacity; FEF, forced expiratory flow; PEFR, peak expiratory flow rate; RPD, restrictive pulmonary disease; N, normal; ↑, increased; ↓, decreased.

expiratory or inspiratory limbs of the flow volume curve also has significance and is indicative of extrathoracic airway obstruction.

In restrictive lung diseases, volumes are decreased whereas flow rates are maintained until late in the disease process. In individuals with restrictive lung diseases, VC and FEV_1 are reduced; however, in contrast to OPD, the decreases are proportional; that is, the FEV_1/FVC ratio is normal (Table 4-3). The shape of the flow volume curve and the spirogram appear normal but are reduced in size, reflecting the reductions in FVC with normal (or even supranormal) expiratory flow rates.

APPROACH TO INTERPRETING LUNG VOLUMES, SPIROGRAMS, AND FLOW VOLUME CURVES

In beginning to examine the reported data, it is first essential to examine the quality and reproducibility of the test (Fig. 4-8). This is especially important in regard to the spirogram and flow volume curve because patient cooperation and maximal effort are required. The test is

TABLE 4-3
Causes of Abnormal Vital Capacity

Pulmonary Lesions
Loss of distensible lung tissue
Pulmonary edema
Pneumonia
Atelectasis
Surgical resection
Bronchogenic carcinoma

Non-pulmonary Lesions
Neuromuscular disease
Thoracic space reduction
   (pleural effusion, pneumothorax, cardiac enlargement)
Diaphragm movement limitation (pregnancy, ascites)
Chest wall movement limitation (scleroderma, kyphoscoliosis, pain)
Central nervous system depression

reproducible if the FVC and FEV_1 on three maneuvers are within 5% to 10% of each other. On inspection, a good test is associated with a rapid rise in expiratory flow with a smooth decline as the RV is approached. On the spirogram, there should be a clear plateau with

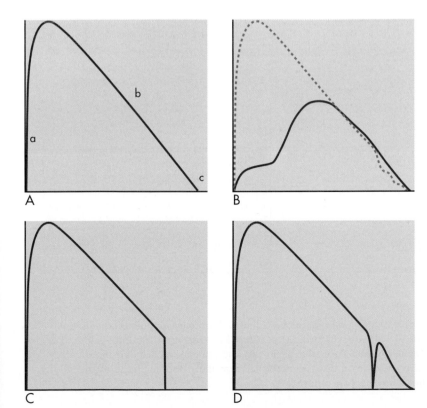

A

B

C

D

FIGURE 4-8 ■ Interpreting the quality of the expiratory flow volume curve. **A,** Excellent effort and test quality. Important elements of an excellent test are a rapid rise (a), a smooth decrease in expiratory flow (b), and a decrease in flow to the baseline (c). **B,** A hesitant start; compare to normal curve as shown by dotted line. This curve is unacceptable. **C,** Good effort at the start, but patient abruptly stopped exhalation before reaching residual volume; this curve is unacceptable. **D,** Good effort at the start, but subject stopped exhaling momentarily, closed glottis and then continued the effort; test should be repeated.

a change of less than 200 mL in exhaled volume over the last 2 seconds of the maneuver and a total expiratory time of 6 seconds or greater in adults (2 seconds or greater in children).

If the spirogram and flow volume curve are reproducible and of high quality, the results can be interpreted. Next, examine the shape of the flow volume curve and its relationship to normal (Fig. 4-9). The greater the discrepancy between the subject's curve and the normal curve, the greater the ventilatory abnormality.

A concave shape with a decreased slope is indicative of an obstructive process. In contrast, a steep slope with a reduced FVC is consistent with restrictive lung disease.

Then examine the numbers. A reduced FEV_1 out of proportion to a change in FVC with low expiratory flow rates and elevated lung volumes with an increase in the RV/TLC ratio due to an increase in RV out of proportion to any change in TLC are indicative of OPD. A reduced FEV_1 with a reduced FVC and a normal

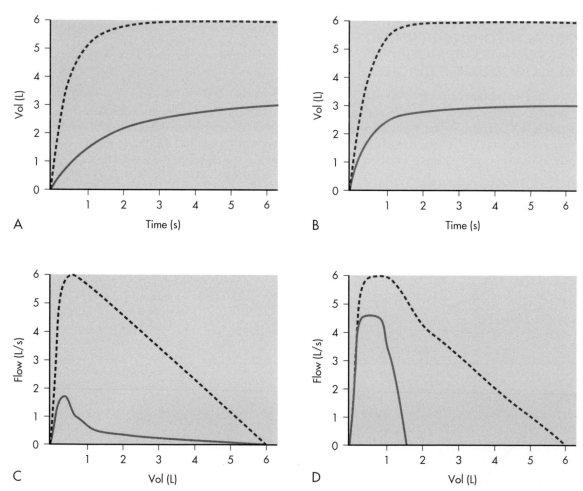

FIGURE 4-9 ■ Spirograms and expiratory flow volume curves for an individual with obstructive pulmonary disease (OPD) (**A** and **C**) and with restrictive pulmonary disease (**B** and **D**). *Dashed lines* represent normal values. For the individual with OPD, note the prolonged time to reach the vital capacity (**A**) and the marked decrease in expiratory flow rates (**C**). For the individual with restrictive pulmonary disease, note the reasonably normal shape of the spirogram (**B**) and the flow volume curve (**D**). Volumes, however, are reduced.

FEV_1/FVC ratio in conjunction with preserved expiratory flow rates (except in severe disease) with reduced lung volumes and an elevated RV/TLC ratio secondary to a reduction in TLC out of proportion to a change in RV are hallmarks of restrictive pulmonary disease. The degree of ventilatory limitation can be defined by the loss of area under the normal curve. An area loss of 25% is defined as mild, 50% as moderate, and 75% as a severe ventilatory limitation.

PEAK EXPIRATORY FLOW RATE

The peak expiratory flow rate (PEFR) can be read directly from the expiratory flow volume curve and also can be measured using a peak flow meter. Peak flow meters are portable, inexpensive, and easy to use. As a result, they are often used at home, especially by individuals with asthma, to monitor airway caliber and disease status. More than other measures, peak expiratory flow is very dependent on patient effort. The individual must exhale as forcefully as possible to obtain reproducible results. Another limitation is that peak expiratory flow measures large airway function; thus, the PEFR can both underestimate and overestimate the overall degree of airway obstruction.

OTHER USEFUL TESTS OF LUNG FUNCTION

Although the VC maneuver is the single most important pulmonary function test, other tests are useful in helping to diagnose underlying lung disease. Some of these clinically important tests are described here.

The diffusion capacity for carbon monoxide (D_{LCO}) is a measure of the surface available for gas diffusion. An abnormal test is indicative of a loss of surface area usually because of destruction of the capillary bed. Carbon monoxide (CO) is used as the test gas in part because it is easier to measure than O_2, and in part because there is no limitation to the diffusion of CO. There are two different ways that the test can be done—either as a single breath or in a steady state. The single breath test is easiest and quickest. In this test, the subject exhales to residual volume and then inhales a gas mixture containing a very low concentration of carbon monoxide and an inert gas (usually helium) to TLC. At TLC, the subject holds his/her breath for 10 seconds and then exhales; the exhaled gas is measured for carbon monoxide and helium. The helium is used to measure TLC, and the difference between the inhaled and the exhaled CO is used to calculate the surface area for diffusion.

The normal value for D_{LCO} is 20 to 30 mL. Because the surface area for diffusion will vary with lung size, dividing D_{LCO} by the total alveolar volume (VA) estimated from the helium concentration normalizes the value for differences in size. The D_{LCO}/VA is called the Krogh constant.

Of the numerous conditions in which the D_{LCO} may be elevated, the most important causes of an abnormal D_{LCO} are those that result in a decrease (Table 4-4). Any process that alters or decreases the surface area for gas diffusion will result in a decrease in the D_{LCO}. Some of these conditions deserve further discussion.

Emphysema

Emphysema produces a contradiction of sorts. Lung volumes in patients with emphysema are increased, but alveolar walls and capillaries are destroyed. Thus, the surface area for gas exchange is reduced. A reduction in

TABLE 4-4
Causes of Abnormal D_{LCO}

Decreased Area for Diffusion
Emphysema
Lung/lobe resection
Bronchial obstruction, as by tumor
Multiple pulmonary emboli
Anemia

Increased Thickness of the Alveolar-Capillary Membrane
Idiopathic pulmonary fibrosis
Sarcoidosis involving parenchyma
Asbestosis
Alveolar proteinosis
Hypersensitivity pneumonitis, including farmer's lung
Histiocytosis X (eosinophilic granuloma)
Congestive heart failure
Collagen vascular disease (scleroderma, lupus erythematosis)
Alveolitis or fibrosis—drug-induced (bleomycin, nitrofurantoin, amiodarone, methotrexate)

Miscellaneous
High carbon monoxide back pressure from smoking
Pregnancy
Ventilation/perfusion mismatch

D_{LCO}, diffusion capacity for carbon monoxide.

the DLCO is the single best test to distinguish between emphysema and chronic bronchitis in an individual with COPD.

Lung Resection

If a significant amount of lung has been removed, the DLCO will be decreased. However, the DLCO/VA, which corrects for lung volume, will be normal.

Bronchial Obstruction

If there is a tumor obstructing a large airway, the DLCO will be reduced, but here again the DLCO corrected for lung volume will be normal.

Multiple Pulmonary Emboli

Emboli in the pulmonary circulation decrease perfusion to alveoli and effectively decrease the surface area for diffusion. Also, pulmonary hypertension causes a decrease in capillary area for diffusion

Anemia

Any condition that lowers capillary blood volume, including conditions that lower the hemoglobin (Hgb) in the capillaries, effectively reduces the area for diffusion. Anemia can be corrected using the following equation:

$$\text{DLCO (corr)} = \frac{\text{DLCO (uncorr)} \times [10.22 + \text{Hgb}]}{[1.7 \times \text{Hgb}]}$$

This is particularly important in individuals who have cancer and are receiving chemotherapeutic drugs that can induce pulmonary toxicity and reduce DLCO. Many of these same individuals are also anemic because of their chemotherapy.

USES OF THE MEASUREMENT OF THE DLCO

The DLCO, as mentioned previously, can help to distinguish between chronic bronchitis and emphysema in individuals with COPD. Pulmonary function abnormalities in individuals with chronic bronchitis and emphysema can look the same, but the DLCO can distinguish between the two. The DLCO is also useful to follow the course of disease progression in a patient with pulmonary fibrosis or the extent of intra-alveolar

hemorrhage in diseases such as Goodpasture's. In individuals with interstitial pulmonary fibrosis, there is an initial alveolar inflammatory response, with subsequent scar formation (connective tissue deposition—collagen) within the interstitial space. The inflammation and scar tissue thicken the interstitial space, making it more difficult for gas diffusion, resulting in decreased DLCO. This is a classic characteristic of a restrictive lung disease process; gas readily enters the alveolus but is restricted in its ability to diffuse into the blood. DLCO can also determine the presence of pulmonary toxicity in patients without respiratory symptoms who are undergoing chemotherapy.

AIRWAY RESISTANCE AND LUNG COMPLIANCE

Airway resistance (Raw) measurements are routinely performed in fully equipped pulmonary function laboratories, whereas measurements of lung compliance (CL) are performed in fully equipped research pulmonary function laboratories at academic institutions. The latter add little to what has already been learned using spirometry and lung volumes coupled with an appropriately taken arterial blood gas.

Raw can be measured in two ways: using a flow meter and by body plethysmography.

In the first method, flow at the mouth is measured with the flow meter (Fig. 4-10). A small balloon is passed into the mid-portion of the esophagus and is connected to a pressure transducer. The pressure in the esophagus, which is a reflection of the pressure in the pleura, is then measured. The difference between the pressure in the pleura (esophageal pressure) and the pressure at the mouth is the driving force for gas flow. This difference is divided by the expiratory flow to give pulmonary resistance (RPULM).

In the second method, body plethysmography, alveolar pressure relative to mouth pressure is measured. For this measurement of resistance, flow is measured with a pneumotachometer. The subject sits in the air-tight box and pants through a mouthpiece with the shutter open. Flow is plotted again box pressure. The shutter is briefly closed, usually at end exhalation, and alveolar pressure is recorded. The difference between alveolar pressure and mouth pressure divided by the flow is the Raw. The esophageal balloon method

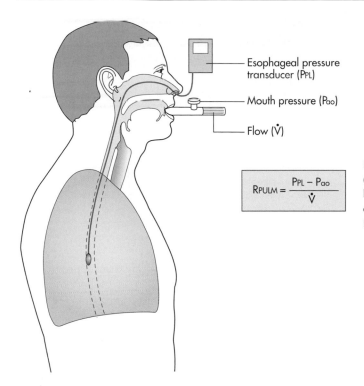

Esophageal pressure
transducer (PPL)

Mouth pressure (Pao)

Flow (V̇)

$$R_{PULM} = \frac{P_{PL} - P_{ao}}{\dot{V}}$$

FIGURE 4-10 ■ Measurement of pulmonary resistance (RPULM) using an esophageal balloon. The esophageal balloon measures pleural pressure (PPL). The difference between the pressure at the mouth (Pao) and the PPL divided by the flow rate (V̇) equals RPULM.

actually measures pulmonary resistance (RPULM), whereas the body box method measures Raw. Because RPULM is composed of both RAW and lung tissue resistance, Raw is always slightly lower than RPULM.

Normal Raw is 1 to 3 cm $H_2O/L \cdot$ sec. Raw varies with lung size. In young infants with smaller airways, Raw is higher than in adults. Raw also varies with lung volume—the greater the lung volume, the lower the resistance, because airway size varies with lung volume. Raw is usually measured at FRC to control for this effect of lung volume. Raw is also increased when the airways are narrowed because of bronchospasm, edema, or infection. Because these processes alter airway caliber, there is a strong negative correlation between Raw and maximal expiratory flow.

MEASUREMENT OF LUNG COMPLIANCE

Clinically, CL can be measured using an esophageal balloon connected to a pressure transducer and a spirometer. Esophageal balloon pressure is a measure of pleural pressure (PPL). When the lung is not moving

(that is, when airflow is zero), PPL is subatmospheric or negative. This is because the lungs are elastic and are always tending to collapse. Because this tendency of the lung to collapse is resisted by the chest wall, the PPL, when volume is not changing, reflects the elastic pressure or recoil of the lung at that volume. If lung volume is increased by a known amount (ΔV) and volume is then held constant, the new PPL is more negative (lung recoil is greater). The ΔV divided by the change in PPL is the CL. Because this compliance is measured in the absence of airflow, it is a measure of static compliance (CLstat).

Dynamic lung compliance, or compliance during breathing, also can be measured. At end inspiration and end exhalation, airflow is zero. The difference between PPL at end inspiration and end exhalation divided by the tidal volume is called the dynamic compliance of the lung (CLdyn) (see Fig. 3-8).

In normal individuals, CLstat and CLdyn are nearly the same (0.150 to 0.250 L/cm H_2O). CL is lower in smaller lungs and is reduced in individuals with pulmonary fibrosis. CLstat is elevated in individuals with emphysema, reflecting the floppy, inelastic lungs.

In emphysema, CL_{dyn} is reduced and CL_{stat} is increased. The reason for this difference is the non-uniform ventilation in this disease. In patients with emphysema, air flows preferentially into and out of the more normal regions of the lung. Because the elasticity of these regions is not as severely impaired, CL_{dyn} is nearer normal volumes. The difference between CL_{stat} and CL_{dyn} is referred to as frequency dependence of compliance. A low CL_{dyn} in patients with emphysema does not mean that the lung is stiff or fibrotic.

USES OF SPIROMETRY AND BODY PLETHYSMOGRAPHY

As previously mentioned, pulmonary function tests are most useful to follow the course of a disease, especially the progression of OPD, and the response to therapy. They quantify defects in function and can sometimes suggest appropriate therapy (bronchodilators). They are least useful to diagnose clinical disease and as a single, isolated test. The reason for this is that pulmonary function tests have greater inter-subject variability than intra-subject variability. Different pulmonary function tests have different levels of variability.

Thus, pulmonary function tests have a wide range of normal values. For example, a patient may have an FVC of 90% of predicted or expected, which is well within the normal range. What you do not know is whether this patient had an FVC of 120% of predicted values 3 months ago (in which case the patient has experienced a significant decline in function) or whether the FVC always been 90% of predicted values. Longitudinal pulmonary function tests are the most useful to follow the course of a disease.

Pulmonary function tests are also helpful in determining surgical risk and can aid in detecting non-symptomatic disease in patients at risk for pulmonary function abnormality. For example, pulmonary function tests can be helpful in diagnosing early COPD in a smoker before the individual becomes symptomatic. In individuals with cystic fibrosis, the development of pulmonary function abnormalities in the absence of symptoms is quite common. When these abnormalities are identified, changes in therapy that may reverse

TABLE 4-5
Normal Values for Lung Volumes and Pulmonary Function Mechanics

Lung Volumes	
Functional residual capacity (FRC)	2.4 L
Total lung capacity	6 L
Tidal volume	0.5 L
Breathing frequency	12/min
Pulmonary Function Mechanics	
Pleural pressure (mean)	−5 cm H_2O
Chest wall compliance (at FRC)	0.2 L/cm H_2O
Lung compliance (at FRC)	0.2 L/cm H_2O
Airway resistance	2.0 cm H_2O/ L·sec

the early abnormalities and delay disease progression can be tried.

Spirometry and lung volume measurements thus can provide important clinical information. Individual results are compared with predicted values derived from tests performed in large numbers of normal individuals. Predicted values vary by age, gender, ethnicity, height, and to a lesser extent weight. Normal ranges vary by test but in general are larger for flow rates than for volumes (Table 4-5). Abnormalities in values are indicative of abnormal pulmonary function and can be used to predict eventual abnormalities in gas exchange. They can detect the presence of abnormal lung function long before the development of respiratory symptoms, determine disease severity, and demonstrate response to therapy. An improved response of >12% in FEV_1 after administration of a bronchodilator, for example, is considered a clinically significant improvement and suggests that bronchodilator administration may be beneficial.

WHEN SHOULD PULMONARY FUNCTION TESTS BE USED?

Because almost all pulmonary function tests require the cooperation of the subject and a trained technician, pulmonary function tests are not useful in all cases. The subject must be instructed in how to perform pulmonary function testing. In general, the subject must have a natural airway (e.g., no tracheostomy), although some experienced laboratories can test individuals who have a tracheostomy or an endotracheal tube. Pulmonary function tests cannot be successfully performed in a person who cannot follow instructions for whatever reason (mental incapacity, age, etc.).

Pulmonary function tests are underused by clinicians. The following groups of individuals should be considered for regular pulmonary function testing: any patient who smokes; any individual with respiratory symptoms; any individual with asthma; and anyone at risk for lung disease because of environmental exposures on the job or at home.

SUMMARY

1. Vital capacity (VC) is the single most important pulmonary function measurement and is the maximal amount of air that an individual can either inspire or exhale.
2. Pulmonary function tests (spirometry, flow volume loop, body plethysmography) can detect abnormalities in lung function before diseases become symptomatic.
3. Obstructive lung disease (OPD) is characterized by increases in lung volumes and airway resistance and decreases in expiratory flow rates. Emphysema, a specific type of COPD, is further characterized by increased lung compliance and decreased diffusion capacity for carbon monoxide (D_{LCO}).
4. In OPD, the FEV_1/FVC ratio is decreased, whereas in restrictive lung disease, the FEV_1 and FVC are reduced proportionately, resulting in a normal FEV_1/FVC ratio.
5. Restrictive lung diseases are characterized by decreases in lung volume, normal expiratory flow rates and resistance, and a marked decrease in lung compliance.
6. The RV/TLC ratio can be increased in both OPD and restrictive lung disease, although for different reasons.
7. Events that occur early in the forced vital capacity (FVC) maneuver reflect large airway function and are effort-dependent. Events that occur later in the FVC maneuver reflect small airway function and are effort-independent.
8. Predicted values for lung volumes and expiratory flow rates vary by age, gender, ethnicity, height, and to a lesser extent weight.

KEY WORDS

- Airway resistance (Raw)
- Body plethysmography
- Boyle's law
- Obstructive pulmonary disease (OPD)
- Diffusion capacity for carbon monoxide (D_{LCO})
- $\dfrac{FEV_1}{FVC}$ ratio
- Flow volume loop
- Forced vital capacity (FVC)
- Lung compliance (CL)
- Pulmonary function tests
- Residual volume/total lung capacity (RV/TLC) ratio
- Restrictive pulmonary disease
- Slow vital capacity (SVC)
- Spirometry

SELF-STUDY PROBLEMS

1. What is your interpretation of each of the following flow volume curves (A through D)?
2. Describe the pulmonary function abnormalities in obstructive pulmonary disease. How would you distinguish emphysema from chronic bronchitis?
3. Describe the pulmonary function test abnormalities in individuals with restrictive lung disease.
4. List the requirements for a normal D_{LCO}.

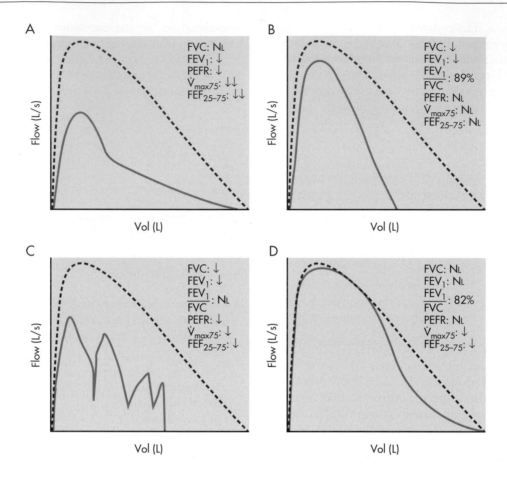

REFERENCES

Altose MD: The physiological basis of pulmonary function testing. Clin Symp 31:1-39, 1979.

Brand PL, Roorda RJ: Usefulness of monitoring lung function in asthma. Arch Dis Child. 88:1021-1025, 2003.

Chetta A, Marangio E, Olivieri D: Pulmonary function testing in interstitial lung diseases. Respiration 71:209-213, 2004.

Contreras G, Gutierrez M, Beroiza T, et al: Ventilatory drive and respiratory muscle function in pregnancy. Am Rev Respir Dis 144:837-844, 1991.

Crapo RO, Jensen RL: Standards and interpretive issues in lung function testing. Respir Care 48:764-772, 2003.

Evans SE, Scanlon PD: Current practice in pulmonary function testing. Mayo Clinic Proc 78:758-763, 2003.

Hyatt RE, Scanlon PD, Nakamura M (eds): Interpretation of Pulmonary Function Tests. A Practical Guide. Philadelphia, Lippincott Williams & Wilkins, 1997.

Ruppel GL: Manual of Pulmonary Function Testing. 7th ed. St. Louis, Mosby, 1998.

Wang JS: Pulmonary function tests in preoperative pulmonary evaluation. Respir Med 98:598-605, 2004.

5

ALVEOLAR VENTILATION

OBJECTIVES

1. Understand the composition of gases from ambient air to the alveoli.

2. Describe the alveolar air equation and its use.

3. Define the alveolar carbon dioxide equation and the relationship between alveolar ventilation and arterial P_{CO_2}.

4. Characterize lung and chest wall interactions in terms of pressure gradients and pressure-volume relationships.

5. Describe the distribution of ventilation at the apex and at the base in upright individuals.

6. Describe how the nitrogen washout test can be used to examine the distribution of ventilation.

7. Define anatomic and physiologic dead space and their measurement.

8. Outline the effects of aging upon lung growth, lung volumes, elastic recoil, expiratory muscle strength, airway closure, and the diffusion capacity for carbon monoxide.

entilation is the process by which fresh gas moves in and out of the lung. Alveolar ventilation is the process by which gas moves between the alveoli and the external environment. It includes both the volume of fresh air entering the alveoli and the (similar) volume of alveolar air leaving the body. Minute (**or total**) **ventilation (MV)**, also referred to as $\dot{V}E$, is the volume of air that enters or leaves the lung per minute and is described by:

$$MV = f \times V_T$$

where f is the frequency or number of breaths/minute, and V_T (also expressed as TV) is the tidal volume or volume of air inspired (or exhaled) per breath. V_T varies with age, gender, body position, and metabolic activity. In an average-sized adult, V_T is 500 mL; in children, V_T is 3 to 5 mL/kg.

COMPOSITION OF A GAS MIXTURE

The process of respiration brings oxygen from the ambient air to the alveoli where oxygen is taken up and carbon dioxide is excreted. Alveolar ventilation thus begins with ambient air. Ambient air is a gas mixture composed of nitrogen and oxygen with minute quantities of carbon dioxide, argon, and other inert gases. The composition of a gas mixture can be described either in terms of the gas fractions or as the corresponding partial pressures. Because ambient air is a gas, it obeys the gas laws. The two most important gas laws governing ambient air and alveolar ventilation are **Boyle's law** and **Dalton's law**. Boyle's law has been described previously (see Chapter 1); it states that when temperature is constant, pressure (P) and volume (V) are inversely related; that is, $P_1V_1 = P_2V_2$. Dalton's law states that the partial pressure of a gas in a gas mixture is the pressure that the gas would exert if it occupied the total volume of the mixture in the absence of the other components.

Using these gas laws and applying them to ambient (or atmospheric) air, two important principles arise. The first is that when viewed in terms of gas fractions (F), the sum of the individual gas fractions of nitrogen [F_N], oxygen [F_O], and argon and other gases [$F_{argon\ and\ other\ gases}$]) must equal 1; that is, for ambient air,

$$1.0 = F_N + F_{O_2} + F_{argon\ and\ other\ gases}$$

When viewed using Boyle's gas law, the sum of the **partial pressures** (in mm Hg) or **tensions** (in torr) of a gas must be equal to the total pressure. (mm Hg also can be expressed as torr, named for Evangelista Torricelli, the inventor of the barometer. The two terms are equal and interchangeable.) Thus, at sea level, where the partial pressure is 760 mm Hg, the partial pressure of the individual gases in ambient air (also known as the barometric partial pressure or P_B) is:

$$P_B = P_{O_2} + P_{N_2} + P_{argon\ and\ other\ gases}$$
$$760\ mm\ Hg = P_{O_2} + P_{N_2} + P_{argon\ and\ other\ gases}$$

The second important principle is that the partial pressure of a gas (P_{gas}) is equal to the fraction of gas in the gas mixture (F_{gas}) times the total or ambient (barometric) pressure.

$$P_{gas} = F_{gas} \times P_B$$

Ambient air is composed of approximately 21% oxygen and 79% nitrogen. Therefore, the partial pressure of oxygen in ambient air (P_{O_2}) is:

$$P_{O_2} = F_{O_2} \times P_B$$
$$= 0.21 \times 760\ mm\ Hg$$
$$= 159\ mm\ Hg\ (or\ 159\ torr)$$

This is the **oxygen tension** (i.e., the partial pressure of oxygen) at the mouth at the start of inspiration. It can be seen that the oxygen tension at the mouth can be altered in one of two ways—by changing the fraction of oxygen or by changing the barometric (atmospheric) pressure. For example, if the fraction of oxygen is increased through the administration of supplemental oxygen, the partial pressure of oxygen will be increased. On the other hand, if the barometric (atmospheric) pressure is decreased—for example, by

high altitude—the partial pressure of ambient oxygen will decrease.

As inspiration begins, the ambient gases are brought into the airways, where they become warmed to body temperature and humidified. By the time the inspired gas reaches the larynx, it has become saturated with water vapor; water vapor is a gas that exerts a partial pressure equal to 47 mm Hg at body temperature. Because the total pressure remains constant at the barometric pressure, water vapor dilutes the total pressure of the other gases. This can be best understood by considering that humidification of a liter of dry gas in a container at 760 torr would increase its total pressure to 807 torr (i.e., 760 torr + 47 torr). In the body, however, barometric pressure remains constant, and therefore the gas simply expands, according to Boyle's law. As a result, the partial pressures of the other gases in the 1 L of gas at 760 torr are diluted by the added water vapor pressure. In order to calculate the partial pressure of a gas in a *humidified* mixture, the water vapor partial pressure must be subtracted from the total barometric pressure. Thus, in the conducting airways, the partial pressure of oxygen is:

$$P_{trachea}O_2 = (P_B - P_{H_2O}) \times F_{O_2}$$
$$= (760 - 47\ mm\ Hg) \times 0.21$$
$$= 150\ mm\ Hg$$

and the partial pressure of nitrogen is:

$$P_{trachea}N_2 = (760 - 47\ mm\ Hg) \times 0.79$$
$$= 563\ mm\ Hg$$

Note that the total pressure has remained at 760 mm Hg (150 + 563 + 47 mm Hg). Water vapor pressure, however, has reduced (diluted) the partial pressures of oxygen and nitrogen. The conducting airways do not participate in gas exchange, and therefore the partial pressures of oxygen, nitrogen, and water vapor remain unchanged in the airways until the gas reaches the alveolus.

ALVEOLAR GAS COMPOSITION

At functional residual capacity, the alveoli contain 2.5 to 3 L of gas; an additional 350 mL of gas will enter and leave the alveoli with each breath (Fig. 5-1). Diffusion of O_2 from the alveoli to the pulmonary capillary blood and of CO_2 from the pulmonary capillary blood

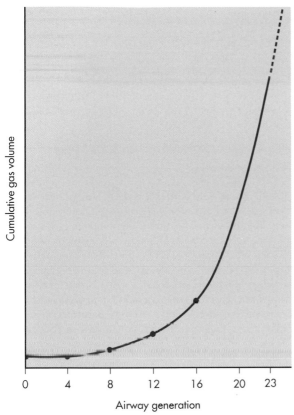

FIGURE 5-1 ■ Cumulative gas volumes in the airways with increasing generation number. The average volume of gas in the conducting airways is approximately 100 to 200 mL, whereas the average volume of gas in the terminal bronchioles, alveolar ducts, and alveoli is approximately 3000 to 4000 mL at functional residual capacity. (*Modified from Leff A, Schumacker P: Respiratory Physiology: Basics and Applications. Philadelphia, WB Saunders, 1993.*)

into the alveoli is a continuous process. Each minute at rest, on average, 300 mL of O_2 are taken up and 250 mL of CO_2 are removed by alveolar ventilation. Thus, the partial pressures of O_2 and CO_2 in the alveolar air are determined by alveolar ventilation, by O_2 consumption, and by CO_2 production. The process by which oxygen is taken up and carbon dioxide is removed by the pulmonary capillary blood is described in Chapter 8.

Here we will describe only alveolar ventilation. At the end of inspiration with the glottis open, the total pressure in the alveolus is atmospheric; the same gas laws apply, namely the partial pressures of the gases in the alveolus must equal the total pressure, which in this case is atmospheric. The composition of the gas mixture however is changed and can be described as:

$$1.0 = F_{O_2} + F_{N_2} + F_{H_2O} + F_{CO_2} + F_{argon\ and\ other\ gases}$$

Nitrogen and argon are inert gases, and therefore the fraction of these gases in the alveolus does not change. The fraction of water vapor also does not change, because the gas is already fully saturated and at body temperature by the time the gas reaches the trachea. As a consequence of gas exchange, the fraction of oxygen in the alveolus decreases and the fraction of carbon dioxide in the alveolus increases. Because of the changes in the fractions of oxygen and carbon dioxide, the partial pressures exerted by these gases also change. The partial pressure of oxygen in the alveolus (P_{AO_2}) is given by the **alveolar gas equation**, sometimes also called the ideal alveolar oxygen equation:

$$P_{AO_2} = P_{IO_2} - \frac{P_{ACO_2}}{R}$$

$$= (P_B - P_{H_2O}) \bullet F_{IO_2} - \frac{P_{ACO_2}}{R}$$

where P_{IO_2} is the inspired partial pressure of oxygen, which is equal to the inspired oxygen fraction (F_{IO_2}) times the difference between barometric pressure (P_B) and water vapor pressure (P_{H_2O}), P_{ACO_2} is the alveolar gas carbon dioxide tension, and R is the respiratory exchange ratio or respiratory quotient.

The **respiratory quotient** is the ratio of carbon dioxide excreted ($\dot{V}_{CO_2}$) to the oxygen taken up ($\dot{V}_{O_2}$) by the lungs. It is the number of carbon dioxide molecules produced relative to the number of oxygen molecules consumed by metabolism and is dependent upon intake. The respiratory quotient varies between 0.7 and 1.0 (Table 5-1). In states of exclusive fatty acid metabolism, R is 0.7, whereas in states of exclusive carbohydrate metabolism, R is 1.0. Because the respiratory quotient is rarely measured, it is considered to be 0.8 under usual circumstances, demonstrating that more oxygen is taken up than carbon dioxide released in the alveoli. *The alveolar air equation is one of the most important equations in respiratory medicine.*

The partial pressures of oxygen, carbon dioxide, nitrogen, and water from ambient air to the alveolus to the blood are shown in Table 5-2.

TABLE 5-1

Oxygen Consumption and Carbon Dioxide Production in the Determination of the Respiratory Quotient (R)

Carbohydrate

$$C_6H_{12}O_6 + 6O_2 \longrightarrow 6CO_2 + 6H_2O + 36ATP$$
$$\underbrace{\phantom{C_6H_{12}O_6 + 6O_2 \longrightarrow}}_{R=1.0}$$

Fat

$$C_{16}H_{32}O_6 + 23O_2 \longrightarrow 16CO_2 + 16H_2O + 130ATP$$
$$\underbrace{\phantom{C_{16}H_{32}O_6 + 23O_2 \longrightarrow}}_{R=0.71}$$

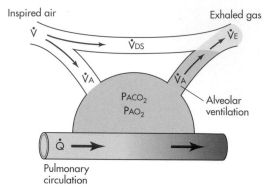

FIGURE 5-2 ■ Relationship between alveolar ventilation, dead space, and perfusion in a continuous flow model of the lung. Even though ventilation is not continuous, it is useful to view it as if it received continuous minute ventilation ($\dot{V}_E$). Alveolar ventilation ($\dot{V}_A$) is that part of the minute ventilation that reaches the alveoli and participates in gas exchange. Anatomic dead space ($\dot{V}_{DS}$) is that part of the ventilation that fills the conducting airways effectively bypassing the alveoli and thus not participating in gas exchange. $\dot{Q}$, pulmonary perfusion. (*Modified from Leff A, Schumacker P: Respiratory Physiology: Basics and Applications. Philadelphia, B Saunders, 1993.*)

The fraction of carbon dioxide in the alveolus is a function of the production of carbon dioxide by the cells during metabolism and the rate at which the carbon dioxide is removed or eliminated from the alveolus, a term known as **alveolar ventilation** (Fig. 5-2). Even though ventilation is episodic (i.e., it occurs only during inspiration), alveolar ventilation is described as a *continuous* gas flow through alveoli that exchange gas with pulmonary capillary blood. The relationship between carbon dioxide production and alveolar ventilation is defined by the **alveolar carbon dioxide equation**:

$$\dot{V}_{CO_2} = \dot{V}_A \times F_{ACO_2}$$

where $\dot{V}_{CO_2}$ is the rate of carbon dioxide production by the body, $\dot{V}_A$ is the alveolar ventilation, and F_{ACO_2} is the dry fraction of carbon dioxide in alveolar gas. This relationship demonstrates that the rate of elimination of CO_2 from the alveolus is related to alveolar ventilation and the fraction of CO_2 in the alveolus (Fig. 5-3).

Because the alveolar P_{ACO_2} is defined by the following equation:

$$P_{ACO_2} = F_{ACO_2} \times (P_B - P_{H_2O})$$

we can substitute for the F_{ACO_2} in the previous equation as follows:

$$P_{ACO_2} = \frac{\dot{V}_{CO_2} \times (P_B - P_{H_2O})}{\dot{V}_A}$$

TABLE 5-2

Total and Partial Pressures of Respiratory Gases in Ideal Alveolar Gas and Blood at Sea Level Barometric Pressure (760 mm Hg)

	AMBIENT AIR (DRY)	MOIST TRACHEAL AIR	ALVEOLAR GAS (R = 0.80)	SYSTEMIC ARTERIAL BLOOD	MIXED VENOUS BLOOD
P_{O_2}	159	150	102	90	40
P_{CO_2}	0	0	40	40	46
P_{H_2O}, 37°C	0	47	47	47	47
P_{N_2}	601	563	571*	571	571
P_{TOT}	760	760	760	760	704†

*P_{N_2} is increased in alveolar gas by 1% because R is <1 normally.

†P_{TOT} is less in venous than in arterial blood because P_{O_2} has decreased more than P_{CO_2} has increased.

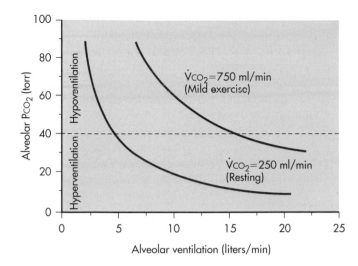

FIGURE 5-3 ■ Alveolar P_{CO_2} as a function of alveolar ventilation in the lung. Each line corresponds to a given metabolic rate associated with a constant production of carbon dioxide ($\dot{V}_{CO_2}$; isometabolic line). Normally, alveolar ventilation is controlled to maintain an alveolar P_{CO_2} of about 40 torr. During hypoventilation, the alveolar ventilation is low relative to $\dot{V}_{CO_2}$, and alveolar P_{CO_2} rises. During hyperventilation, the alveolar ventilation is excessive relative to $\dot{V}_{CO_2}$, and thus the alveolar P_{CO_2} falls. *(From Berne RM, Levy ML, Koeppen BM, Stanton BA (eds): Physiology, 5th ed. St. Louis, Mosby, 2004.)*

This equation demonstrates a number of interesting and important relationships. The first is that there is an inverse relationship between the partial pressure of carbon dioxide in the alveolus (P_{ACO_2}) and alveolar ventilation ($\dot{V}_A$) irrespective of exhaled CO_2. Specifically, if you double your alveolar ventilation, you will halve the P_{ACO_2}; and if you halve the alveolar ventilation, you will double the partial pressure of CO_2 in the alveolus. Second, if you maintain a constant alveolar ventilation ($\dot{V}_A$) and double your metabolic production of carbon dioxide ($\dot{V}_{CO_2}$), such as with an increase in body temperature, you will double the partial pressure of CO_2 in the alveolus (P_{ACO_2}). This relationship is with alveolar ventilation and not with tidal volume, of which alveolar ventilation is a part (see discussion of dead space later in this chapter).

Clinically, this principle is used in individuals who are being mechanically ventilated and cannot self-regulate their breathing. If the partial pressure of carbon dioxide increases in their blood, it is an indication that the partial pressure of carbon dioxide in the alveolus has increased. You can decrease the P_{ACO_2} (and thus, the arterial P_{CO_2}) by increasing alveolar ventilation ($\dot{V}_A$). If this same individual now develops a fever and cannot increase alveolar ventilation, the arterial P_{CO_2} will increase as a result of the increase in CO_2 production.

In normal individuals, the alveolar P_{CO_2} is tightly regulated to remain constant around 40 mm Hg. Specialized chemoreceptors monitor the P_{CO_2} in arterial blood and in the brainstem with changes in minute ventilation in accordance with the level of P_{CO_2}. Increases or decreases in arterial P_{CO_2}, particularly when associated with changes in pH, have profound effects upon cell functions including enzyme and transport functions. Because of this, the body tightly regulates arterial P_{CO_2}.

Because of its high diffusibility (see Chapter 8), alveolar P_{CO_2} is the same as arterial P_{CO_2} (P_{aCO_2}). Thus, $P_{ACO_2} = P_{aCO_2}$, and the two terms are used interchangeably. An increase in P_{aCO_2} due either to an increase in CO_2 production or to a decrease in alveolar ventilation results in an (respiratory) acidosis (pH < 7.35), whereas a decrease in P_{aCO_2} results in an (respiratory) alkalosis (pH > 7.45) (see Chapter 9). Hypercapnia is an elevation in P_{aCO_2} and is secondary to inadequate alveolar ventilation (hypoventilation) relative to CO_2 production. Conversely, hyperventilation is present when alveolar ventilation exceeds CO_2 production and results in a low P_{aCO_2} (hypocapnia).

DISTRIBUTION OF VENTILATION

Ventilation is not evenly distributed in the lung. There are regional differences in ventilation due in large part to the effects of gravity. When an individual is in the upright position, ventilation per unit of volume is greatest in the lower regions of the lungs, compared with the upper lung regions.

In order to understand the reasons for regional differences in ventilation, we need to re-examine

TABLE 5-3

Pleural (PPL) and Transpulmonary (PL) (cm H₂O) Pressure at FRC at the Top and Bottom of the Lung

POSITION	TOP OF LUNG		BOTTOM OF LUNG	
	P_{PL}	P_L	P_{PL}	P_L
Upright	− 8	8	− 2	2
Supine	− 4	4	0	0
Prone	− 3.5	3.5	0	0

From Agostoni E: Mechanics of the pleural spaces. Physiol Rev 52:57-128, 1972. FRC, functional residual capacity.

pleural pressures. In describing pleural pressure, we previously assumed that it was uniform throughout the chest. This, however, is not the case. When a person is in the upright position, the intrapleural surface pressure is less negative in the lower, gravity-dependent regions of the chest than in the upper nondependent regions (Table 5-3). The pleural surface pressure increases approximately +0.2 cm H₂O for every centimeter of vertical displacement from the top of the lung to the most dependent part of the lung. This pressure gradient is due to a combination of gravity and the effects of lung weight. This vertical pressure gradient creates a transpulmonary (PL) gradient (recall that $P_L = P_A − P_{PL}$), and this in turn affects alveolar size (Fig. 5-4). When an individual is in the upright position, alveoli near the apex of the lung are more expanded than alveoli at the base. This is because the pleural surface pressure is decreased (more negative) at the apex relative to the base because of gravity and the weight of the lung pulling down or away from the chest wall. If the pleural pressure is decreased (more negative), the static translung pressure ($P_L = P_A − P_{PL}$) is increased, and the alveolar volume in this area is increased.

As inspiration begins, alveoli at the apex and at the base of the lung have different volumes and are therefore at different locations on the pressure-volume curve. Alveoli at the base are at the steeper portion of the pressure-volume curve and receive more of the ventilation (i.e., they have a greater compliance). In contrast, the expanded alveoli at the apex are closer to the top of the pressure-volume curve, have a lower compliance, and thus receive proportionately less of the tidal volume.

In the absence of gravity, such as when astronauts are in space, this type of non-uniformity disappears. The effect is also less pronounced when an individual is supine compared with upright, and is less when a person is supine compared with prone. (This is because the diaphragm is pushed cephalad when one is supine and affects the size of all of the alveoli.)

In addition to gravitational effects on the distribution of ventilation, there is local non-uniform ventilation among terminal respiratory units. This is caused by variable airway resistance (R) or compliance (C) and it may be described by the following equation:

$$\tau = R \times C$$

in which the τ is the time constant.

Alveolar units with long time constants fill and empty slowly. Thus, a unit with increased resistance, increased compliance, or both will take longer to fill and longer to empty (see Fig. 3-9). In normal adults, the respiratory rate is ~12 breaths per minute, with an inspiratory time of approximately 2 seconds and an expiratory time of about 3 seconds. In normal individuals, this is sufficient time to almost reach equilibrium (Fig. 5-5). However, in the presence of an increased resistance (or an increased compliance), equilibrium is not reached. This contributes to the air trapping seen in diseases associated with increased resistance (e.g., chronic bronchitis) or increased compliance (e.g., emphysema).

TESTS OF DISTRIBUTION OF VENTILATION

Several methods have been used to examine the distribution of ventilation in patients. One of these is the single-breath nitrogen test. The subject exhales to residual volume and then takes a single maximal inspiration of 100% O₂. During the subsequent exhalation, the nitrogen concentration of the exhaled air is measured. Air (100% O₂, 0% nitrogen) initially exits from the conducting airways; the nitrogen concentration then begins to rise as alveolar emptying occurs. Finally, there is a plateau concentration of nitrogen as only alveoli containing nitrogen empty (Fig. 5-6).

Understanding the single-breath nitrogen test is an exercise in pulmonary physiology and the distribution of ventilation. At RV, the alveoli in the dependent portions of the lung are at a smaller volume than those in the

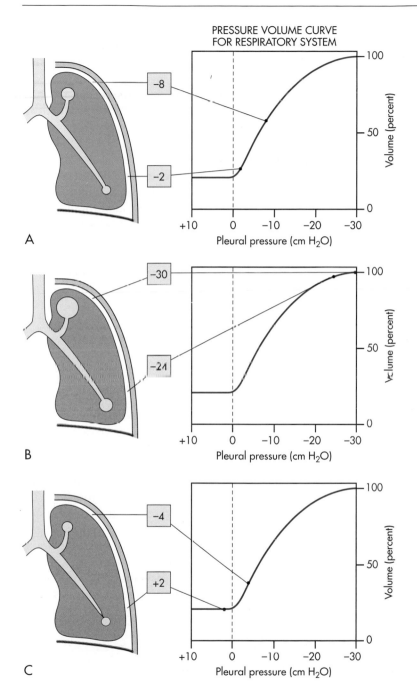

PRESSURE VOLUME CURVE
FOR RESPIRATORY SYSTEM

A

B

C

FIGURE 5-4 ■ The vertical transpulmonary pressure gradient in the upright lung at different lung volumes. **A,** At functional residual capacity, alveoli at the base are at the steeper portion of the pressure-volume curve and receive proportionately more ventilation **B,** At total lung capacity, alveoli both at the base and at the apex are at the top of the pressure-volume curve and have a lower compliance. **C,** At residual volume, alveoli at the base are compressed and could even close. *(Redrawn from Hinshaw HC, Murray JF: Diseases of the Chest, 4th ed. Philadelphia, WB Saunders, 1979.)*

apical portion. Thus, the apical alveoli contain a larger volume of nitrogen. As the subject inhales 100% oxygen, the superior alveoli receive proportionately less oxygen than the more dependent alveoli that sit at the steeper part of the pressure-volume curve. Therefore, the nitrogen concentration is higher in the apically located alveoli and there is a gradual decrease in nitrogen concentration farther down the lung, with the most diluted gas at the base. At the end of inspiration, the trachea and upper airways contain only oxygen.

A

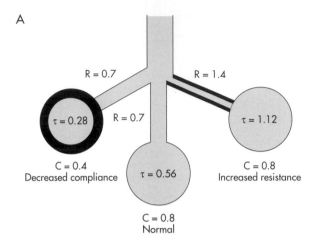

B

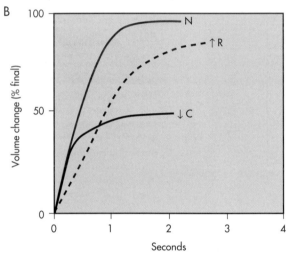

FIGURE 5-5 ■ Examples of local regulation of ventilation due to variation in resistance (R) or compliance (C) of individual lung units. **A,** In the unit at the *center*, the normal lung has a time constant (τ) of 0.56 second. This unit reaches 97% of final equilibrium in 2 seconds, the normal inspiratory time (N, shown in the graph in **B**). The unit at the *right* has a twofold increase in resistance; hence, its time constant is doubled. This unit is underventilated and fills more slowly, reaching only 80% equilibrium during a normal breath. The unit on the *left* has reduced compliance (stiff), which acts to reduce its time constant. This unit fills faster than the normal unit but receives only half the ventilation of a normal unit. **B,** Volume-time curve for normal lung (N), for lung with increased resistance (R) and for lung with decreased compliance (C). *(From Berne RM, Levy ML, Koeppen BM, Stanton BA (eds): Physiology, 5th ed. St. Louis, Mosby, 2004.)*

As exhalation begins, the gas in the trachea and upper airways exits first, and this gas has no nitrogen. Thus, phase I shows 0% nitrogen. As exhalation continues, alveolar gas begins to mix with the dead space oxygen, and the nitrogen concentration begins to slowly rise (phase II). Phase III consists entirely of alveolar gas. Initially, the gas comes predominantly from the dependent alveolar regions, where the nitrogen concentration is the lowest. As exhalation proceeds, increasing amounts of gas come from the apical regions, where nitrogen concentrations are highest. During phase III there is a gradual increase in nitrogen concentration; the normal slope of this phase is 1% to 2.5% nitrogen per liter exhaled.

The onset of phase IV is associated with an abrupt increase in nitrogen concentration. This occurs when dependent lung units have completely emptied, and more of the final portion of exhalation comes from the apical regions with the highest concentration of nitrogen. The onset of phase IV has been said to indicate the onset of airway closure in the dependent regions of the lung, and it is often called the "closing volume." Phase IV normally begins with approximately 15% of the vital capacity still remaining to be exhaled. This increases to 25% in older individuals. With disease, both the slope of phase III and the location of the phase IV slope increase. This occurs because the normal pattern of gas distribution, including the vertical gradient of nitrogen concentration, is abolished. Disease occurs unevenly throughout the lung; regions with greater disease with high resistance empty less completely and hence receive less oxygen; in addition, they empty more slowly, and this results in the elevated slope of phase III (Fig. 5-7). Today, phase IV has proved to be less sensitive than previously thought, but phase III is an excellent index of nonuniform ventilation.

DEAD SPACE

Anatomic Dead Space

Alveolar ventilation is less than tidal volume and minute ventilation because part of every breath fills and remains in the conducting airways and does not reach the alveoli. This air within the conducting airways does not participate in gas exchange. The volume of air present in the conducting airways is called the

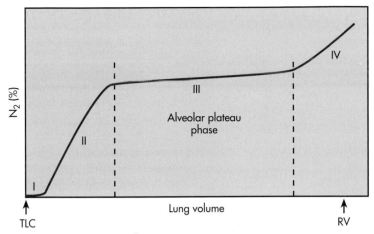

FIGURE 5-6 ■ The single-breath nitrogen washout curve is a simple and useful pulmonary function test of regional ventilation distribution. It clearly shows that all lung units do not have the same ventilation to perfusion ratio. The well-ventilated units (short time constant) empty faster than less well-ventilated units (long time constant). The portion of the curve up to the first vertical dashed line (phase I and II) represents the washout of dead space air mixed with alveolar gas. In phase III, the long alveolar plateau (between the vertical dashed lines) rises slowly (<2%) if ventilation distribution is relatively uniform, as shown here. The final phase (phase IV), after the second vertical line, shows very late, slowly emptying alveoli. This phase is accentuated with age. *(From Berne RM, Levy ML, Koeppen BM, Stanton BA (eds): Physiology, 5th ed. St. Louis, Mosby, 2004.)*

anatomic dead space (V_{DS}). The volume of air in the anatomic dead space is determined by the anatomy (size and number) of the conducting airways. When the letter V is used to denote volume, the letters T, DS, and A are used to denote tidal, dead space, and alveolar volume, respectively. The "dot" above the letter V denotes volume per unit of time (n). Thus,

$$V_T = V_{DS} + V_A$$

Therefore,

$$V_T \times n = V_{DS} \times n + V_A \times n$$

Or

$$\dot{V}_E = \dot{V}_{DS} + \dot{V}_A$$

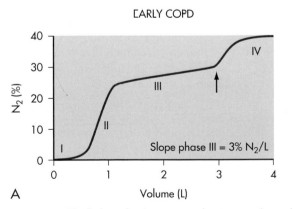

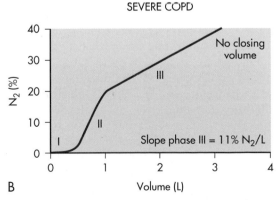

FIGURE 5-7 ■ Single-breath nitrogen washout curve in an individual with early (**A**) and severe (**B**) chronic obstructive pulmonary disease (COPD). Closing volume is noted by the arrow in **A**. *(Modified from Hyatt RE, Scanlon PD, Nakamura M: Interpretation of Pulmonary Function Tests: A Practical Guide. Philadelphia, Lippincott Williams & Wilkins, 1997.)*

Where $\dot{V}_E$ is the exhaled minute volume and $\dot{V}_{DS}$ and $\dot{V}_A$ are the dead space and alveolar ventilation per minute, respectively.

In the normal adult, at functional residual capacity (FRC), the volume of gas contained in the conducting airways is approximately 100 to 200 mL, compared with the 3000 mL of gas in the entire lung (see Fig. 5-1). With each tidal breath (approximately 500 mL), fresh gas moves first into the conducting airways and then into the alveoli. The ratio of the volume of the conducting airways (dead space) to tidal volume describes the fraction of each breath that is wasted in "ventilating" the conducting airways. This volume (V_{DS}) is related to the tidal volume (V_T) and to the exhaled ventilation (V_E) in the following way:

$$V_{DS} = \frac{V_{DS}}{V_T} \times V_E$$

As can be seen, dead space ventilation (V_{DS}) varies inversely with tidal volume (V_T). The larger the tidal volume, the smaller the dead space ventilation.

Normally, dead space ventilation represents 20% to 30% of the minute ventilation. This dead space is called the **anatomic dead space** because it is due to wasted ventilation of airways that do not and cannot participate in gas exchange (see Fig. 5-2). Another type of dead space, known as physiologic dead space, is discussed next.

Physiologic Dead Space Ventilation

Imagine a diseased lung in which some alveoli are not perfused but continue to be ventilated. These ventilated but not perfused areas of the lung, in a sense, are just like the conducting airways that are also ventilated but do not participate in gas exchange. The *total* volume of gas in each breath that does not participate in gas exchange is called the **physiologic dead space ventilation**. It includes the anatomic dead space and the dead space secondary to ventilated, but not perfused, alveoli or alveoli overventilated relative to the amount of perfusion. Thus, the physiologic dead space is always as large as the anatomic dead space, and in the presence of disease, it may be considerably larger. In healthy individuals, the physiologic dead space normally represents 25% to 30% of the minute ventilation.

MEASUREMENTS OF DEAD SPACE

Dead space usually is not measured clinically. However, dead space can be determined in two ways: using **Bohr's dead space equation,** originally described by the physiologist Christian Bohr at the turn of the 19th century, and **Fowler's method**.

Fowler's method and Bohr's equation do not measure exactly the same thing. Fowler's method measures the volume of the conducting airways down to the level where rapid dilution of inspired gas occurs with gas already in the lung. Thus, Fowler's method measures anatomic dead space. In contrast, Bohr's equation measures the volume of the lung that does not eliminate CO_2. Thus, Bohr's equation measures physiologic dead space. In normal individuals, there is very little difference between anatomic and physiologic dead space. In people with lung disease, however, the difference can be very large.

Bohr's Dead Space Equation

Bohr's equation measures the P_{CO_2} in alveolar gas and in mixed expired gas ($P_{E_{CO_2}}$) (Fig. 5-8). The dilution of CO_2 in the $P_{E_{CO_2}}$ relative to alveolar gas is measured and is a function of the amount of wasted ventilation relative to the minute ventilation. This is because conducting airways and ventilated, but not perfused, alveoli do not contribute to the CO_2 in expired gas. Exhaled gas is collected in a bag over a period of time, and the P_{CO_2} in the arterial blood (which is the same as the $P_{A_{CO_2}}$ in the alveolus) and in the bag ($P_{E_{CO_2}}$) is measured. Any volume of CO_2 in the $P_{E_{CO_2}}$ must come from both ventilated and perfused alveoli, because ambient air contains negligible amounts of CO_2. The dead space ventilation as a function of the tidal volume ($\dot{V}_{DS}/\dot{V}_T$) is described by the following equation:

$$\frac{\dot{V}_{DS}}{\dot{V}_T} = 1 - \frac{P_{E_{CO_2}}}{P_{A_{CO_2}}}$$

This equation can be derived from Boyle's law as follows:

$$P_1 V_1 = P_2 V_2 \text{ (Boyle's law)}$$

where P_1 is the partial pressure of CO_2 in the bag ($P_{E_{CO_2}}$) and V_1 is the exhaled tidal volume (V_T). Because all of the CO_2 was generated in alveoli that were perfused, P_2 is the arterial (alveolar) partial

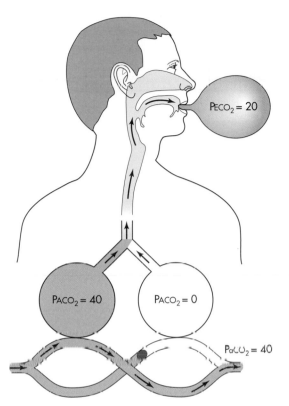

FIGURE 5-8 ■ Measurement of physiologic dead space using the dilution of carbon dioxide in mixed expired gas (P_{ECO_2}) and Bohr's dead space equation. In this example, dead space is 50% (0.5). *(Redrawn from Leff A, Schumacker P: Respiratory Physiology: Basics and Applications. Philadelphia, WB Saunders, 1993.)*

pressure of CO_2 and V_2 is the alveolar ventilation (V_A); that is,

$$P_{BCO_2} \cdot V_T = P_{ACO_2} \cdot V_A$$

Alveolar ventilation cannot be measured directly, but $V_A = V_T - V_{DS}$. Substituting for V_A,

$$P_{ECO_2} \cdot V_T = P_{ACO_2} \cdot (V_T - V_{DS})$$

Dividing by V_T,

$$P_{ECO_2} = P_{ACO_2} - \frac{V_{DS}}{V_T} \cdot P_{ACO_2}$$

Solving for V_{DS}/V_T,

$$\frac{V_{DS}}{V_T} = 1 - \frac{P_{BCO_2}}{P_{ACO_2}}$$

Fowler's Method

Dead space ventilation also can be measured using **Fowler's method** (Fig. 5-9). The subject takes a single breath of 100% oxygen and then exhales into a tube that continuously measures the nitrogen concentration in the exhaled gas. As the subject exhales, the volume of the anatomic dead space empties first. This volume has 100% oxygen in it and 0% nitrogen because it has not participated in any gas exchange. As the alveoli begin to empty, the oxygen level falls and the nitrogen level begins to rise. Finally, an almost uniform gas concentration of nitrogen is seen, representing entirely alveolar gas. This phase is called the **alveolar plateau**. The volume with initially 0% nitrogen plus half of the rising nitrogen volume is equal to the anatomic dead space.

AGING

Aging affects both the structure and the function of the respiratory system. Lung growth, best measured by the forced expiratory volume after 1 second (FEV_1), occurs throughout childhood and reaches a peak or maximum level at approximately 18 years of age in women and 27 years of age in men. Lung function then declines, with a loss in FEV_1 of approximately 30 mL/year (Fig. 5-10). This loss occurs due to the progressive loss of alveolar elastic recoil combined with costal cartilage calcification, decreased intervertebral space, and greater spinal curvature.

FRC increases with age in association with the decrease in elastic recoil and dynamic compression. Expiratory muscle strength also decreases and the combination results in decreased expiratory airflow rates. Airway closure occurs in dependent airways. As a result, there is greater ventilation to the apices of the lung—regions that are normally less well ventilated. This results in decreased arterial oxygen tension (see Chapter 7) as a result of ventilation:perfusion inequality (Fig. 5-11). Finally, there is a loss of alveolar surface area and decreased pulmonary capillary blood flow, resulting in decreased diffusion capacity that also contributes to the decrease in arterial oxygen tension in older individuals.

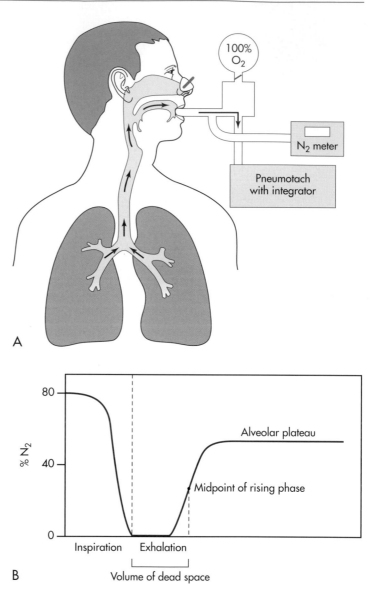

FIGURE 5-9 ■ Fowler's method for measuring anatomic dead space. **A,** The subject takes a single breath of 100% oxygen, holds his breath for a second, and then exhales. Nitrogen concentration is measured continuously during a steady rate of expiratory gas flow. **B,** At the beginning of exhalation, gas empties from the conducting airways that have been filled with 100% oxygen. Thus, the nitrogen concentration in the exhaled air is 0. As gas begins to empty from alveoli, the nitrogen concentration rises and then plateaus when only gas from previously filled alveoli empties. The volume of gas exhaled to the midpoint of the rising phase of the exhaled nitrogen concentration trace is the anatomic dead space. *(Modified from Levitzky M: Pulmonary Physiology, 4th ed. McGraw-Hill, 1995.)*

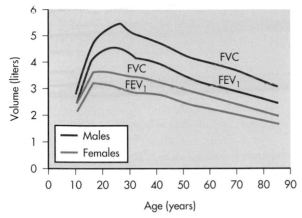

FIGURE 5-10 ■ Changes in forced vital capacity (FVC) and forced expiratory volume after 1 second (FEV₁) with age in normal men and women. Peak lung function occurs around 18 years of age for women and 27 years of age for men. *(Redrawn from Knudson RJ, Slatin RC, Lebowitz MD, Burrows B: The maximal expiratory flow-volume curve. Normal standards, variability and the effects of age. Am Rev Respir Dis 113:587-600, 1976.)*

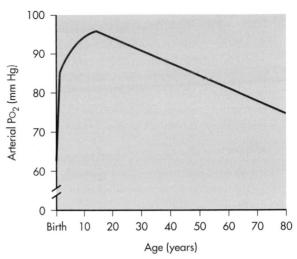

FIGURE 5-11 ■ Effect of age on arterial levels of oxygen. *(Data from Mansell A, Bryan C, Levison H: Airway closure in children. J Appl Physiol 33:711-714, 1972; Nelson NM: Neonatal pulmonary function. Pediatr Clin North Am 13:769-799, 1966; and Sorbini CA, Grassi V, Solinas E, Muiesan GI: Arterial oxygen tension in relation to age in healthy subjects. Respiration 25:3-13, 1968)*

SUMMARY

1. The sum of the partial pressures of a gas must be equal to the total pressure. The partial pressure of a gas (P_{gas}) is equal to the fraction of gas in the gas mixture (F_{gas}) times the total pressure (P_{TOT}).

2. By the time inspired gas reaches the trachea, it is fully saturated with water vapor, which exerts a pressure of 47 mm Hg at body temperature and dilutes the partial pressures of nitrogen and oxygen.

3. The conducting airways do not participate in gas exchange, and therefore the partial pressures of oxygen, nitrogen, and water vapor remain unchanged in the airways until the gas reaches the alveolus.

4. The partial pressure of oxygen in the alveolus is given by the *alveolar air equation*. This is the partial pressure of oxygen in the ideal situation—that is, in the absence of disease.

5. The respiratory quotient is defined as the ratio of carbon dioxide production to oxygen consumption. It is 0.8 under usual circumstances.

6. The relationship between carbon dioxide production and alveolar ventilation is defined by the *alveolar carbon dioxide equation*. There is an inverse relationship between the partial pressure of carbon dioxide in the alveolus (P_{ACO_2}) and alveolar ventilation (V_A) irrespective of exhaled CO_2. In normal individuals, the alveolar P_{ACO_2} is tightly regulated to remain constant at about 40 mm Hg.

7. There are regional differences in ventilation due in large part to the effects of gravity. In an individual in the upright position (compared with the supine position), alveoli at the apex of the lung are larger and less compliant and receive less of each tidal volume breath than alveoli at the base or dependent portion of the lung.

8. Alveolar units in the lung with long time constants ($\tau = R \times C$) fill and empty slowly.

9. In the single-breath nitrogen test, the slope of phase III is an excellent index of non-uniform ventilation.

10. The volume of air in the conducting airways is called the anatomic dead space. Dead space ventilation ($\dot{V}_{DS}$) varies inversely with tidal volume (V_T). The total volume of gas in each breath that does not participate in gas exchange is called the physiologic dead space. It includes the anatomic dead space and the dead space secondary to ventilated, but not perfused, alveoli or alveoli over-ventilated relative to the amount of perfusion.

11. Dead space ventilation can be measured using Bohr's equation and Fowler's method.

12. Aging results in a loss of lung elastic recoil, decreased expiratory muscle strength, airway closure in dependent lung units, decreased chest wall compliance, decreased arterial oxygen tension, loss of alveolar surface area and decreased pulmonary capillary blood flow with decreased diffusion capacity.

KEY WORDS

- Aging lung
- Alveolar carbon dioxide equation
- Alveolar gas equation
- Alveolar ventilation
- Anatomic dead space
- Bohr's dead space equation
- Boyle's law
- Carbon dioxide production
- Dalton's law
- Dead space
- Distribution of ventilation
- Fowler's method
- Gas fraction
- Gas tension
- Minute ventilation
- Oxygen consumption
- Partial pressure
- Physiologic dead space
- Pressure-volume curve
- Respiratory quotient
- Single-breath nitrogen test
- Tidal volume (V_T, or TV)
- Time constant (τ)
- Torr
- Water vapor pressure

SELF-STUDY PROBLEMS

1. If the dead space is 150 mL and the tidal volume increases from 500 to 600 mL, with the same minute ventilation, what is the effect on dead space ventilation?

2. A patient is breathing into a spirometer at a tidal volume of 500 mL and a respiratory frequency of 12 breaths/minute. The inspired gas is switched to 100% O_2 at the end of a full exhalation (residual volume), and the nitrogen concentration is monitored at the lips during the following exhalation. The nitrogen concentration is zero for the first 130 mL and then increases to a constant level of 50% at 170 mL of exhaled gas and remains at this level for the duration of exhalation. What is the dead space?

3. At Pike's Peak (445 mm Hg), what is the partial pressure of inspired air? Of air in the conducting airways?

4. What is the effect of an increased Pa_{CO_2} on alveolar P_{O_2}?

5. If alveolar ventilation is held constant, what is the effect of increased CO_2 production on alveolar P_{O_2}?

6. What is the effect of standing on your head on the distribution of ventilation?

REFERENCES

Agostoni E: Mechanics of the pleural space. Physiol Rev 52:57-128, 1972.

Anthonisen NR, Fleetham JA: Ventilation: Total, alveolar, and dead space. In Farhi LE, Tenney SM (eds): Gas Exchange. Handbook of Physiology, Section 3: The Respiratory System, vol 4. Bethesda, American Physiological Society, 1987.

Burrows B, Lebowitz MD, Camilli AE, Knudson RJ: Longitudinal changes in forced expiratory volume in one second in adults: Methodologic considerations and findings in healthy nonsmokers. Am Rev Respir Dis 133:974-980, 1986.

Ferrannini E. The theoretical basis of indirect calorimetry: a review. Metabolism 37:287-301, 1988.

Gattinoni L, Vagginelli F, Carlesso E, et al: Decrease in Pa_{CO_2} with prone position is predictive of improved outcome in acute respiratory distress syndrome. Crit Care Med 31:2727-2733, 2003.

Lucangelo U, Blanch L: Dead space. Intensive Care Med 30:576-579, 2004.

Lum L, Saville AL, Venkataraman ST: Accuracy of physiologic dead space measurement in intubated pediatric patients using a metabolic monitor: Comparison with the Douglas bag method. Crit Care Med 26:760-764, 1998.

Mummery HJ, Stolp BW, deL Dear G, et al: Effects of age and exercise on physiological dead space during simulated dives at 2.8 ATA. J Appl Physiol 94:507-517, 2003.

Shadick NA, Sparrow D, O'Connor GT, et al: Relationship of serum IgE concentration to level and rate of decline of pulmonary function; the Normative Aging Study. Thorax 51:787-792, 1996.

Wagner PD, West JB, Ventilation, blood flow and gas exchange. In Murray JF, Nadel JA (eds): Textbook of Respiratory Physiology, vol 1, 4th ed. St. Louis, WB Saunders, 2005, pp 51–87.

THE PULMONARY CIRCULATION

OBJECTIVES

1. Describe the two circulations in the lung in terms of anatomy, function, physiology, and regulation.
2. Describe the distribution of pulmonary blood flow.
3. Explain pulmonary vascular resistance in alveolar and extra-alveolar vessels and the effect of lung volume on these resistances.
4. List the anatomic components of the alveolar-capillary network.
5. Describe lymphatic flow and its components.
6. Explain the mechanisms of pulmonary edema formation.

The systemic circulation is composed of the vascular system supplied by the left ventricle that pumps blood into the aorta for distribution to the rest of the body. In contrast, the **pulmonary circulation** is composed of the vascular system that conducts blood from the right side of the heart through the lungs. These two vascular systems exist in parallel and both receive the entire **cardiac output** each minute.

The lung is the only organ in the body that receives blood from two separate sources. The pulmonary circulation brings deoxygenated blood from the right ventricle to the gas-exchanging units. At the gas-exchanging units, oxygen is transported across the alveolar and capillary endothelium into the red blood cell and carbon dioxide is transferred from the blood into the alveolus before it is returned to the left atrium for distribution to the rest of the body. The second blood supply is the **bronchial circulation**, which arises from the aorta and provides nourishment to the lung parenchyma. The blood supply to the lung is unique in its dual circulation and, as we will see later, in its

ability to accommodate large volumes of blood at low pressure.

PULMONARY BLOOD FLOW

Pulmonary blood flow consists of the entire output of the right ventricle. All of the mixed venous blood from all of the tissues in the body is pumped out of the right ventricle into the pulmonary circulation. As a result, pulmonary blood flow is equal to cardiac output—about 3.5 L/min/m² of body surface area at rest. At rest, the volume of blood contained in the lung (from the main pulmonary artery to the left atrium) is approximately 500 mL, or 10% of the circulating blood volume. Of this 500 mL, 70 mL of blood is contained in the pulmonary capillary bed. Approximately 280 billion capillaries supply the approximately 300 million alveoli, resulting in a surface area for gas exchange of 70 to 80 m².

The pulmonary capillary bed has the largest surface area of any vascular bed in the body. Many of these pulmonary capillaries are closed at rest and open periodically during periods of increased pulmonary blood flow. The network of capillaries is so dense that it may be considered to be a sheet of blood interrupted by small, vertical, connective-tissue supporting posts (see Fig. 1-7). At rest it takes a red cell about 4 to 5 seconds to travel through the pulmonary circulation with 0.75 seconds of this time spent in the pulmonary capillaries. The pulmonary capillaries have diameters of about 6 μm, slightly smaller than the diameter of a red blood cell (8 μm). Thus red blood cells must change their shape as they pass through the pulmonary capillaries. This shape change ensures the smallest possible distance between oxygen in the alveolus and the hemoglobin in the red cell.

During **exercise**, cardiac output and thus pulmonary blood flow can increase to as much as 25 L/min/m^2 and the pulmonary capillary volume increases and approaches about 200 mL. This increase in the pulmonary capillary volume during exercise occurs through two different processes (Fig. 6-1). First, closed or compressed capillary segments are recruited and open as the increase in cardiac output raises the pulmonary vascular pressure. Second, previously open capillaries enlarge as their internal pressure rises. Enlargement of open capillaries also occurs in individuals with left-sided heart failure, which is associated with an elevated left atrial pressure and an increase in pulmonary capillary volume.

The pulmonary veins are situated within loose interlobular connective tissue septae and receive blood from many lung units. They return blood to the left atrium through conventional and supernumerary branches. Because of their large numbers and thin walls, the pulmonary veins provide a large reservoir for blood, and these veins can either increase or decrease their capacitance in order to provide a constant left ventricular output in the face of a variable pulmonary arterial flow.

Pulmonary arteries and veins with diameters larger than 50 μm contain smooth muscle and have a motor supply through the sympathetic branch of the

FIGURE 6-1 ■ There are two processes responsible for increased pulmonary capillary volume with exercise in the lung. At rest, many pulmonary capillaries are not perfused; with exercise and increased pulmonary blood flow, previously closed capillaries can fill with blood (recruitment) secondary to an increase in perfusion pressure or already-open capillaries can increase in volume (distention). Both processes occur during exercise and neither results in a significant increase in pulmonary vascular resistance. *(Modified from Levitzky MG: Pulmonary Physiology, 4th ed. New York, McGraw-Hill, 1995.)*

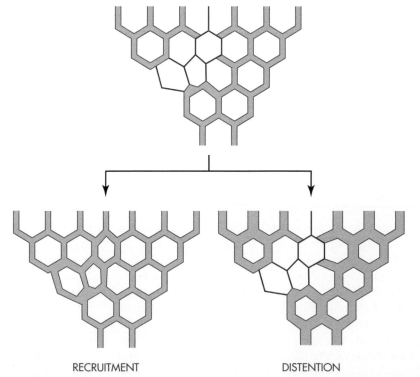

RECRUITMENT   DISTENTION

autonomic nervous system. Their extensive sensory innervation, located in the outer connective tissue layer (adventitia) of the vessel wall, can be stimulated by changes in vascular pressure (stretch) and various chemical substances. These vessels actively regulate their diameter and thus alter resistance to blood flow.

BRONCHIAL BLOOD FLOW

The existence of a second, separate circulatory system in the lung with oxygenated blood from the systemic circulation was first observed by Frederich Ruysch in the latter half of the 17th century. This second circulatory system is the bronchial circulation, and it provides systemic arterial perfusion to the trachea, upper airways, surface secretory cells, glands, nerves, visceral pleural surface, lymph nodes, pulmonary arteries, and pulmonary veins (Fig. 6-2). The bronchial circulation perfuses the respiratory tract to the level of the terminal bronchioles. Lung structures distal to the terminal bronchioles, including the respiratory bronchioles, alveolar ducts, alveolar sacs, and alveoli, are directly oxygenated by diffusion from the alveolar air and receive their nutrients from the mixed venous blood in the pulmonary circulation.

Bronchial blood flow comprises only 1% to 3% of the output of the left ventricle. The bronchial arteries, usually three in number, arise either from the aorta or from the intercostal arteries and accompany the bronchial tree and divide with it (see Fig. 1-14). The pressure in the bronchial arteries is equal to the systemic pressure and is therefore much higher than the pressure in the pulmonary circulation.

The return of venous blood from the capillaries of the bronchial circulation to the heart occurs either through true bronchial veins or through bronchopulmonary veins. True bronchial veins are present in the area of the hilum and flow into the azygos, hemiazygos, or intercostal veins before entering the right atrium. The bronchopulmonary veins are formed through a network of tributaries composed of both bronchial and pulmonary circulatory vessels, which anastomose and form vessels with an admixture of blood from both circulatory systems (see Fig. 6-2). Blood from these anastomosed vessels returns to the left atrium through pulmonary veins. It is estimated that about two thirds of the total bronchial circulation is returned to the

heart via the pulmonary veins and this anastomosis route. This deoxygenated blood, which mixes with oxygen-enriched blood in the pulmonary veins, contributes to the small alveolar-arterial oxygen difference in normal individuals.

The physiologic function of the bronchial circulation remains somewhat of an enigma; lung transplant studies have shown that adult lungs can function normally in the absence of a bronchial circulatory system. Thus, in healthy individuals, these anastomoses are probably of little importance. They may, however, be important in neonates and young children in bringing nutrients to the developing lung and in disease states in which reciprocal changes in flow in the two circulations provide a steady supply of nutrients. For example, in individuals with a pulmonary embolus, the bronchial circulation increases to the areas of the lung normally supplied by the pulmonary arteries; as a result, **pulmonary infarction** (death of the lung tissue) rarely occurs even with large pulmonary emboli. Similarly, in individuals who have undergone lung transplantation in which the bronchial circulation has been removed, necrosis (death) of the airway cells and other structures supplied by the bronchial circulation does not occur because of an increase in pulmonary circulation to these areas.

In contrast to the pulmonary circulation, the bronchial circulation has angiogenesis capabilities. These capabilities are particularly important for repair when tissue damage occurs; however, this property can be detrimental, as in the case of tumor angiogenesis. The major pathway for tumor angiogenesis in the lung is via the bronchial circulation. Although the bronchial arteries normally receive only a very small percentage of the cardiac output, in the presence of diseases such as cystic fibrosis the bronchial arteries are capable of increasing in size (hypertrophy), and they can receive as much as 10% to 20% of the cardiac output. Erosion into these vessels secondary to infection is responsible for the hemoptysis (coughing up blood) that can occur in this disease.

PRESSURES AND FLOWS IN THE PULMONARY CIRCULATION

The pulmonary circulation begins in the right atrium. Deoxygenated blood from the right atrium enters

FIGURE 6-2 ■ The anatomic features of the bronchial circulation are shown. The bronchial circulation supplies blood to the trachea and airways to the level of the terminal bronchioles as well as to the pulmonary blood vessels, visceral pleura, hilar lymph nodes, and vagus nerve and its branches. *Inset* depicts a bronchopulmonary anastomosis. Venous drainage in the lung is to both the right side of the circulation via the azygos and hemiazygos veins and to the left side of the circulation via the pulmonary veins *(Redrawn from Deffebach ME, Charan NB, Lakshminarayan S, Butler J: The bronchial circulation: Small but a vital attribute of the lung. Am Rev Respir Dis 135:463, 1987.)*

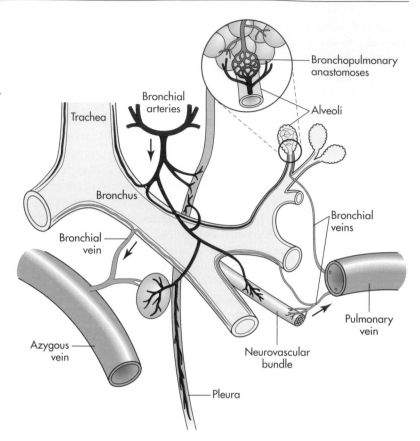

the right ventricle via the tricuspid valve and is then pumped *under low pressure* (9-24 mm Hg) into the pulmonary artery through the pulmonic valve (Fig. 6-3). The main pulmonary artery, also known as the pulmonary trunk, is about 3 cm in diameter; it branches quickly (5 cm from the right ventricle) into the right and left main pulmonary arteries, which supply blood to the right and left lungs, respectively. *The arteries of the pulmonary circulation are the only arteries in the body that carry deoxygenated blood.* The deoxygenated blood passes through a progressively smaller series of branching vessels (vessel diameters: arteries >500 μm, arterioles 10-200 μm, capillaries <10 μm) ending in a complex, mesh-like network of capillaries with very thin walls and large internal diameters relative to their wall thickness. The sequential branching pattern of the pulmonary arteries follows a pattern similar to airway branching, such that there are supporting vascular structures for each airway (see Fig. 1-14). The pulmonary

circulatory system functions to a) reoxygenate the blood and remove CO_2; b) aid in maintenance of fluid balance in the lung; c) distribute the metabolic products of the lung.

Oxygenation of red blood cells occurs in the alveolus where the pulmonary capillary bed and the alveoli come together in the alveolar wall in a configuration that achieves optimal gas exchange. Gas exchange occurs through this **alveolar-capillary network**.

Oxygenated blood leaves the alveolus through a network of small pulmonary venules (15-500 μm in diameter) and veins, which quickly coalesce to form larger pulmonary veins (>500 μm in diameter) in which the oxygenated blood returns to the left atrium of the heart. In contrast to arteries, arterioles, and capillaries, which closely follow the branching patterns of the airways, venules and veins run quite distant from the airways.

Unlike systemic arteries, the arteries of the pulmonary circulation are thin-walled with minimal

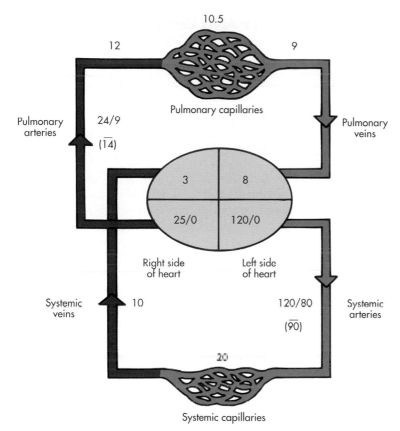

10.5

12

9

Pulmonary capillaries

Pulmonary arteries

24/9
(14̄)

Pulmonary veins

3 | 8

25/0 | 120/0

Right side of heart | Left side of heart

Systemic veins

10

120/80
(90̄)

Systemic arteries

20

Systemic capillaries

FIGURE 6-3 ■ Schematic representation of the phasic and mean pressures within the systemic and pulmonary circulations in a normal, resting human adult lying supine (dorsal recumbency). The units are millimeters of mercury (mm Hg) for easy comparison. The driving pressure in the systemic circuit is the difference between the pressure in the aorta (Pao) and the pressure in the right atrium (PRA), and is represented as (Pao − PRA) = 90 − 30 = 87 mm Hg, whereas the driving pressure in the pulmonary circuit is the differences between the pressure in the pulmonary artery (PPA) and the pressure in the left atrium (PLA), which is represented as (PPA − PLA) = 14 − 8 = 6 mm Hg. Cardiac output must be the same in both circuits in the steady state because they are in series; thus the resistance to flow through the lungs is less than 10% than the rest of the body. Note also that the pressures in the left heart chambers are higher than those in the right heart. Any congenital openings between the right and left sides of the heart favor left-to-right flow. (From Berne RM, Levy ML, Koeppen BM, Stanton BM (eds): Physiology, 5th ed. St. Louis, Mosby, 2004.)

smooth muscle. This has important physiologic consequences, including less resistance to blood flow. Pulmonary arteries also more distensible and compressible than systemic arterial vessels, and they are seven times more compliant. This highly compliant state requires much less work (lower pressures throughout the pulmonary circulation) for blood flow through the pulmonary circulation compared to the more muscular, noncompliant arterial walls of the systemic circulation. Furthermore, the vessels in the pulmonary circulation, under normal circumstances, are in a dilated state and have larger diameters compared with similar arteries in the systemic circulation. All of these factors contribute to a very compliant, low-resistance circulatory system, which aids in the flow of blood through the pulmonary circulation via the "weak" pumping action of the right ventricle.

This low-resistance, low-work system is also why the right ventricle is less muscular than the left ventricle. The pressure gradient differential for the pulmonary circulation from the pulmonary artery to the left atrium is only 6 mm Hg (14 mm Hg in the pulmonary artery minus 8 mm Hg in the left atrium) (see Fig. 6-3). It is almost 15 times less than the pressure gradient differential of 87 mm Hg present in the systemic circulation (90 mm Hg in the aorta minus 3 mm Hg in the right atrium).

PULMONARY VASCULAR RESISTANCE

Four factors influence blood flow in the lung: pulmonary vascular resistance (PVR), gravity, alveolar pressure, and the arterial to venous pressure gradient. Blood flows through the pulmonary circulation in a pulsatile manner following the pressure gradient in this low resistance system. PVR cannot be measured directly but is most often calculated using Poiseuille's law, in which R equals the difference in pressure between the beginning of the tube (P_1) and the end of the tube (P_2) divided by the flow (Q); that is,

$$R = \frac{P_1 - P_2}{Q}$$

In the pulmonary circulation, PVR is the change in pressure from the pulmonary artery (Ppa) to the left atrium (PLA) divided by the flow (QT), which is the cardiac output; that is,

$$PVR = \frac{P_{Pa} - P_{LA}}{Q_T}$$

Under normal circumstances, with normal cardiac output,

$$PVR = \frac{14 \text{ mm Hg} - 8 \text{ mm Hg}}{6 \text{ L} / \text{min}}$$
$$= 1.0 \text{ mm Hg} / \text{L} / \text{min}$$

This resistance is approximately 10 times less than the resistance in the systemic circulation. As previously mentioned, the low resistance in the pulmonary circulation system has two unique features, recruitment and distention, which allow for increased blood flow upon demand with little or no increase in PVR (Fig. 6-4). All of the available vessels are not utilized under normal resting conditions; this allows for compensation and recruitment of new vessels upon increased demand such as during exertion or exercise with little or no increase in pulmonary artery pressure. The distensibility of the blood vessels in the pulmonary circulation enables the vessels to increase their diameter with only a minimal increase in pulmonary arterial pressure.

At rest, about one third of the resistance to blood flow is located in the pulmonary arteries, one third is located in the pulmonary capillaries and one third is located in the pulmonary veins. In contrast, in the systemic circulation, most (70%) of the resistance to blood flow is located in the highly muscular systemic arterioles.

GRAVITY AND EFFECTS ON PULMONARY BLOOD FLOW

Because the pulmonary circulation is a low-pressure/low-resistance system, it is influenced by gravity much more dramatically than is the systemic circulation. This gravitational effect contributes to an uneven distribution of blood flow in the lung. In an individual in the upright position, under normal resting conditions there is a linear increase in blood flow from the apex of the lung (lowest flow; can approach zero under various conditions) to the base of the lung, where it is greatest but with no difference anterior to posterior (Fig. 6-5). Similarly, when a person is supine, blood flow is less in the uppermost (anterior) regions and greater in the lower (posterior) regions but equal in the apical and basal regions of the lung. Under conditions of stress, such as exercise, the difference in blood flow

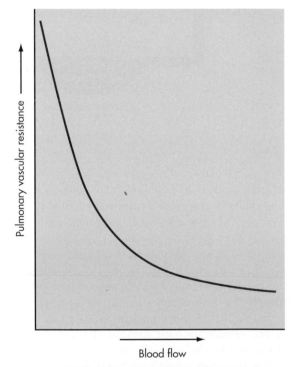

FIGURE 6-4 ■ Effect of pulmonary blood flow on pulmonary vascular resistance. With exercise, pulmonary blood flow increases and pulmonary vascular resistance decreases due to distention and recruitment of pulmonary vessels. *(Borst HG, et al: Influence of pulmonary arterial and left atrial pressure on pulmonary vascular resistance. Circ Res 4:393, 1956.)*

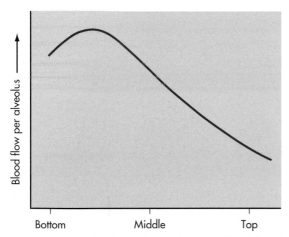

FIGURE 6-5 ■ Gravity-dependent pulmonary blood flow in the lung. In general, blood flow to alveoli at the bottom of the lung is greater than blood flow at the top at total lung capacity when an individual is in the upright position, even though at the very bottom of the lung there is a small decrease in blood flow per alveolus. *(Redrawn from Hughes JMB, Glazier JB, Maloney JE, West JB: Effect of lung volume on the distribution of pulmonary blood flow in man. Respir Physiol 4:58, 1968.)*

in the upright position in the apical and basal regions becomes less, due mainly to the increase in flow and the increase in arterial pressure.

Upon leaving the pulmonary artery, blood must travel up to the apex of the lung, against gravity, in the upright position. It is estimated that for every increase of 1 cm in height above the heart, there is a corresponding decrease in hydrostatic pressure relative to the change in height. Thus a change of 1 cm in height is equivalent to a change in hydrostatic pressure of 0.74 mm Hg, and a segment of lung that is 10 cm above the heart will have a decrease in arterial pressure of 7.4 mm Hg. At this point, the arterial pressure would be 6.6 mm Hg (arterial pressure at level of the heart equals 14 mm Hg minus 7.4 mm Hg). Conversely, a segment of lung 5 cm below the heart will experience an increase in arterial pressure of 3.7 mm Hg and thus have an arterial pressure of 17.7 mm Hg. The effect of gravity on blood flow equally affects arteries as well as veins. It is obvious from these two examples that there are wide variations in arterial and venous pressures from the apex to the base of the lung. These variations not only influence flow but also ventilation/perfusion relationships (see Chapter 7).

In addition to the arterial pressure (Pa) and venous pressure (Pv) gradients, differences in the pulmonary alveolar pressure (PA) influence blood flow in the lung. When referring to blood flow, the lung has been classically divided into three zones based on the different physiologic aspects of function in each zone or region (Fig. 6-6). Zone 1 represents the apex, where it is possible to have no blood flow. This could occur at the very top of the lung where the Pa is so low that it can be exceeded by PA. The capillaries collapse because

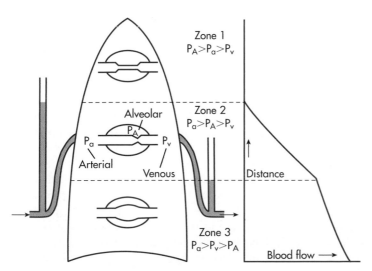

FIGURE 6-6 ■ Model depicting the uneven distribution of blood flow in the lung, based on the pressures affecting the capillaries. *(From West JB, Dollery CT, Naimark J: Distribution of blood flow in isolated lung: Relation to vascular and alveolar pressure. J Appl Physiol 19:713, 1964.)*

of the greater external P_A that prevents blood flow. Under normal conditions, this zone does not exist; however, this state may be reached during positive-pressure mechanical ventilation or if a physiologic alteration sufficiently decreases Pa. Under conditions of decreased arterial pressure, the blood flow rises only to the level at which the arterial and alveolar pressures are equal; above this, there is no flow.

Under normal circumstances, and when a person is in the upright position, most of the lung functions in what is referred to as Zones 2 and 3. In Zone 2, which comprises the upper one third of the lung, Pa is greater than P_A, which also is greater than Pv. Because P_A is greater than Pv, the greater external P_A partially collapses the downstream capillaries, causing a "damming" effect before the blood flows to the venous system. This phenomenon is often referred to as the "waterfall" effect. In Zone 3, Pa is greater than Pv, which is greater than P_A, and blood flow in this area follows the pressure gradients. Because the effect of gravity is equal on both arteries and veins, there is no change in the pressure differential at the base of the lung compared with the apex. Flow is increased in the basal area due to an increase in transmural pressure, which has the effect of distending the vessels and thus lowering resistance.

EFFECTS OF PRESSURE CHANGES ON EXTRA-ALVEOLAR AND ALVEOLAR VESSELS

Changes in alveolar and intrapleural pressure can also influence pulmonary blood flow, but the effects are different depending on the location of the vessels. The vessels in the pulmonary circulation can be divided into three categories—**extra-alveolar, alveolar, and microcirculation**. These three categories of pulmonary vessels are not well defined anatomically, but they have marked differences in physiologic properties that change under various conditions such as stress and exercise.

The extra-alveolar vessels are generally larger vessels (arteries, arterioles, veins, and venules); these vessels are not influenced by alveolar pressure changes but are affected by intrapleural and interstitial pressure changes (Fig. 6-7). As the transmural pressure gradient (which is equal to the pressure inside minus the

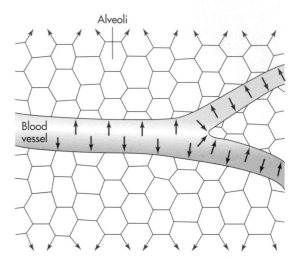

FIGURE 6-7 ■ Influence of alveolar pressure on extra-alveolar blood vessels. By virtue of their location, extra-alveolar blood vessels are not influenced directly by alveolar pressure. The extra-alveolar blood vessels are, however, tethered to the surrounding alveoli, and thus their caliber changes with changes in lung volume. Resistance to blood flow is higher at low lung volumes because the traction on the vessel walls is decreased. *(Redrawn from Jeff A, Schumacker P: Respiratory Physiology Basics and Applications. Philadelphia, WB Saunders, 1993.)*

pressure outside the vessel) increases, the vessel diameter increases and resistance decreases. Changes in either the intrapleural pressure or the interstitial pressure as a result of changes in lung volume and the retractive force generated by elastin (radial traction) greatly influence vessel caliber. For example, at high lung volumes, the decrease in pleural pressure increases the transmural pressure and increases the caliber of (dilates) extra-alveolar vessels, resulting in a decrease in resistance. In contrast, at low lung volumes, an increase in pleural pressure decreases transmural pressure and has a constricting effect with an increase in resistance.

Alveolar vessels are the capillaries within the interalveolar septa. These vessels are very sensitive to shifts in alveolar pressure but not to changes in pleural or interstitial pressure (Fig. 6-8). During inspiration, alveoli increase in volume; this increase is associated with elongation and compression of the vessels located in the interalveolar septae. As a result, at high lung

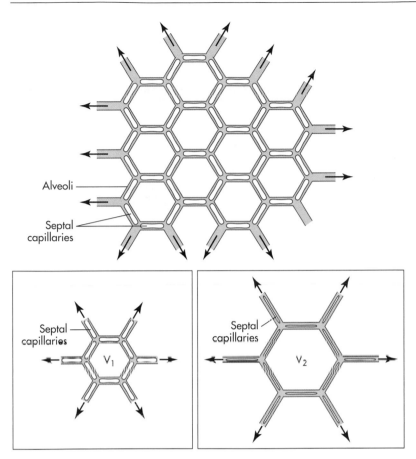

Alveoli

Septal
capillaries

Septal
capillaries V_1

Septal
capillaries V_2

FIGURE 6-8 ■ Influence of alveolar pressure on intra-alveolar or septal capillaries. These capillaries are very thin-walled and lack significant structural features. Their size and shape are highly dependent upon the pressures across their walls (inside-outside pressure difference). As a result, increases in alveolar pressure secondary to increases in lung volume distort and distend these capillaries and increase their resistance to blood flow. *(Redrawn from Levitzky MG: Pulmonary Physiology, 4th ed. New York, McGraw-Hill, 1995.)*

volumes the resistance to blood flow within these alveolar vessels increases; similarly, at low lung volumes, compression is less and resistance to blood flow decreases.

It should be clear from the previous discussion that changes in lung volume affect PVR through their influence on alveolar and extra-alveolar vessels. Thus, at end inspiration, the fully distended, air-filled alveoli apply pressure on the alveolar capillaries, increasing PVR. This stretching effect during inspiration has an opposite effect on the larger extra alveolar vessels, which increase in diameter due to radial traction and elastic recoil influences. During exhalation, the deflated alveoli apply the least resistance, and PVR is diminished.

The resistances of the alveolar and extra-alveolar vessels are additive at any lung volume because the alveolar and extra-alveolar vessels exist in series with each other. This results in the U-shaped curve of the total **pulmonary vascular resistance** (Fig. 6-9). Total PVR is lowest near FRC and increases at both high and low lung volumes.

With positive-pressure mechanical ventilation, there is both an increase in alveolar pressure and a decrease in the transmural pressure gradient in the extra-alveolar vessels. This results in compression of both the extra-alveolar and the alveolar capillaries and can block blood flow to the area. This can create Zone 1 blood flow.

The **pulmonary microcirculation** is a term used to describe the small vessels—usually pulmonary capillaries, but arterioles and venules to some extent—that participate in liquid and solute exchange in the maintenance of fluid balance in the lung.

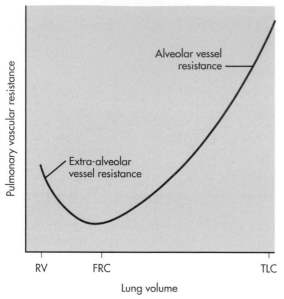

FIGURE 6-9 ■ Total pulmonary vascular resistance and lung volume. Total pulmonary vascular resistance is the sum of the resistances of the extra-alveolar and the alveolar or septal capillaries. At low lung volumes, resistance increases because of the increased resistance originating from the extra-alveolar vessels, whereas at total lung capacity (TLC), resistance increases because of the increase in resistance in the alveolar vessels. Total pulmonary vascular resistance is lowest at functional residual capacity (FRC). RV, residual volume. *(Modified from Levitzky MG: Pulmonary Physiology, 4th ed. New York, McGraw-Hill, 1995.)*

THE ALVEOLAR-CAPILLARY NETWORK

Gas exchange in the lung occurs in the alveolar-capillary unit. The alveolar-capillary unit results from the sequential branching pattern of the pulmonary arteries, which culminates with the branching of the small arterioles into the alveolar wall. This unique pattern establishes a dense, mesh-like network of capillaries and alveoli with little structure other than the thin epithelial lining cells of the alveolus, the endothelial cells of the vessels, and their supportive matrix. There can be nearly 1000 pulmonary capillaries per alveolus, resulting in an **alveolar-capillary network** with a surface area of approximately 70 m^2 (about the size of a tennis court) (see Fig. 1-3). The structural matrix and the tissue components of this

alveolar-capillary network are composed of type I alveolar epithelial cells, capillary endothelial cells, and their respective basement membranes that are organized back-to-back (Fig. 6-10). The distance for gas exchange through this basement membrane barrier is only about 1 to 2 μm in thickness. Surrounded mostly by air, this network creates an ideal environment for gas exchange. Red blood cells pass through this network in less than 1 second, sufficient time for CO_2 and O_2 gas exchange.

In addition to gas exchange, this network also functions in transcapillary exchange and fluid regulation within the lung. Solvents and solutes move across the capillary endothelial wall by diffusion, filtration, and/or pinocytosis. Diffusion is the most important means for solute transfer across the capillary endothelium; small molecules such as water, NaCl, urea, and glucose move freely; their net movement is limited only by the rate at which blood flow transports them. Thus their transport is **flow-limited**. For larger molecules, diffusion across the capillary pores (clefts) limits exchange; for these large molecules, exchange is **diffusion-limited**. Lipid-soluble molecules such as O_2 and CO_2 move across the capillary wall through pores by diffusion and directly through the capillary endothelium. O_2 diffuses across both the arterioles and venules. At low blood flow rates, this gas exchange may limit the supply of O_2 to the tissue. Pinocytosis is capable of moving large (30 nm) lipid-insoluble molecules between the blood and interstitial space.

Capillary filtration is regulated by the hydrostatic and osmotic forces across the endothelium. An increase in the intracapillary hydrostatic pressure favors the movement of fluid from the vessel to the interstitial space. Conversely, an increase in the concentration of osmotically active particles within the vessel favors movement of fluid into the vessels from the interstitial space.

All capillaries in the body have a variable degree of leakiness. At the pulmonary capillary level, the balance between hydrostatic pressure and oncotic pressure results in a small net movement of fluid (liquid, electrolytes, and protein) out of the vessels into the interstitial space. Fluids that leak into the interstitial space are inhibited from entering the airspace by the alveolar epithelium (type I and type II epithelial cells) that establishes a tight restrictive barrier and thus

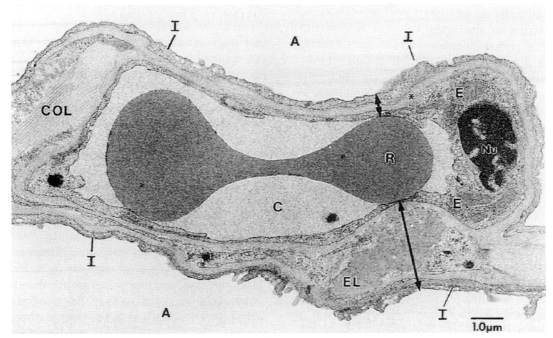

FIGURE 6-10 ■ Cross section of an alveolar wall showing the path for oxygen and carbon dioxide diffusion. The thin side of the alveolar wall barrier *(short double arrow)* consists of type I epithelium (I), interstitium (*) formed by the fused basal laminae of the epithelial and endothelial cells, capillary endothelium (E), plasma in the alveolar capillary (C), and finally by the cytoplasm of the red blood cell (R). The thick side of the gas-exchange barrier *(long double arrow)* has an accumulation of elastin (EL), collagen (COL), and matrix that jointly separate the alveolar epithelium from the alveolar capillary endothelium. As long as the red blood cells are flowing, oxygen and carbon dioxide diffusion probably occurs across both sides of the gas-exchange barrier. A, Alveolus; Nu, nucleus of the capillary endothelial cell. (Human lung specimen, transmission electron microscopy.) *(From Berne RM. Levy ML, Koeppen BM, Stanton BM (eds): Physiology, 5th ed. St. Louis, Mosby, 2004.)*

contains them in the interstitium. This barrier is highly advantageous, because any fluid in the airspace will interfere with gas diffusion.

The alveolar-capillary network is also very fragile and susceptible to a wide variety of injurious agents and events. The type I cell is the site of gas diffusion from the air into the capillaries but is quite susceptible to injury, perhaps because of its thin elongated shape and large surface area. In certain disease states, such as interstitial lung diseases, the type I cell dies, leaving a denuded alveolar epithelium that is associated with increased permeability. The cuboidal-shaped type II epithelial cell then proliferates and differentiates into type I cells in an attempt to restore the normal lung architecture.

THE PULMONARY LYMPHATIC SYSTEM

Fluid that leaks out of the vascular compartment enters the interstitium surrounding the capillaries. From there it travels to the alveolar corners and then to the peribronchial interstitial space surrounding the bronchi and small arteries. Fluid then enters the lymphatic system, which is responsible for moving fluid out of the lung. The terminal lymphatic vessels are a closed-end network of highly permeable lymph capillaries. They lack tight junctions between endothelial cells and are anchored to connective tissue by fine filaments. Skeletal muscle contraction distorts the filaments and opens spaces between the endothelial cells.

Blood capillary filtrate and the protein and cells that have passed from the vascular to the interstitial space enter the lymphatic capillaries. Lymph flows in an extensive system of one-way (monocuspid) valves, aided by skeletal muscle and lymphatic vessel contraction through thin-wall vessels of increasing diameter, and finally enters the subclavian veins at the junction with the internal jugular veins. The thoracic duct, which is the largest lymphatic vessel in the body, drains the lower extremities and the gastrointestinal tract and liver.

Fluid in the interstitium is removed from the lung by the lymphatic system and enters the circulation via the vena cava in the area of the hilum. In normal adults, it is estimated that an average of 30 mL of fluid/hour is returned to the circulation via this route. In 24 hours, a person's total plasma volume flows through the lymphatic system. Approximately one fourth to one half of the circulating plasma proteins are returned by the lymphatics to the blood. This is the system for returning albumin to the circulation. The lymphatic system also filters lymph through the lymph nodes and removes foreign particles such as bacteria.

The Starling equation describes the movement of liquid across the capillary endothelium:

$$\text{Flux (flow in mL/min)} = Kfc \left[(Pjv - Pis) - sd \, (\pi jv - \pi is) \right]$$

Where

Kfc = capillary filtration coefficient

Pjv = intravascular (capillary) hydrostatic pressure

Pis = interstitial hydrostatic pressure

sd = reflection coefficient (reflects the permeability of the membrane to protein)

πjv = intravascular colloid osmotic pressure

πis = interstitial colloid osmotic pressure

In principle, the Starling equation illustrates the forces creating the net flux of fluid out of the pulmonary capillaries (Fig. 6-11). However, in practice it is not possible to actually calculate this flux. Many of the parameters needed cannot be measured. For instance, the Kfc is dependent on the number of capillaries actually being perfused, which is not possible to determine.

PULMONARY EDEMA

Increases in extravascular fluid accumulation in the lung can occur resulting in a condition called **pulmonary edema**. This fluid accumulation can occur either because of an increase in outward fluid filtration or because of a decrease in fluid removal. Causes of pulmonary edema have been categorized on the basis of the Starling equation.

Increased capillary permeability resulting in increased outward fluid filtration can occur when the integrity of the capillary endothelium is destroyed. For example, the capillary endothelium can be damaged by infections, toxins, and oxygen toxicity.

Under normal conditions, the capillary hydrostatic pressure is 10 mm Hg. Increases in capillary hydrostatic pressure result in greater outward fluid filtration. If the rate of outward fluid filtration exceeds lymphatic drainage, fluid accumulates in the interstitium. This is the most common cause of pulmonary edema. It is seen in individuals with left-sided cardiac dysfunction either from cardiac infarction, left ventricular failure or mitral valve stenosis. As pressures in the left atrium rise, the pulmonary capillary hydrostatic pressure increases and more fluid leaks into the interstitium.

The other major and common cause of pulmonary edema is a decrease in colloid osmotic pressure of the plasma. This can occur in individuals who are hypoproteinemic or after overzealous administration of intravenous fluids. Less common causes of pulmonary edema are listed in Table 6-1.

ACTIVE REGULATION OF BLOOD FLOW

Although the passive mechanisms of blood flow regulation discussed earlier in this chapter represent the major factors influencing blood flow in the lung, there are also several active mechanisms of blood flow regulation in the lung. The smooth muscle around the pulmonary vessels is much thinner than the musculature around the systemic vessels, but it is sufficient to have a measurable impact on vessel caliber. This is especially true in capillaries in which blood flow depends chiefly on the contractile state of the arterioles. This contractile state is determined by the contraction and relaxation of the smooth muscle in the

PULMONARY CAPILLARY
FLUID BALANCE

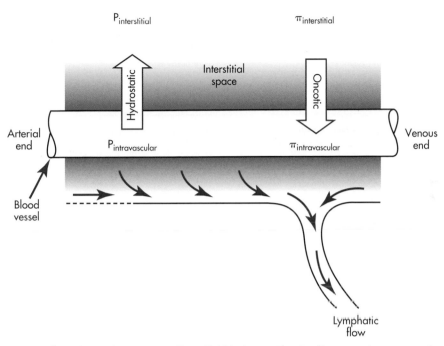

FIGURE 6-11 ■ Factors influencing pulmonary capillary fluid balance. The Starling equation summarizes the balance of forces favoring fluid flux into or out of the pulmonary vessels. Normally there is a net flux of fluid out of the vessels, which are drained from the interstitial space by the lymphatic system. *(From Berne RM, Levy ML, Koeppen BM, Stanton BM (eds): Physiology, 5th ed. St. Louis, Mosby, 2004.)*

pre-capillary vessel (arteriole) and the transmural pressure gradient (discussed previously). In contrast, true capillaries are devoid of smooth muscle and are incapable of active contraction. Changes in their diameter are passive and are caused by alterations in pre-capillary and post-capillary resistance.

Low and high oxygen levels have a major impact on pulmonary capillary blood flow. **Hypoxic vasoconstriction** occurs in small arterial vessels in response to decreased arterial Po_2. The response is local and is believed to be a protective response by shifting the blood flow from the hypoxic areas to normal areas in an effort to enhance gas exchange. Isolated, local hypoxia does not alter PVR; it is estimated that approximately 20% of the vessels need to be hypoxic before a change in PVR can be measured. Low levels of inspired oxygen due to exposure to high altitudes will have a greater and broader effect and can increase PVR (see

Chapter 12). High concentrations of inspired oxygen can dilate pulmonary vessels and decrease PVR.

In addition to alterations in oxygen, there are a wide range of factors and mediators that can influence vessel caliber (Table 6-2). Several of these mediators warrant further discussion.

Endothelin is a potent vasoconstrictor that is released by pulmonary endothelial cells in response to sheer stress and hypoxia. Increased levels of endothelin are thought to play a major role in the development of pulmonary hypertension; the recent development of endothelin antagonist drugs represents a major advance in the treatment of this progressive group of diseases.

Thromboxane A_2, a product of arachidonic acid metabolism, is one of the most potent vasoconstrictors of airway and vascular smooth muscle. It is released from white blood cells, macrophages and platelets.

TABLE 6-1	
Factors Predisposing to Pulmonary Edema	
FACTORS	CLINICAL PROBLEMS
Starling Equation	
Increased capillary permeability (K_τ; σ)	Adult respiratory distress syndrome
	Oxygen toxicity
	Inhaled or circulating toxins
Increased capillary hydrostatic pressure (P_c)	Increased left atrial pressure resulting from left ventricular infarction or mitral stenosis
	Overadministration of intravenous fluids
Decreased interstitial hydrostatic pressure (P_k)	Too rapid evacuation of pneumothorax or hemothorax
Decreased colloid osmotic pressure (π_{pt})	Protein starvation
	Dilution of blood proteins by intravenous solutions
	Renal problems resulting in urinary protein loss (proteinuria)
Other Etiologies	
Insufficient pulmonary lymphatic drainage	Tumors
Unknown etiology	Interstitial fibrosing diseases
	High-altitude pulmonary edema
	Pulmonary edema after head injury (neurogenic pulmonary edema)
	Drug overdose

Source: Reproduced with permission from Levisky MG, Cairo JM, Hall SM: Introduction to Respiratory Care. Philadelphia, Saunders, 1990.

TABLE 6-2
Compounds with Active Regulatory Properties in Pulmonary Blood Flow
Pulmonary Vasoconstrictors
Low P_{AO_2}
Thromboxane A_2
α-Adrenergic catecholamines
Angiotensin
Leukotrienes
Neuropeptides
Serotonin
Endothelin
Histamine
Prostaglandins
High CO_2
Pulmonary Vasodilators
High P_{AO_2}
Prostacyclin
Nitric oxide
Acetylcholine
Bradykinin
Dopamine
β-Adrenergic catecholamines

The capillary endothelium is also capable of producing potent vasodilators. One of these is endothelium-derived relaxing factor, which has been shown to be the gas **nitric oxide** (NO). NO is formed and released by the endothelium in response to various agents including acetylcholine, adenosine triphosphate (ATP), serotonin, bradykinin, histamine, and substance P. Most of these vasoconstricting and vasodilating factors are released by local cells or by inflammatory cells. They have a short half-life and their effect is usually local.

MEASUREMENT OF PULMONARY VASCULAR PRESSURES

The pressures in the pulmonary circulation can be measured during a procedure known as right heart catheterization (Fig. 6-12). In this procedure, a small, fluid-filled catheter (tube) is inserted into a vein and advanced toward the heart. A balloon at the tip of the catheter is inflated with air; as a result, the catheter is carried with the blood into the right atrium and then into the right ventricle. The catheter has been connected to a pressure transducer, and the pressure in the right atrium and right ventricle can be measured. The catheter is then passed through the pulmonic valve and floated into the pulmonary trunk, where pressure measurements are made. Finally, the catheter lodges in a pulmonary vessel and occludes that vessel. The balloon at the tip of the catheter is inflated, and all blood flow to the area ceases.

The pressure that is measured at the point of occlusion is approximately the same as the pressure in the left atrium because there is a static column of blood in the area. The left atrial pressure measured by inflating the balloon around the tip of the catheter in the pulmonary artery and occluding blood flow is called the *pulmonary capillary wedge pressure* (Fig. 6-12). This measurement is particularly useful in sorting out cardiac from pulmonary causes of pulmonary edemas. It is, however, an invasive procedure and can be done only in the cardiac catheterization laboratory or in the intensive care unit.

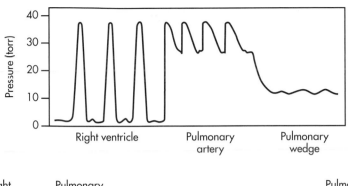

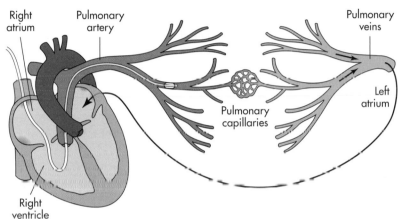

FIGURE 6-12 ■ Measurement of pulmonary capillary pressures in the lung. The right side of the heart is catheterized and a water-filled balloon is floated out into the pulmonary artery. The tip of the catheter is wedged into a branch of the pulmonary artery. When the balloon is inflated, all blood flow ceases; the pressure recorded at the balloon tip (pulmonary capillary wedge pressure) is approximately equal to the pressure in the left atrium. The recording of the various pressures as the catheter is advanced can be used to measure pulmonary artery pressure and right ventricular pressure and is very useful in the intensive care unit to discriminate between pulmonary and cardiac disease. *(Redrawn from Leff A, Schumacker P: Respiratory Physiology: Basics and Applications. Philadelphia, WB Saunders, 1993.)*

This same catheter, however, when equipped with a temperature sensor near the distal tip, can also be used to measure pulmonary blood flow, and thus cardiac output. In this procedure, called **thermodilution**, ice-cold water is injected into the right atrium and the temperature is measured by the sensor located in the pulmonary artery. The temperature-time curve is integrated, and the volume and temperature of the injected bolus is recorded and used to determine the cardiac output. It can be seen that large decreases in the temperature of the fluid noted by the sensor reflect high cardiac outputs, because energy is conserved and the drop in temperature reflects a rapid movement of the fluid bolus with little time to warm to body temperature. The computations are complex and computer programs are used to generate the results.

SUMMARY

1. The lung is the only organ in the body with two separate blood supplies. The first is the pulmonary circulation, which brings deoxygenated blood from the right ventricle to the gas-exchanging units. In these units, oxygen is picked up and carbon dioxide is removed before the blood returns to the left atrium for distribution to the rest of the body.

2. The second blood supply is the bronchial circulation, which arises from the aorta and provides nourishment to the lung parenchyma.

3. The pulmonary circulation is a low-pressure, low-resistance system with a driving pressure almost 16 times less than that of the systemic circulation.

4. The arteries of the pulmonary circulation are the only arteries that carry deoxygenated blood.

5. The recruitment of new capillaries and the distensibility of pulmonary capillaries are unique features of the lung and allow for stress adjustments, as in the case of exercise. The arteries of the pulmonary circulation are thin-walled with minimal smooth muscle. They are seven times more compliant than systemic vessels and are easily distensible.

6. Pulmonary vascular resistance is the change in pressure from the pulmonary artery (Ppa) to the left atrium (PLA) divided by the flow (QT), or cardiac output. This resistance is approximately 10 times less than in the systemic circulation.

7. When an individual is in the upright position, under normal resting conditions there is a linear increase in blood flow from the apex of the lung (lowest flow; can approach zero under various conditions) to the base of the lung, where it is the greatest.

8. The lung classically has been divided into three zones. Zone 1 represents the apex region, where it is possible to have no blood flow. In Zone 2, which constitutes the upper one third of the lung, arterial pressure (Pa) is greater than alveolar pressure (PA), which is greater than venous pressure (Pv). In Zone 3, Pa is greater than Pv, which is greater than PA, and blood flow in this area follows the pressure gradients.

9. The extra-alveolar vessels are generally larger vessels (arteries, arterioles, veins, and venules) that are not influenced by alveolar pressure changes but are affected by intrapleural and interstitial pressure changes. Alveolar vessels are the capillaries within the inter-alveolar septa and are very sensitive to shifts in alveolar pressure but not to changes in pleural or interstitial pressure. Pulmonary microcirculation is a term used to describe small vessels that participate in liquid and solute exchange in the maintenance of fluid balance in the lung.

10. The alveolar-capillary network is composed of a dense mesh-like network of capillaries and alveoli separated only by their basement membranes.

11. The balance between hydrostatic and osmotic forces regulates fluid filtration, resulting in a net outward movement of fluid into the interstitium.

12. The lymphatics clear fluid from the interstitium. The fluid volume moved through the lymphatics in 24 hours is equal to an individual's total plasma volume, and 1/4 to 1/2 of the total plasma proteins are returned to the circulation through the lymphatics in 24 hours.

13. Pulmonary edema occurs when there is an increase in extravascular fluid accumulation in the lung, either because of an increase in outward fluid filtration or because of a decrease in fluid removal.

14. Hypoxic vasoconstriction occurs in small arterial vessels in response to decreased P_{O_2}. Local hypoxia does not alter pulmonary vascular resistance (PVR). Other important vasoconstrictors are endothelin and thromboxane A_2; nitric oxide (NO) is a potent vasodilator of the pulmonary endothelium.

KEY WORDS

- Alveolar vessels
- Alveolar-capillary network
- Bronchial circulation
- Capillary filtration
- Cardiac output
- Endothelin
- Exercise
- Extra-alveolar vessels
- Hypoxic vasoconstriction
- Nitric oxide
- Pulmonary circulation
- Pulmonary edema
- Pulmonary lymphatic system
- Pulmonary microcirculation
- Pulmonary vascular resistance
- Starling equation
- Thermodilution
- Thromboxane A_2

SELF-STUDY PROBLEMS

1. What is the relationship between lung volume and vascular resistance in the entire lung? In the alveolar vessels? In the extra-alveolar vessels?

2. What is the distribution of pulmonary blood flow in individuals in outer space under zero gravity conditions?

3. How would a drop in pulmonary artery pressure affect the distribution of blood flow in the three zones of the lung?

4. What is the effect of high altitude on pulmonary artery pressure?

5. During cardiac catheterization, what is the effect of oxygen on pulmonary artery pressure and pulmonary vascular resistance?

REFERENCES

Bongartz G, Boos M, Scheffler K, Steinbrich W: Pulmonary circulation. Eur Radiol 8:698-706, 1998.

Glenny RW: Blood flow distribution in the lung. Chest 114:8S-16S, 1998.

Leff AR. Schumacker PT: Respiratory Physiology: Basics and Applications. Philadelphia, WB Saunders, 1993.

Murray JP: The Normal Lung, 2nd ed. Philadelphia, WB Saunders, 1986.

Weibel ER: The Pathway for Oxygen: Structure and Function of the Mammalian Respiratory System. Cambridge, MA, Harvard University Press, 1984.

Weir EK, Archer SL: The mechanism of acute hypoxic pulmonary vasoconstriction: The tale of two channels. FASEB J 9:183-189, 1995.

VENTILATION ($\dot{V}$), PERFUSION ($\dot{Q}$) & RELATIONSHIPS

O B J E C T I V E S

1. Describe the significance of a normal ventilation-perfusion ratio ($\dot{V}/\dot{Q}$).

2. Characterize the $\dot{V}/\dot{Q}$ at the apex and at the base of the lung in upright individuals.

3. Calculate the alveolar-arterial oxygen difference ($AaDo_2$) and describe how to use it.

4. List the four major causes of hypoxemia and describe their anatomy and physiology.

5. List the two major causes of hypercarbia and describe their anatomy and physiology.

6. Distinguish pathophysiologic processes associated with hypoxemia using 100% oxygen.

Although ventilation and pulmonary blood flow (perfusion) are important individual components in the primary function of the lung, the relationship between ventilation and perfusion—specifically the ratio of ventilation to perfusion—(defined as ($\dot{V}/\dot{Q}$) is the major determinant of normal gas exchange. Before reading about ventilation-perfusion relationships, review ventilation (Chapter 5) and perfusion (Chapter 6).

VENTILATION-PERFUSION RATIO

Up to this point, we have examined ventilation ($\dot{V}$) and lung perfusion ($\dot{Q}$) in isolation. Both are essential elements in the normal functioning of the lung, but they are insufficient to ensure normal **gas exchange**. For example, consider the situation in which blood is perfusing an area of the lung that has no ventilation (Fig. 7-1). Overall ventilation and overall perfusion in the lung may be normal, but in this specific area of the lung, normal gas exchange cannot occur because there is no ventilation. Thus, without ventilation, the blood entering and leaving the area would be unchanged and would remain deoxygenated. Similarly, imagine an area of the lung with normal ventilation but no perfusion. Gas entering and leaving the alveoli in this area would be unchanged; that is, it would not participate in gas exchange because there is no blood flow to the area.

The ventilation-perfusion ratio ($\dot{V}/\dot{Q}$) is the ratio of ventilation to blood flow. It can be defined for a single alveolus, for a group of alveoli, or for the entire lung. At the level of a single alveolus, it is defined as the alveolar ventilation ($\dot{V}A$) divided by the capillary blood flow ($\dot{Q}c$). At the level of the lung, it is defined as the total alveolar ventilation divided by the cardiac output.

In normal individuals, alveolar ventilation and blood flow are uniformly distributed to the gas-exchanging units with slightly less alveolar ventilation relative to pulmonary blood flow. At rest, in normal individuals, alveolar ventilation is ~4.0 L/min and pulmonary blood flow is ~5.0 L/min. Thus, in the normal lung,

FIGURE 7-1 ■ Alveolar O_2 and CO_2 levels in relation to the ventilation-perfusion ratio ($\dot{V}/\dot{Q}$). **A,** Normally ventilated and perfused alveoli. **B,** $\dot{V}/\dot{Q}$ equal to 0 secondary to absent ventilation. O_2 and CO_2 levels in the alveolus are equal to those in the mixed venous blood. **C,** $\dot{V}/\dot{Q}$ equal to infinity secondary to absent perfusion. Note that in this alveolar unit the O_2 and CO_2 levels are equal to those in ambient air, because no gas exchange occurs. *(Modified and reproduced with permission from West JB: Ventilation-perfusion relationships. Am Rev Respir Dis 116:919, 1977.)*

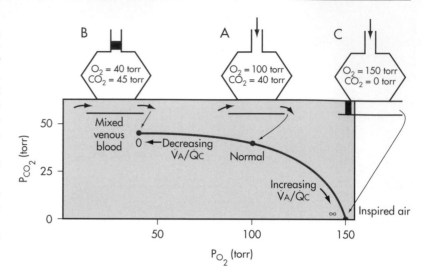

the overall ventilation-perfusion ratio is ~0.8; however, there is a wide range of ventilation-perfusion ratios in different lung units (Fig. 7-2). If ventilation and blood flow are mismatched, impairment of both O_2 and CO_2 transfer occurs. When ventilation exceeds perfusion, then $\dot{V}/\dot{Q}$ is greater than 1; when perfusion exceeds ventilation, then $\dot{V}/\dot{Q}$ is less than 1. Ventilation-perfusion mismatching occurs with increasing age (see Fig. 7-2) and with various lung diseases. *In individuals with cardiopulmonary disease, mismatching of pulmonary blood flow and alveolar ventilation is the most frequent cause of systemic arterial hypoxemia.*

A normal ventilation-perfusion ratio does not mean that ventilation and perfusion to that lung unit are normal; it simply means that the *relationship* between ventilation and perfusion is normal. The following example may clarify this point.

In the presence of a lobar pneumonia, ventilation to the affected lobe is decreased. If perfusion to this area remained unchanged, there would be perfusion in excess of ventilation—an example of an abnormal ventilation-perfusion ratio ($\dot{V}/\dot{Q} = <1$). However, as a result of decreased ventilation to this area, hypoxic vasoconstriction occurs in the pulmonary capillary bed supplying this lobe. The result is a decrease in perfusion to the affected area and a more "normal" ventilation-perfusion ratio. However, neither the ventilation to this area nor the perfusion to this area is normal (both are decreased); but the relationship between the two is (approaches) "normal."

REGIONAL DIFFERENCES IN VENTILATION AND PERFUSION

Because of regional differences in ventilation and perfusion. due largely to gravity effects, even in the normal lung, the $\dot{V}/\dot{Q}$ in different areas of the lung is greater than or less than the "ideal" normal value of 0.8. When a person is in the upright position, from the top to the bottom of the lung, ventilation increases more slowly than blood flow increases. As a consequence, the $\dot{V}/\dot{Q}$ at the top of the lung is high (increased ventilation relative to very little blood flow in the pulmonary circulation because of gravity effects), whereas the $\dot{V}/\dot{Q}$ at the bottom of the lung is "abnormally" low. The relationship between ventilation and perfusion from the top to the bottom of the lung is shown in Figure 7-3. The important point here is that although the overall $\dot{V}/\dot{Q}$ in the normal lung is 0.8, it is composed of a wide range of localized ventilation-perfusion ratios (Fig. 7-4).

ALVEOLAR-ARTERIAL DIFFERENCE

Before examining ventilation-perfusion ratios in greater depth, we need to examine the relationship between

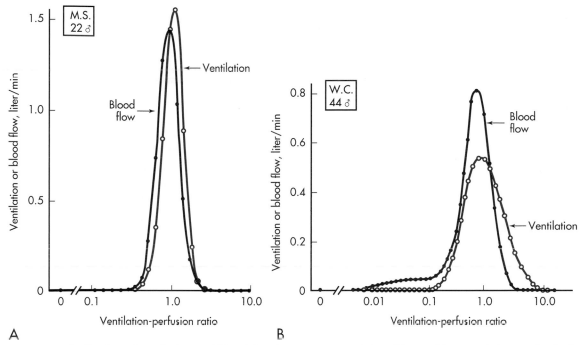

FIGURE 7-2 ■ Distributions of ventilation and blood flow in a young man (**A**) and in an older man (**B**). In **A**, both distributions are positioned about a ventilation-perfusion ratio ($\dot{V}/\dot{Q}$) close to 1.0; the curves are symmetric on a log scale with no areas of high or low ventilation-perfusion ratios, and there is no shunt (i.e. $\dot{V}/\dot{Q} = 0$). In **B**, there are areas where perfusion exceeds ventilation and the $\dot{V}/\dot{Q}$ is less than 1, and areas where ventilation exceeds perfusion and the $\dot{V}/\dot{Q}$ is greater than 1 but there are no areas of shunt ($\dot{V}/\dot{Q} = 0$). *(Redrawn from Wagner PD, Laravuso RB, Uhl RR, West JB: J Clin Invest 54: 54, 1974. The Society of Clinical Investigation.)*

alveolar O_2 and arterial O_2. In a perfect situation, there would be no difference between alveolar and arterial O_2. Even in normal individuals, a small difference in alveolar and arterial O_2 occurs. The difference between the alveolar O_2 (P_{AO_2}) and the arterial PO_2 (PaO_2) is called $AaDO_2$. An increase in the $AaDO_2$ is one of the hallmarks of abnormal O_2 exchange. The small difference between alveolar and arterial O_2 is not the result of imperfect gas exchange but rather is due to a small number of veins (carrying deoxygenated blood) that bypass the lung and empty directly into the arterial circulation. The thebesian vessels of the left ventricular myocardium drain directly into the left ventricle (rather than into the coronary sinus in the right atrium) while some **bronchial veins** and mediastinal veins drain into **pulmonary veins** (bronchopulmonary anastomoses; see Fig. 6-2). This results in a **venous admixture** and a decrease in arterial PaO_2 (this is an example of an anatomic shunt; see page 105). It is estimated that approximately 2% to 3% of the cardiac output is shunted in this way.

Clinically, we measure the effectiveness of gas exchange by measuring the oxygen and carbon dioxide in arterial blood. This can be done simply by inserting a needle into either the radial or the brachial artery (other peripheral arteries can also be used) and measuring the PaO_2 and $PaCO_2$. By knowing the barometric pressure (P_B), the fraction of oxygen in the inspired air, the water vapor pressure (P_{H_2O}), the alveolar CO_2 (which is equal to the arterial CO_2), and the respiratory quotient (usually considered to be 0.8), we can calculate the alveolar P_{AO_2} using the alveolar

VENTILATION-PERFUSION RELATIONSHIPS

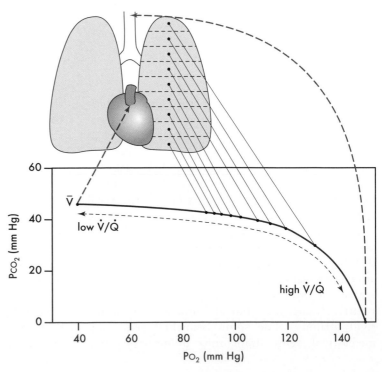

Vol (%)	$\dot{V}$ (L/min)	$\dot{Q}$ (L/min)	$\dot{V}/\dot{Q}$	P_{O_2} (mmHg)	P_{CO_2} (mmHg)	P_{N_2} (mmHg)	O_2 content (mL/100 mL)	CO_2 content (mL/100 mL)	pH	O_2 in (mL/min)	CO_2 out (mL/min)
7	.24	.07	3.3	132	28	553	20.0	42	7.51	4	8
13	82	1.29	0.63	89	42	582	19.2	49	7.39	60	39

FIGURE 7-3 ■ Regional differences in gas exchange down the normal lung. Only the apical and basal values are shown for clarity. *(From Berne RM, Levy ML, Koeppen BM, Stanton BM (eds): Physiology, 5th ed. St. Louis, Mosby, 2004.)*

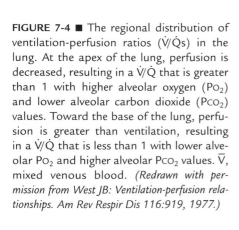

FIGURE 7-4 ■ The regional distribution of ventilation-perfusion ratios ($\dot{V}/\dot{Q}$s) in the lung. At the apex of the lung, perfusion is decreased, resulting in a $\dot{V}/\dot{Q}$ that is greater than 1 with higher alveolar oxygen (P_{O_2}) and lower alveolar carbon dioxide (P_{CO_2}) values. Toward the base of the lung, perfusion is greater than ventilation, resulting in a $\dot{V}/\dot{Q}$ that is less than 1 with lower alveolar P_{O_2} and higher alveolar P_{CO_2} values. $\overline{V}$, mixed venous blood. *(Redrawn with permission from West JB: Ventilation-perfusion relationships. Am Rev Respir Dis 116:919, 1977.)*

air equation. The difference between the alveolar P_{AO_2} and the measured arterial Pa_{O_2} is the AaD_{O_2}. In normal individuals breathing room air, the AaD_{O_2} is less than 15 mm Hg. It rises approximately 3 mm Hg per decade of life. For this reason, an AaD_{O_2} less than 25 mm Hg is considered the upper limit of normal.

As we will see later, abnormalities in arterial Pa_{O_2} can occur in the presence or absence of an abnormal AaD_{O_2}. The relationship between Pa_{O_2} and AaD_{O_2} is useful in determining the cause of an abnormal Pa_{O_2} and in predicting response to therapy (particularly supplemental oxygen administration). Thus, *the AaD_{O_2} should be calculated as part of every arterial blood gas analysis*. This information can then be used to determine the cause of an abnormal arterial O_2. Causes of a reduction in arterial Pa_{O_2} (arterial hypoxemia) and its effect on AaD_{O_2} are shown in Table 7-1. Each cause is discussed in greater detail later.

ARTERIAL BLOOD GAS ABNORMALITIES

Arterial hypoxemia is said to be present when the arterial Pa_{O_2} is below the normal range. In general, an arterial Pa_{O_2} of less than 80 mm Hg in an adult breathing room air at sea level is abnormal. **Hypoxia** occurs when there is insufficient oxygen to carry out normal metabolic functions, and thus hypoxia and hypoxemia mean different things but are frequently used interchangeably. Hypocarbia is defined as an increase in arterial Pa_{CO_2} above the normal range (40 ± 2 mm Hg) and hypocapnia is a lower than normal arterial Pa_{CO_2} (usually less than 35 mm Hg).

VENTILATION-PERFUSION RATIO IN A SINGLE ALVEOLUS

A useful way to examine the interaction and relationship between ventilation and perfusion is the two-lung unit model first described by Comroe in 1962. In Figure 7-5, ventilation is seen going to two alveoli, each of which is supplied by a part of the cardiac output. When there is uniform ventilation, half of the inspired gas goes to each of the alveoli; when there is uniform perfusion, half of the cardiac output goes to each alveolus. In this normal unit, the V̇/Q̇ in each of the alveoli is the same and equals 1. The alveoli are perfused by mixed venous blood that is deoxygenated and contains increased Pa_{CO_2}. Alveolar O_2 is higher than mixed venous O_2, and this provides a gradient for the movement of oxygen into the blood. In contrast, mixed venous CO_2 is increased relative to alveolar CO_2, and this provides a gradient for the movement of CO_2 into the alveolus. Note that in this ideal model, there is no alveolar-arterial O_2 difference.

ANATOMIC SHUNT

Now imagine that a certain amount of mixed venous blood bypasses the gas exchange unit and goes directly into the arterial blood (Fig. 7-6). In this instance, alveolar ventilation and the distribution and composition of alveolar gas are normal. The distribution of the cardiac output is changed, however. Some of it goes through the pulmonary capillary bed supplying the two gas exchange units, whereas the rest bypasses

TABLE 7-1*			
Causes of Hypoxemia			
CAUSE	ARTERIAL Pa_{O_2}	AaD_{O_2}	ARTERIAL Pa_{O_2} RESPONSE TO 100% O_2
Anatomic shunt	Decreased	Increased	No Change in Pa_{O_2}
Decreased F_{IO_2}	Decreased	Normal	Increased Pa_{O_2}
Physiologic shunt	Decreased	Increased	Increased Pa_{O_2}
Low ventilation-perfusion ratio	Decreased	Increased	Increased Pa_{O_2}
Hypoventilation	Decreased	Normal	Increased Pa_{O_2}

*Diffusion abnormalities are an extremely uncommon cause of decreased arterial Pa_{O_2} at rest but have greater significance during exercise; when associated with decreased Pa_{O_2}, the AaD_{O_2} is increased.
AaD_{O_2}, alveolar-arterial oxygen difference; F_{IO_2}, fraction of inspired oxygen; Pa_{O_2}, partial pressure of arterial oxygen.

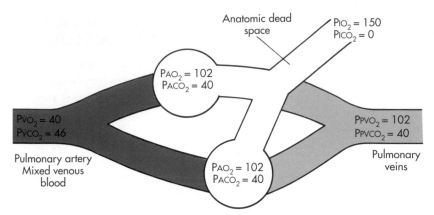

FIGURE 7-5 ■ Simplified model showing two normal parallel lung units. Both units receive equal quantities of fresh air and blood flow for their size. The blood and alveolar gas partial pressures (P) are normal values in a resting person. Pa_{O_2}, partial pressure of arterial oxygen; Pa_{CO_2}, partial pressure of arterial carbon dioxide; PA_{O_2}, partial pressure of alveolar oxygen; PA_{CO_2}, partial pressure of alveolar carbon dioxide; PI_{O_2}, partial pressure of inspired oxygen; PI_{CO_2}, partial pressure of inspired carbon dioxide; Ppv_{O_2}, partial pressure of pulmonary venous oxygen; Ppv_{CO_2}, partial pressure of pulmonary venous carbon dioxide. *(From Berne RM, Levy ML, Koeppen BM, Stanton BM (eds): Physiology, 5th ed. St. Louis, Mosby, 2004.)*

the gas exchange units and goes directly into the arterial blood. The blood that bypasses the gas exchange unit is said to be "shunted," and because it is deoxygenated blood, this is said to be a right-to-left shunt. Most often anatomic shunts occur within the heart and occur when deoxygenated blood from the *right* atrium or ventricle crosses the septum and mixes with blood from the *left* atrium or ventricle. The effect of this right-to-left shunt is to mix deoxygenated blood with oxygenated blood, and it results in varying degrees of arterial hypoxemia.

An important feature of an anatomic shunt is that the hypoxemia cannot be abolished by giving the individual 100% oxygen to breathe. This is because

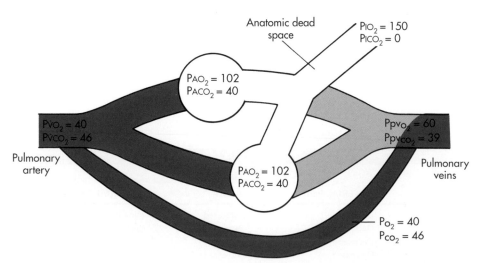

FIGURE 7-6 ■ Right-to-left shunt. Alveolar ventilation is normal, but a portion of the cardiac output bypasses the lung and mixes with oxygenated blood. The Pa_{O_2} will vary depending on the size of the shunt. (See Fig. 7-5 for definitions of symbols.) *(From Berne RM, Levy ML, Koeppen BM, Stanton BM (eds): Physiology, 5th ed. St. Louis, Mosby, 2004.)*

the blood that bypasses ventilation is never exposed to the enriched oxygen, so that it continues to be deoxygenated. Since the blood that is *not* being shunted is exposed to the enriched oxygen and *does* increase its arterial PaO_2, some elevation of the arterial PaO_2 occurs in the presence of an anatomic shunt. Because normally, hemoglobin in the blood that perfuses the ventilated alveoli is almost fully saturated, most of the added O_2 is in the form of dissolved O_2, which is not an effective way to substantially increase PaO_2 (see Chapter 8).

An anatomic shunt does not usually cause an increase in $PaCO_2$ even though the shunted blood has an elevated level of CO_2. This is because central chemoreceptors respond to any increase in CO_2 in the blood with an increase in ventilation. This increase reduces the arterial $PaCO_2$ to the normal range. When the $PaCO_2$ is below the normal range, this is occurs because, if the hypoxemia is severe, the increased respiratory drive secondary to the hypoxemia further increases ventilation and further decreases $PaCO_2$.

PHYSIOLOGIC SHUNT

Next, imagine a circumstance in which the ventilation to one of the lung units is cut off (Fig. 7-7). As a result, all of the ventilation now goes to the other lung unit, while the perfusion is equally distributed between both of the lung units. The lung unit without ventilation but with perfusion has a V̇/Q̇ of zero. The blood perfusing this unit is mixed venous blood; because

there is no ventilation, there is no gas exchange in the unit, and the blood leaving this unit remains mixed venous. This is called a physiologic shunt (or venous admixture); it is similar in its effect to an anatomic shunt; that is, deoxygenated blood bypasses a gas-exchanging unit and admixes with arterial blood. In this instance, however, the problem is a reduction in ventilation to an area of the lung that is being perfused. Clinically, atelectasis is the most common cause of a physiologic shunt (V̇/Q̇ = 0). Atelectasis occurs when there is obstruction to ventilation of a gas-exchanging unit with subsequent loss of volume and can be caused by obstruction to ventilation by a mucus plug, airway edema, a foreign body, or a tumor in the airway.

VENTILATION-PERFUSION MISMATCHING

Ventilation-perfusion mismatching is the most common cause of arterial hypoxemia in patients with disorders affecting the respiratory system. In most cases, the composition of mixed venous blood, the total volume of blood flow (cardiac output), and the distribution of blood flow are normal. However, the same total alveolar ventilation is now distributed unevenly between the two gas exchange units (Fig. 7-8). Because blood flow is equally distributed, the unit with the decreased ventilation has a V̇/Q̇ less than 1, and the unit with the increased ventilation has a V̇/Q̇ greater than 1. This causes variation in the alveolar and end-capillary gas compositions. Both arterial oxygen

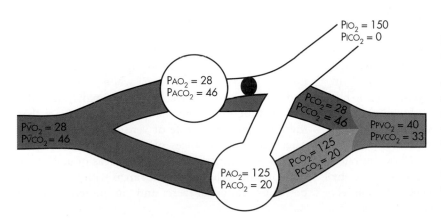

FIGURE 7-7 ■ Physiologic shunt (venous admixture). Notice the marked decrease in PaO_2 compared with PCO_2. The alveolar-arterial oxygen difference (AaDO$_2$) is 85 mm Hg $PP\bar{V}O_2$ = 40, $PP\bar{V}CO_2$ = 33. (See Fig. 7-5 for definitions of other symbols.) *(From Berne RM, Levy ML, Koeppen BM, Stanton BM (eds): Physiology, 5th ed. St. Louis, Mosby, 2004.)*

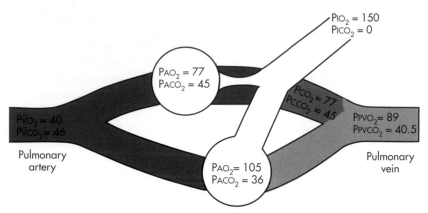

FIGURE 7-8 ■ Effects of ventilation-perfusion mismatching on gas exchange. The decrease in ventilation to the one lung unit could be due to mucus obstruction, airway edema, bronchospasm, a foreign body, or a tumor. Po_2, partial pressure of oxygen; Pco_2, partial pressure of pulmonary capillary O_2; $P\bar{v}o_2$, partial pressure of mixed venous oxygen; $P\bar{v}co_2$, partial pressure of mixed venous carbon dioxide; $Pcco_2$, partial pressure of pulmonary capillary CO_2. (See Fig. 7-5 for definitions of other symbols.) *(From Berne RM, Levy ML, Koeppen BM, Stanton BM (eds): Physiology, 5th ed. St. Louis, Mosby, 2004.)*

and arterial carbon dioxide will be abnormal in the blood that has come from the unit with the decreased ventilation ($\dot{V}/\dot{Q} = <1$). The unit with the increased ventilation ($\dot{V}/\dot{Q} = >1$) will have a lower $Paco_2$ and a higher Pao_2 because it is being overventilated. The actual Pao_2 and $Paco_2$ values will vary depending on the relative contribution of each of these units to the arterial blood.

In this instance, there will be a difference in the alveolar-arterial oxygen gradient ($AaDo_2$). This difference occurs because the relative overventilation of one unit does not fully compensate (either by adding extra O_2 or by removing extra CO_2) for the disturbances created by underventilating the other unit. The failure to compensate is greater in the case of O_2 than in that of CO_2, owing to the flatness of the upper part of the oxyhemoglobin dissociation curve compared with the CO_2 dissociation curve (see Chapter 8). In other words, increased ventilation raises Pao_2 but adds little extra O_2 content to the blood, whereas the steeper slope of the CO_2 curve allows more CO_2 to be eliminated when ventilation increases. This is because hemoglobin is close to being 100% saturated in these overventilated areas, whereas CO_2 moves by diffusion, and as long as a CO_2 gradient is maintained, CO_2 diffusion will occur.

HYPOVENTILATION

Alveolar oxygen is determined by a balance between the rate of oxygen removal (determined by the blood flow through the lung and the metabolic demands of the tissues) and the rate of oxygen replenishment by ventilation. If ventilation decreases, then Pao_2 will decrease and Pao_2 will subsequently decrease. In addition, there is a direct relationship between alveolar ventilation and $Paco_2$. When ventilation is halved, alveolar and thus arterial carbon dioxide doubles (see Fig. 5-3). This process of decreased ventilation is called **hypoventilation**. Hypoventilation always decreases Pao_2 (except when the subject breathes an enriched source of oxygen) and increases $Paco_2$.

One of the hallmarks of hypoventilation is a normal $AaDo_2$. This occurs when gas exchange and perfusion to the alveolus are normal; that is, the lung is functioning normally. The problem is that there is a decreased rate of ventilation to the unit. There are few instances of "pure" hypoventilation because, as ventilation decreases, areas of atelectasis develop, and atelectasis creates areas with ventilation-perfusion ratios of zero and an increase in the $AaDo_2$.

DIFFUSION ABNORMALITIES

Abnormalities in the diffusion of oxygen across the alveolar-capillary barrier may also result in arterial hypoxia. Because equilibration between alveolar and capillary oxygen and carbon dioxide occurs rapidly and in a fraction of the time it takes for red blood cells to go through the pulmonary capillary network, diffusion equilibrium almost always occurs in normal subjects, even during exercise when transit time through the lung of red blood cells increases significantly. An alveolar-arterial oxygen difference that has been attributable to incomplete diffusion (**diffusion disequilibrium**) has been observed in normal individuals only during exercise at high altitudes (≥10,000 ft). Diffusion disequilibrium is an unusual and uncommon cause of hypoxemia. Even in individuals with abnormal diffusing capacities, diffusion disequilibrium at rest is unusual. In contrast, abnormalities of diffusion are more likely to affect arterial blood gas composition during exercise, and the effects are magnified at higher altitudes.

Alveolar capillary block, or thickening of the air-blood barrier, is not nearly as common a cause of decreased diffusing capacity as is a reduction in the volume of pulmonary capillary blood. In this disorder, the mechanism of hypoxemia is different. As capillaries are progressively destroyed or obstructed, previously unperfused capillaries are progressively recruited until finally the velocity of blood flow through the remaining vessels increases. (Recall that the lung "accepts" the entire cardiac output; flow remains normal even with destruction of capillaries until all capillaries have been recruited. At this point, flow through the remaining capillaries increases.) When this process is severe, the time available for gas exchange in these patients at rest may be similar to that observed in normal individuals during exercise. In these individuals who are experiencing increased flow at rest, during exercise transit time may be too short to permit equilibration to occur.

DISEASES ASSOCIATED WITH HYPOXIA

There are several types of congenital heart disease that cause cyanosis (a bluish discoloration of the lips and fingers that occurs when 5 g of reduced hemoglobin are present). In most of these disorders, anatomic shunts are the mechanism of hypoxemia. The most common of the cyanotic congenital heart diseases is **Tetralogy of Fallot** (Fig. 7-9), characterized by pulmonary valve stenosis and a ventricular septal defect (a hole in the septum between the right and left ventricles). As a result, the pressure in the right ventricle increases to supersystemic levels, and deoxygenated blood is shunted from the right ventricle to the left ventricle (anatomic shunt) bypassing the lung.

Guillain-Barré syndrome is an acute neuromuscular disease associated with ascending muscle weakness. When respiratory muscles are involved, particularly the diaphragm, minute ventilation (tidal volume × frequency) decreases, PaO_2 decreases, and $PaCO_2$ increases. Guillain-Barré syndrome thus causes hypoxemia through hypoventilation.

Asthma is a chronic inflammatory lung disease characterized by exacerbations interspersed with periods of inactive disease. When the disease is inactive,

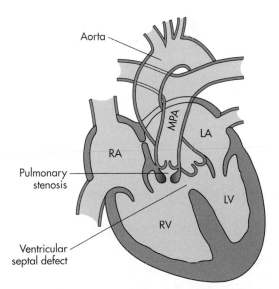

FIGURE 7-9 ■ Anatomy of Tetralogy of Fallot. Features include pulmonary valve stenosis, ventricular septal defect (VSD) and an overriding aorta. As a result, right ventricular pressure increases and deoxygenated blood is shunted across the VSD into the left ventricle. LA, left atrium; LV, left ventricle; MPA, main pulmonary artery; RA, right atrium; RV, right ventricle.

pulmonary function tests and arterial blood gases are normal. During an exacerbation, there is evidence of airway inflammation, bronchospasm, and airway edema. This results in airflow obstruction, areas of poor ventilation ($\dot{V}/\dot{Q}$ mismatch), and hypoxemia.

MECHANISMS OF HYPERCARBIA

There are two major mechanisms for the development of hypercarbia (excess of carbon dioxide in the blood): **hypoventilation** and **wasted ventilation**. As previously noted, there is a direct relationship between alveolar ventilation and alveolar carbon dioxide (see Fig. 5-3). When ventilation is halved, alveolar and thus arterial P_{CO_2} doubles. Hypoventilation always decreases Pa_{O_2} (except when the subject breathes an enriched source of oxygen) and increases Pa_{CO_2}.

Wasted ventilation occurs when there is a marked reduction in pulmonary blood flow in the presence of normal ventilation ($\dot{V}/\dot{Q} = >1 \rightarrow \infty$). This most often occurs because of obstruction of blood flow by a pulmonary embolus. In the presence of a pulmonary embolus, there is absent pulmonary blood flow to areas with normal ventilation ($\dot{V}/\dot{Q} = \infty$). In this situation, the ventilation is "wasted" because it fails to oxygenate any of the mixed venous blood, and the ventilation to the now perfused lung is less than ideal (i.e., there is relative "hypoventilation" to this area because this area now receives all of the pulmonary blood flow with "normal" ventilation). If compensation did not occur, the Pa_{CO_2} would increase and the Pa_{O_2} would decrease. Compensation after a pulmonary embolus, however, begins almost immediately with a shift in the distribution of ventilation to areas being perfused. As a result, changes in Pa_{CO_2} and Pa_{O_2} are minimized.

EFFECT OF 100% OXYGEN ON ARTERIAL BLOOD GAS ABNORMALITIES

One of the ways that a right-to-left shunt can be distinguished from other causes of hypoxemia is by having an individual breathe 100% oxygen through a non-rebreathing facemask for approximately 15 minutes. When a person is breathing 100% oxygen, all of the nitrogen in the alveolus is replaced by oxygen.

Thus alveolar oxygen can be derived using the alveolar air equation:

$$P_{AO_2} = 1.0\ (P_B - P_{H_2O}) - Pa_{CO_2}/0.8$$

$$= 1.0\ (760 - 47) - 40/0.8$$

$$= 663\ mm\ Hg$$

In the normal lung, the alveolar oxygen rapidly increases and provides the gradient for oxygen transfer into the capillary blood. This is associated with a marked increase in arterial oxygen (see Table 7-1). Similarly, during the 15- to 20-minute period of breathing enriched oxygen, even areas with very low ventilation-perfusion ratios will develop a high alveolar oxygen pressure as the nitrogen is replaced by oxygen; in the presence of normal perfusion to these areas, there is a gradient for gas exchange and the end capillary gas is highly enriched in oxygen. In contrast, in the presence of a right-to-left shunt, oxygenation is not corrected because mixed venous blood continues to flow through the shunt and mix with blood that has perfused normal units. The poorly oxygenated blood from the shunt lowers the arterial oxygen level and maintains (and even augments) the AaD_{O_2}. An elevated AaD_{O_2} value during a properly conducted 100% O_2 study signifies the presence of a right-to-left shunt; the magnitude of the difference can be used to quantify the proportion of the cardiac output that is shunted.

EFFECT OF CHANGING CARDIAC OUTPUT

Changes in cardiac output are the only nonrespiratory factor that affects gas exchange. Decreasing cardiac output causes a decrease in O_2 content and an increase in CO_2 content in mixed venous blood. Increasing the cardiac output has the opposite effect. This change in O_2 and CO_2 content will have little effect on Pa_{O_2} and Pa_{CO_2} in individuals with normal lungs unless cardiac output is extremely low. In the presence of lung disease secondary to ventilation-perfusion mismatching or in the presence of an anatomic shunt, the composition of mixed venous blood will have a significant effect on Pa_{O_2} and Pa_{CO_2} levels. For any level of $\dot{V}/\dot{Q}$ abnormality, a decrease in cardiac output is associated with an increasingly abnormal Pa_{O_2}.

EFFECT OF VENTILATION-PERFUSION REGIONAL DIFFERENCES

Up to this point we have examined regional differences in ventilation and in perfusion and in the relationship between ventilation and perfusion. We have also examined the effect of various physiologic abnormalities (shunts, $\dot{V}/\dot{Q}$ mismatch, and hypoventilation) on arterial oxygen and carbon dioxide levels. Before leaving this area, however, it should be apparent to the student that because there are ventilation-perfusion differences in different regions of the lung, end capillary blood coming from these regions will have different oxygen and carbon dioxide levels. These differences are shown in Figure 7-10 (also see Fig. 7-3) and demonstrate the complexity of the lung. First, recall that the volume of the lung at the apex is larger than the volume at the base. As previously described, ventilation and perfusion are less at the apex than at the base but the differences in perfusion are greater than the differences in ventilation. Thus, the $\dot{V}/\dot{Q}$ is abnormally high at the apex and abnormally low at the base, and the $\dot{V}/\dot{Q}$ decreases from the apex to the base of the lung. This difference in ventilation-perfusion ratios is associated with a difference in P_{AO_2} and P_{ACO_2} between the apex and the base; that is, the P_{AO_2} is higher and the P_{ACO_2} is lower in the apex than in the base. This results in differences in end-capillary contents for these gases, with a lower P_{O_2} and consequently a lower oxygen content for end capillary blood at the base compared to the apex. In addition, there is significant variation in the pH of the end capillaries in these areas because of the variation in carbon dioxide content in the presence of a constant base excess (see Chapter 9).

Because of the decreased blood flow at the apex, the oxygen consumed and the carbon dioxide produced are also decreased in this area. Because the carbon dioxide produced is more closely linked to ventilation, and the oxygen consumed is more closely linked to perfusion, the carbon dioxide produced is higher because ventilation relative to perfusion is higher. As a result, the respiratory quotient (CO_2 produced/O_2 consumed) is higher at the apex than the base. During exercise when blood flow to the apex increases and becomes more uniform in the lung, the differences between the apex and the base of the lung diminish.

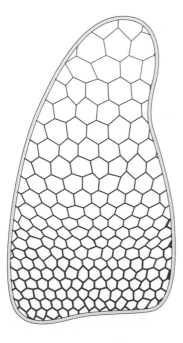

VENTILATION

Intrapleural pressure
more negative

Greater transmural
pressure gradient

Alveoli larger,
less compliant

Less ventilation

Intrapleural pressure
less negative

Smaller transmural
pressure gradient

Alveoli smaller,
more compliant

Greater ventilation

PERFUSION

Lower intravascular
pressures

Less recruitment,
distention

Higher resistance

Less blood flow

Greater intravascular
pressures

More recruitment,
distention

Lower resistance

Greater blood flow

FIGURE 7-10 ■ Regional differences in ventilation *(left)* and perfusion *(right)* in the normal, upright lung. *(Redrawn from Levitzky MG: Pulmonary Physiology, 4th ed. New York, McGraw-Hill, 1995.)*

SUMMARY

1. Regional differences in ventilation and perfusion are due in large part to the effects of gravity.
2. The alveolar air equation is used to calculate the alveolar-arterial oxygen difference (AaD_{O_2}), the most useful measurement of abnormal arterial oxygen. In normal individuals breathing room air, the AaD_{O_2} is less than 15 mm Hg.
3. The ventilation-perfusion ratio ($\dot{V}/\dot{Q}$) is defined as the ratio of ventilation to blood flow. In the normal lung, the average ventilation-perfusion ratio is approximately 0.8. When ventilation exceeds perfusion, the ventilation-perfusion ratio is greater than 1 ($\dot{V}/\dot{Q} = >1$); when perfusion exceeds ventilation, the ventilation-perfusion ratio is less than 1 ($\dot{V}/\dot{Q} = <1$).
4. The ventilation-perfusion ratio at the top of the lung is high (increased ventilation relative to very little blood flow in the pulmonary circulation because of gravity effects), whereas the ventilation-perfusion ratio at the bottom of the lung is abnormally low.
5. There are four mechanisms of hypoxemia: anatomic shunt, physiologic shunt, ventilation-perfusion mismatching and hypoventilation.
6. There are two mechanisms of hypercarbia: increase in dead space and hypoventilation.
7. Changes in cardiac output are the only nonrespiratory factors that affects gas exchange.

KEY WORDS

- Alveolar-arterial oxygen difference (AaD_{O_2})
- Alveolar capillary block
- Anatomic shunt
- Asthma
- Cardiac output
- Diffusion disequilibrium
- Guillain-Barré syndrome
- Hypoventilation
- Physiologic shunt
- Tetralogy of Fallot
- Ventilation-perfusion ratio ($\dot{V}/\dot{Q}$)
- Wasted ventilation

SELF-STUDY PROBLEMS

1. How can you distinguish between the four causes of hypoxemia?
2. What factors determine alveolar P_{AO_2} in a single alveolus?
3. What is responsible for the greater decrease in Pa_{O_2} compared to Pa_{CO_2} in the presence of ventilation-perfusion inequality?

REFERENCES

Bongartz G, Boos M, Scheffler K, Steinbrich W: Pulmonary circulation. Eur Radiol 8:698-706, 1998.

Comroe JH, Jr., et al. The lung. Clinical Physiology and Pulmonary Junction Tests, 2nd ed. Chicago, Year Book Medical Publishers, inc., 1962 pp. 1–390.

Cutaia M, Rounds S: Hypoxic pulmonary vasoconstriction: Physiologic significance, mechanism and clinical relevance. Chest 97: 706-718, 1982.

Glenny RW: Blood flow distribution in the lung. Chest 114:8S-16S, 1998.

Henig NR, Pierson DJ: Mechanisms of hypoxemia. Respir Care Clin N Am 6:501-521, 2000.

Lenfant C: Measurement of ventilation/perfusion distribution with alveolar arterial differences. J Appl Physiol 18:1090-1094, 1963.

Milic-Emili J, Henderson JA, Dolovich MB, et al: Regional distribution of inspired gas in the lung. J Appl Physiol 21:749-759, 1966.

Weir EK, Archer SL: The mechanism of acute hypoxic pulmonary vasoconstriction: The tale of two channels. FASEB J 9:183-189, 1995.

West JB, Dollery CT, Naimark A: Distribution of blood flow in isolated lung: Relation to vascular and alveolar pressures. J Appl Physiol 19:713-724, 1964.

West JB: State of the art: Ventilation-perfusion relationships. Am Rev Respir Dis 116:919-943, 1977.

8 OXYGEN AND CARBON DIOXIDE TRANSPORT

■ ■ ■ ■ ■ ■ ■ ■ ■ ■ ■ ■ ■ ■

OBJECTIVES

1. Explain the concepts of diffusion limitation and perfusion limitation.
2. Apply Fick's law to the alveolar-capillary surface.
3. Describe the diffusion of oxygen and carbon dioxide across the alveolar-capillary membrane.
4. Describe the structure and function of hemoglobin in gas exchange.
5. Explain the oxyhemoglobin dissociation curve, factors that shift the curve, and the effect of these shifts on oxygen uptake and oxygen delivery.

6. Understand the difference between oxygen content, oxygen saturation, and Pa_{O_2}.
7. Outline the effect of carbon monoxide on oxygen content, oxygen saturation, Pa_{O_2}, and stimulation of peripheral chemoreceptors.
8. Describe oxygen consumption.
9. Describe the four types of tissue hypoxia.
10. Explain carbon dioxide production, metabolism, diffusion, and the carbon dioxide dissociation curve.

The maintenance of cell integrity and normal organ function is dependent on energy expenditure. The major source of energy in cells and organs is provided by the intracellular metabolism of oxygen (O_2). In a process known as **oxidative metabolism**, molecular oxygen is consumed within the mitochondrial electron transport system and adenosine triphosphate (ATP) is generated. Energy is subsequently produced by the hydrolysis of ATP to adenosine diphosphate (ADP) and inorganic phosphate.

O_2 is carried in the blood from the lungs to the tissues in two forms: physically dissolved in the blood and chemically combined to hemoglobin. As O_2 is transported into the tissue, carbon dioxide (CO_2), a by-product of cellular metabolism, is transported from the tissues to the blood and eventually to the lungs by the pulmonary circulation. CO_2 is carried in

three forms: physically dissolved in blood, as bicarbonate, and chemically combined to blood proteins as carbamino compounds. O_2 loading and unloading and CO_2 loading and unloading not only occur simultaneously but also facilitate each other. This interdependence is demonstrated both in the lung and in the tissues. Specifically, the uptake of O_2 into the tissues enhances the elimination of CO_2 from the tissues into the blood (Fig. 8-1). Similarly, the uptake of O_2 into the blood through the pulmonary capillaries is facilitated by the simultaneous unloading of CO_2 by the blood. In order to understand the mechanisms involved in the transport of these gases, three processes must be considered: the gas diffusion properties of gases, O_2 and CO_2 transport processes, and O_2 and CO_2 delivery processes.

113

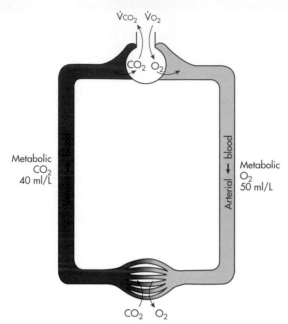

FIGURE 8-1 ■ Oxygen and carbon dioxide transport occur in both arterial and venous blood. However, the extracted or utilized oxygen is present in arterial blood, where it is transferred from arterial capillaries to the tissue. Only ~25% of transported oxygen is actually taken up by the tissue. The source of exhaled carbon dioxide is venous blood; it is expired via the pulmonary capillaries. The flow rates for oxygen ($\dot{V}O_2$) and carbon dioxide ($\dot{V}CO_2$) shown are for 1 liter of blood. The ratio of CO_2 production to O_2 consumption is the respiratory exchange ratio, R, which at rest is ~0.80. *(From Berne RM, Levy ML, Koeppen BM, Stanton BM (eds): Physiology, 5th ed. St. Louis, Mosby, 2004.)*

GAS DIFFUSION

Diffusion of a gas is defined as the net movement of gas molecules from an area in which the particular gas exerts a higher partial pressure to an area in which the gas exerts a lower partial pressure. Diffusion is different from **"bulk flow,"** which occurs in the conducting airways and is due to mass movement or convection. In bulk flow, gas movement occurs when there are differences in **total pressure** with molecules of different gases moving together along the pressure gradients. In diffusion, different gases move according to their **individual pressure** gradients. In diffusion, gas transport is random, occurs in all directions and is

temperature dependent. Net movement, however, is dependent on the difference in the individual gas's partial pressure. Diffusion continues until there is no longer a pressure gradient. In the lung and at the level of the tissues, diffusion is the major mechanism of gas movement. It is important both for gas movement within the alveoli (air → air) as well as for gas movement across the alveoli into the blood (air → liquid) and for gas movement from the blood into the tissue (liquid → tissue).

O_2 is delivered to the alveoli by bulk flow in the conducting airways. The inspired gas velocity decreases as the alveoli are approached because of the dramatic increase in cross-sectional area of the airways due to the multiple bifurcations. Once in the alveolus, gas movement occurs by diffusion. The process of gas diffusion is passive, non–energy-dependent, and similar whether in a gas or liquid state. O_2 moves through the gas phase in the alveoli according to its own pressure gradient, crosses the approximate 1-μm alveolar-capillary interface, and enters the blood. In moving from a gas phase in the alveolus to a liquid phase in the blood, O_2 obeys **Henry's law,** which states that the amount of a gas absorbed by a liquid to which it is not chemically combined is directly proportional to the positive pressure of the gas to which the liquid is exposed and the solubility of the gas in the liquid. Both O_2 and CO_2 maintain their molecular characteristics in blood, and both establish a partial pressure in the blood, according to Henry's law. It is this partial pressure that is measured in an arterial blood gas sample. O_2 and CO_2 in the blood are then carried out of the lung by bulk flow and distributed to the tissues in the body. In the tissues, O_2 diffuses out of the blood, across the interstitium and into the tissue cell and its mitochondrial membrane.

Fick's law of diffusion describes the factors that influence the rate of diffusion of O_2 and CO_2 through the alveolar-capillary barrier and through the capillary-tissue barrier. The transport and delivery of O_2 from the lungs into the blood and from the blood into the tissue (and vice versa for CO_2) are dependent on the gas diffusion laws. Fick's law states that the diffusion of a gas ($\dot{V}gas$) across a sheet of tissue is *directly* related to the surface area of the tissue (A), the diffusion constant of the specific gas (D), and the partial pressure difference of the gas on each side of the tissue ($P_1 - P_2$)

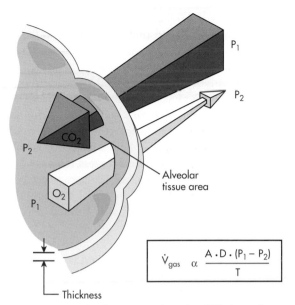

$$\dot{V}_{gas} \ \alpha \ \frac{A \cdot D \cdot (P_1 - P_2)}{T}$$

FIGURE 8-2 ■ Fick's law states that the diffusion of a gas ($\dot{V}_{gas}$) across a sheet of tissue is directly related to the surface area of the tissue (A), the diffusion constant of the specific gas (D), and the partial pressure difference of the gas on each side of the tissue ($P_1 - P_2$) and is inversely related to tissue thickness (T). *(From Berne RM, Levy ML, Koeppen BM, Stanton BM (eds): Physiology, 5th ed. St. Louis, Mosby, 2004.)*

and is *inversely* related to tissue thickness (T) (Fig. 8-2). That is,

$$\dot{V}_{gas} \ \alpha \ \frac{A \cdot D \cdot (P_1 - P_2)}{T}$$

D, or the diffusion constant for a gas, is directly proportional to the solubility of the gas and inversely proportional to the square root of the molecular weight of the gas.

$$D = \frac{\text{solubility}}{\sqrt{\text{molecular weight}}}$$

A number of interesting and important concepts arise from these two equations. Normally, the thickness of the alveolar-capillary diffusion barrier is only about 0.2 to 0.5 μm. The thickness of the barrier, however, is increased in diseases such as interstitial fibrosis and interstitial edema, and the increased thickness of

the alveolar—capillary barrier interferes with diffusion. Increased partial pressure of oxygen in the alveoli increases O_2 transport by increasing the pressure gradient, and this is why supplemental O_2 therapy is used to treat many lung diseases. At the blood capillary–tissue barrier (liquid → tissue), Fick's equation demonstrates that the major rate-limiting step for diffusion from the air to the tissue is at the liquid-tissue interface. This is because at this step, the tissue thickness (T) from the capillaries to the mitochondria is far greater than in the alveolus.

The diffusion constants (D) for CO_2 and O_2 favor CO_2 diffusion. This is because the solubility of CO_2 in blood is about 24 times the solubility of O_2. CO_2, however, has a higher molecular weight. When both the solubility and the molecular weight are considered together, CO_2 diffuses about 20 times more rapidly through the alveolar-capillary membrane than O_2. Clinically, this is demonstrated in patients with diseases resulting in changes in diffusion in which decreases in blood O_2 occur much earlier than CO_2 increases in blood.

PERFUSION LIMITATION

On average, a red blood cell spends between 0.75 and 1.2 sec in the pulmonary capillaries. Some red blood cells spend more time than this and others spend less. Depending on the initial concentration of a gas in inspired air and how rapidly it is removed by the pulmonary capillaries, different gases will have different alveolar partial pressures. This is illustrated in Figure 8-3 for nitrous oxide (N_2O), O_2, and carbon monoxide (CO). The major factors responsible for the difference in the shapes of these relationships are the solubility of the gases in the alveolar-capillary membrane and the solubility of the gases in the blood and their ability to chemically bind to hemoglobin.

Different gases have different solubility factors, which results in different diffusion coefficients. **Solubility** is defined as the volume of gas in milliliters that must be dissolved in 100 mL of the barrier liquid to raise the partial pressure by 1 torr. Gases such as N_2O, nitrogen, and helium have low solubility, whereas ether has high solubility (Fig. 8-4). In general, when the solubility of a gas in the membrane is large, gas will diffuse at a faster rate through the membrane. This is because the

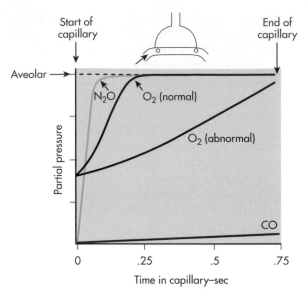

FIGURE 8-3 ■ Uptake of nitrous oxide (N₂O), carbon monoxide (CO), and oxygen (O₂) in blood relative to their partial pressures and the transit time of the red blood cell in the capillary. For gases that are perfusion-limited (N₂O and O₂), their partial pressures have equilibrated with alveolar pressure before exiting the capillary. In contrast, for CO, a gas that is diffusion-limited, its partial pressure does not reach equilibrium with alveolar pressure. Oxygen uptake in various disease conditions can become diffusion-limited. *(From Berne RM, Levy ML, Koeppen BM, Stanton BM (eds): Physiology, 5th ed. St. Louis, Mosby, 2004.)*

highly soluble gas will become dissolved in the barrier more readily than the insoluble gas. N₂O, ether, and helium move through the alveolar-capillary barrier easily, are insoluble in blood, and do not combine chemically with blood. As a result, the partial pressure gradient across the alveolar-capillary barrier is rapidly abolished (see Fig. 8-3). From that point on, no further gas transfer occurs and there is no net diffusion. For these gases, equilibration between alveolar gas and blood occurs rapidly (significantly less than the 0.75 sec that the red blood cell spends in the capillary bed) and is driven by the difference in partial pressure. This type of gas exchange is **perfusion-limited** because blood leaving the capillary has reached equilibrium with alveolar gas. As illustrated in Figure 8-3, the partial pressure of N₂O peaks quickly and is maximal by 0.1 sec, at which point no further N₂O is transferred.

DIFFUSION LIMITATION

In contrast, the partial pressure of CO in the pulmonary capillary blood rises very slowly compared with N₂O and O₂ (see Fig. 8-3). This is because carbon monoxide has a low solubility in the alveolar-capillary membrane but a high solubility in blood. As a result, equilibration between alveolar gas and blood occurs very slowly (significantly greater than the 0.75-second

FIGURE 8-4 ■ Relationship between the content of dissolved gas and its partial pressure in blood. The solubility of the gas in the liquid is the slope of the line. A linear relationship (i.e., constant solubility at a given temperature) is seen for gases that do not combine chemically with the liquid. Note the high solubility of ether and the very low solubility of oxygen. *(Redrawn from Leff A and Schumacker P: Respiratory Physiology: Basics and Applications. Philadelphia, WB Saunders, 1993.)*

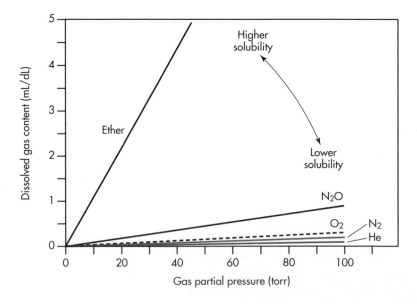

transit time of the red blood cell in the capillary). However, CO solubility varies with CO partial pressure. At partial pressures below 1 to 2 torr, CO solubility is very high, whereas at partial pressures greater than 2 torr, CO solubility is very small, because CO content increases only by adding dissolved CO. For CO, equilibration is not reached during the transit time, resulting in only a minimal increase in the partial pressure. Even though there is only a small increase in partial pressure, if you measured the **CO content** in the blood (mL of CO/mL blood) it would be rising very rapidly. The reason for this rapid rise is that CO binds chemically with hemoglobin with an affinity that is about 10 times that of oxygen for hemoglobin. The CO that is combined with the hemoglobin does not contribute to the partial pressure of CO because it is no longer physically dissolved in the blood. As a result, the partial pressure gradient for CO is maintained throughout the capillary bed, and exchange of CO is still occurring as the red blood cell leaves the end of the capillary because its rate of equilibration is slow relative to the time spent in the capillary. This type of gas transfer is **diffusion-limited.** For CO, this occurs because its solubility in the membrane is very low, whereas its solubility in blood is very high. In the absence of red blood cells, CO uptake would be perfusion-limited because now both the "blood" and the membrane have a similar low solubility to CO.

DIFFUSION OF O₂ AND CO

O_2 (and CO_2 and CO) combines chemically with blood. As a result, the relationship between gas content in the blood and partial pressure is nonlinear (Fig. 8-5). The slope of the relationship for any gas is its effective solubility. The effective solubility of oxygen varies with partial pressure and is greatest at lower partial pressures. O_2 has a relatively low solubility in the membrane of the blood-gas barrier but a high effective solubility in blood because of its combining with hemoglobin. O_2 does not combine with hemoglobin as quickly as CO binds, and so the partial pressure of O_2 in the blood rises more rapidly than does the partial pressure of CO (see Fig. 8-3). Once bound to hemoglobin, O_2 no longer exerts a partial pressure and so the partial pressure gradient across the alveolar-capillary membrane is maintained, and O_2

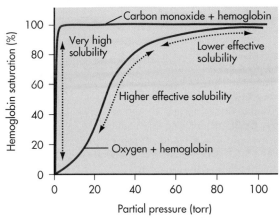

FIGURE 8-5 ■ Oxygen and carbon monoxide content as a function of their partial pressure in blood. The effective solubility of each gas in blood is equivalent to the slope of the line at any point. Thus, oxygen is highly soluble at partial pressures of 20 to 60 torr but relatively insoluble above 100 torr (where most of the hemoglobin sites are occupied). In contrast, carbon monoxide solubility is extremely large at a partial pressure of less than 1 torr. At partial pressures greater than 1 torr, carbon monoxide content increases by adding dissolved carbon monoxide only and its solubility is small. *(Redrawn from Leff A and Schumacker P: Respiratory Physiology: Basics and Applications. Philadelphia, WB Saunders, 1993.)*

transfer continues. Hemoglobin, however, quickly becomes saturated with O_2. When this happens, the partial pressure of O_2 in the blood rises rapidly and is equal to the alveolar partial pressure. At this point, no further O_2 transfer from the alveolus to the equilibrated blood can occur. Thus, under normal conditions, O_2 transfer from the alveolus to the pulmonary capillary is perfusion-limited. That is, the rate of equilibration is sufficiently rapid (usually within 0.25 sec) for complete equilibration to occur during the transit time of the red blood cell within the capillary.

DIFFUSION OF CO₂

The time course of CO_2 equilibration in the pulmonary capillary is shown in Figure 8-6. In a normal individual, equilibrium is reached in about 0.25 sec, the same time period for O_2. The effective solubility of CO_2 is higher than that of O_2 because CO_2 is more soluble in blood than O_2, and its solubility is less variable

FIGURE 8-6 ■ Partial pressure of carbon dioxide as a function of the duration of time that the red blood cell spends in the capillary. Under normal conditions, the P_{CO_2} of blood entering the capillary is 45 torr and decreases to 40 torr by the time the blood leaves the capillary. When the diffusion through the alveolar-capillary barrier is reduced to one-fourth and one-eighth of normal, the P_{CO_2} approaches but is not normal by the time the blood leaves the capillary. With exercise, the time spent in the capillary is reduced to 0.25 sec. This is sufficient in the normal lung but can result in an abnormal Pa_{CO_2} in the lung with abnormal diffusion. *(Redrawn from Wagner PD, Wess JB. Effects of diffusion impairment on O_2 and CO_2 time courses in pulmonary capillaries. J Appl Physiol 33:62, 1972.)*

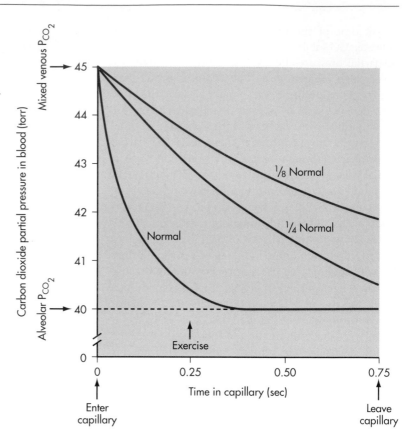

because the partial pressure varies (Fig. 8-7). If the diffusivity of CO_2 is 20 times higher than that of O_2 and the solubility is higher, why is the time to equilibrium the same? It is the same because the partial pressure gradient for CO_2 is much less than the gradient for O_2, and CO_2 has a lower membrane-blood solubility ratio. As a consequence, O_2 and CO_2 take approximately the same amount of time to reach equilibration, and CO_2 transfer, like that of O_2, is usually perfusion-limited.

Diffusion limitation for both O_2 and CO_2 could occur if the red blood cell spent less than 0.25 sec in the capillary bed. Occasionally, this can be seen in very fit athletes during vigorous exercise and in healthy subjects who exercise at high altitude. It may also be present during exercise in individuals with an abnormally thickened barrier due to fibrosis or interstitial edema and at rest in individuals with very severe disease.

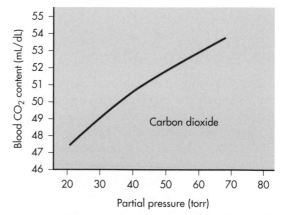

FIGURE 8-7 ■ Carbon dioxide content as a function of its partial pressure in blood. Carbon dioxide is much more soluble in blood than is oxygen (compare with Fig. 8-5 and note the steeper slope). Unlike oxygen, its solubility is relatively constant as a function of partial pressure (the solubility is the slope of the line). *(Redrawn from Leff A and Schumacker P: Respiratory Physiology: Basics and Applications. Philadelphia, WB Saunders, 1993.)*

OXYGEN TRANSPORT

Oxygen is carried in the blood in both the dissolved gaseous state in plasma and bound to hemoglobin (Hgb) as oxyhemoglobin ($HgbO_2$) within red blood cells. O_2 transport occurs primarily through $HgbO_2$, with a minimal contribution of dissolved O_2. As we will see later, at a PaO_2 of 100 mm Hg, only 3 mL of O_2 is dissolved in 1 liter of plasma. The contribution of hemoglobin within the red blood cell enhances the O_2-carrying capacity of blood by about 65-fold. Non–O_2-bound hemoglobin is referred to as **deoxyhemoglobin,** or reduced hemoglobin.

HEMOGLOBIN STRUCTURE

Hemoglobin has a molecular weight of 66,500 kDa and consists of four nonprotein O_2-binding **heme groups** and four polypeptide chains, which make up the **globin protein** portion of the Hgb molecule (Fig. 8-8). The four polypeptide chains of adult Hgb (hemoglobin Type A, or HgbA) are composed of two alpha chains and two beta chains. Iron is present in

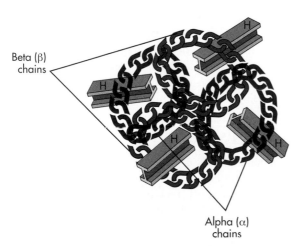

FIGURE 8-8 ■ Schematic illustration of a hemoglobin molecule showing the globin (protein) component with two alpha and two beta chains and the four iron-containing heme groups (oxygen-binding) positioned in the center of each globin portion. Each hemoglobin molecule can bind four oxygen molecules. *(From Berne RM, Levy ML, Koeppen BM, Stanton BM (eds): Physiology, 5th ed. St. Louis, Mosby, 2004.)*

each heme group in the reduced ferrous (Fe^{+2}) form and is the site of O_2-binding. Each of the polypeptide chains can bind one molecule of oxygen to the iron-binding site on its own heme group. Both the globin component and the heme group with its iron atom in the reduced or ferrous state must be in a proper spatial orientation for the chemical reaction with oxygen to occur.

Variations in the amino acid sequence of the globin subunits have significant physiologic consequences. For example, **fetal Hgb (HgbF)** is produced by the fetus to meet the oxygen demands of its specialized environment. HgbF is composed of two alpha chains and two gamma chains. This change in structure in HgbF increases its affinity for O_2 and aids in the transport of O_2 across the placenta. In addition, as discussed later in this chapter, HgbF is not affected or inhibited by the glycolysis product 2,3-diphosphoglycerate (2,3 DPG) in red blood cells, thus further enhancing O_2 uptake. During the first year of life, HgbF is replaced by HgbA.

Genetic substitutions of various amino acids results in a number of abnormal hemoglobins. These changes usually occur in the alpha and beta chains. More than 125 abnormal hemoglobins have been reported. The most important and most common of these is HgbS, which results in the disease called **sickle cell anemia.** Sickle cell anemia is an inherited, homozygous, recessive condition in which individuals have an amino acid substitution (valine for glutamic acid) on the beta chain of the hemoglobin molecule. This creates sickle cell hemoglobin (HgbS), which when unbound (deoxyhemoglobin) forms a gel that distorts the normal biconcave shape of the red blood cell to create a crescent or "sickle" form. This change in shape increases the tendency of the red blood cell to form thrombi or clots that obstruct small vessels and results in a clinical condition known as a *sickle cell crisis.* The symptoms of this condition vary, depending on the site of the obstruction. If it occurs in the central nervous system, patients suffer a stroke. If it occurs in the lung, patients can suffer a pulmonary infarction with death of the lung tissue. Although in its homozygous form sickle cell anemia is a life-shortening, clinical condition, individuals with the heterozygous form (sickle cell trait) are resistant to malaria. Thus there is a survival advantage in regions in the world where malaria is prevalent.

The binding of O_2 to hemoglobin alters the light absorption characteristics of hemoglobin; this is responsible for the change in color of oxygenated arterial blood ($HgbO_2$) and deoxygenated venous blood (Hgb). The binding of O_2 to hemoglobin is readily reversible, and this ready reversibility is a critical component that facilitates the delivery of O_2 to the tissue from the blood. The binding and dissociation of O_2 with Hgb occurs in milliseconds, which is well suited for the average capillary transit time of 0.75 sec for the red blood cell.

There are ~280 million Hgb molecules per red blood cell, which provides a unique and efficient mechanism to transport O_2. Since the amount of hemoglobin present in each red blood cell is relatively equal, the amount of hemoglobin in blood is directly proportional to the percentage of blood volume occupied by red blood cells (**hematocrit**). It should be noted that **myoglobin,** the O_2-carrying and storage protein of muscle tissue, is similar to hemoglobin in structure and function except that it has only 1 subunit of the hemoglobin molecule; thus its molecular weight is about one fourth that of hemoglobin. Myoglobin aids in the transfer of O_2 from blood to the muscle cells and in the storage of O_2, which is especially critical in O_2-deprived conditions.

When oxygen combines with hemoglobin, the iron usually remains in the ferrous state. In a condition known as *methemoglobinemia*, compounds such as nitrites and various cyanides (released in the environment during the burning of plastics or in the workplace from photo supplies, electroplating, and mining) can oxidize the iron molecule in the heme group changing it from the reduced ferrous state to the ferric state (Fe^{+3}). Hemoglobin with iron in the ferric state is brown instead of red. Methemoglobin blocks the release of O_2 from hemoglobin, which inhibits delivery of O_2 to the tissues, a critical aspect of reversible O_2 transport. Under normal conditions, ~1% to 2% of hemoglobin-binding sites are in the ferric state. Intracellular enzymes such as glutathione reductase can reduce the methemoglobin back to the functioning ferrous state. Patients with methemoglobinemia have an absence of glutathione reductase.

DISSOLVED OXYGEN

Oxygen diffuses passively from the alveolus to the plasma, where it dissolves. In its dissolved form,

O_2 maintains its molecular structure and gaseous state. It is this form that is measured clinically in an arterial blood gas sample as the PaO_2. The dissolved O_2 in blood is the product of the oxygen solubility (0.00304 mL O_2/dL · torr) times the oxygen tension (torr). In a healthy normal adult, approximately 0.3 mL O_2 is dissolved in 100 mL blood. This is commonly expressed as 0.3 volumes percent (vol%), where the vol% is equal to the mL O_2/100 mL blood. It can be seen that the O_2 dissolved in plasma is insufficient to meet the body's O_2 demands. In particular, the resting oxygen consumption of an adult is 200 to 300 mL O_2/min. For dissolved oxygen to meet this resting O_2 consumption, a cardiac output of almost 67 L/min would be required; that is,

$$\frac{200 \text{ mL } O_2/\text{min}}{0.3 \text{ mL } O_2/100 \text{ mL blood}} = \frac{66,666 \text{ mL blood}}{\text{min}} = \frac{66.7 \text{ L}}{\text{min}}$$

During exercise, this cardiac output would need to increase 10- to 15-fold. Normal individuals can achieve a cardiac output with vigorous exercise in the range of 25 L/min. Clearly, dissolved oxygen in the blood cannot meet the metabolic needs of the body even at rest, much less during exercise. Thus, the contribution of dissolved oxygen to total O_2 transport is small. In fact, when calculating the O_2 content in blood, the dissolved O_2 is frequently ignored. This small amount of additional dissolved O_2 becomes significant, however, in individuals with severe hypoxemia being treated with high levels of inspired oxygen.

OXYGEN SATURATION

Each hemoglobin molecule can bind up to four O_2 atoms, and each gram of hemoglobin can bind up to 1.34 mL (range of 1.34 to 1.39 mL depending on methemoglobin levels) of O_2. The term **oxygen saturation (SO_2)** refers to the amount of O_2 bound to hemoglobin relative to the maximal amount of O_2 (100% O_2 capacity) that can bind hemoglobin. It is equal to the O_2 content in the blood (minus the physically dissolved O_2) divided by the O_2-carrying capacity of hemoglobin in the blood times 100%.

$$\%\text{Hgb saturation} = \frac{O_2 \text{ bound to Hgb}}{O_2 - \text{carrying capacity of Hgb}} \times 100\%$$

Both O_2 content and O_2-carrying capacity are dependent on the amount of hemoglobin in the person's blood and both are expressed as mL O_2/100 mL blood. In contrast, hemoglobin saturation is only a percentage. Thus, $HgbO_2$ saturation is not interchangeable with the O_2 content. Individuals with different Hgb levels will have different O_2 content levels but can have the same hemoglobin saturation.

At 100% saturation (100% SO_2), the heme group is fully saturated with oxygen. Correspondingly, at 75% SO_2, three of the four heme groups are occupied by O_2. The binding of O_2 to each heme group increases the affinity of the hemoglobin molecule to bind additional O_2. Thus, when three of the heme groups are O_2-bound, the affinity of the fourth heme group to bind O_2 is increased. Because there are about 14 g Hgb/100 mL blood, the normal O_2 capacity is 18.76 mL (1 g Hgb binds 1.34 mL O_2 × 14 g Hgb) of O_2/100 mL blood. A mildly anemic individual with an Hgb concentration of 10 g/100 mL blood and normal lungs would only have an O_2 capacity of 13.40 mL O_2/100 mL blood; a severely anemic individual with an Hgb concentration of 5 g would have an O_2 capacity of 6.70 mL O_2/100 mL blood—one third of normal.

OXYGEN CONTENT (CONCENTRATION) OF BLOOD

The O_2 content in blood is the volume of O_2 contained per unit volume of blood. The total O_2 content is the sum of the O_2 bound to hemoglobin and the dissolved O_2. The hemoglobin-bound O_2 content is determined by the concentration of hemoglobin (in g/dL), the O_2-binding capacity of the hemoglobin (1.34 mL O_2/g Hgb), and the percent saturation of the hemoglobin. The dissolved O_2 content is the product of the O_2 solubility (0.00304 mL O_2/dL · torr) times the O_2 tension

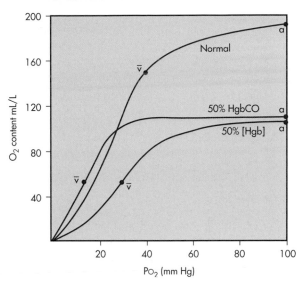

FIGURE 8-9 ■ Comparison of oxygen content curves under three conditions shows why HgbCO is so toxic to the oxygen transport system. Fifty percent [Hgb] represents a reduction in circulating hemoglobin by half; 50% HgbCO represents binding of half the circulating hemoglobin with CO. The 50% [Hgb] and 50% HgbCO curves show the same decreased oxygen content in arterial blood. However, CO has a profound effect in lowering venous PO_2. The arterial (a) and mixed venous ($\bar{v}$) points of constant cardiac output are indicated. *(From Berne RM, Levy ML, Koeppen BM, Stanton BM (eds): Physiology, 5th ed. St. Louis, Mosby, 2004.)*

(torr). Oxygen content decreases with increased CO_2 and CO and in individuals with anemia (Fig. 8-9).

As an example, consider an arterial blood gas with a PaO_2 of 60 torr and an arterial O_2 saturation (SaO_2) of 90%. The patient's hemoglobin is 14 g/dL. What would the total (Hgb-bound and dissolved) O_2 content be?

$$\text{Hgb} - \text{bound } O_2 \text{ content} = \frac{1.34 \text{ mL}}{\text{g Hgb}} \times \frac{14 \text{g Hgb}}{\text{dL blood}} \times \frac{0.90\% \text{ saturation}}{100}$$

$$= 16.88 \text{ mL} / \text{dL blood}$$

$$\text{Dissolved } O_2 \text{ content} = PaO_2 \times O_2 \text{ solubility}$$

$$= 60 \text{ torr} \times 0.00304 \text{ mL } O_2 / \text{dL} \cdot \text{torr}$$

$$= 0.18 \text{ mL } O_2 / \text{dL}$$

$$\text{Total } O_2 \text{ content} = 16.88 \text{ mL} / \text{dL} + 0.18 \text{ mL} / \text{dL}$$

$$= 17.06 \text{ mL} / \text{dL blood}$$

How would the total O_2 content change if the individual is treated with 30% supplemental O_2 and a repeat arterial blood gas reveals a PaO_2 of 95 torr with an SO_2 saturation of 97%?

$$\text{Hgb } O_2 \text{ content} = 1.34 \text{ mL/dL} \times 14 \text{ gm/dL} \times 0.97$$
$$= 18.20 \text{ mL/dL}$$

$$\text{Dissolved } O_2 \text{ content} = 95 \text{ torr} \times 0.00304 \text{ mL } O_2/\text{dL} \cdot \text{torr}$$
$$= 0.29 \text{ mL/dL}$$

$$\text{Total } O_2 \text{ content} = 18.20 \text{ mL/dL} + 0.29 \text{ mL/dL}$$
$$= 18.49 \text{ mL/dL}$$

Oxygen therapy has significantly increased the total O_2 content. Note, again, the very small contribution of dissolved O_2 to the total O_2 content.

THE OXYHEMOGLOBIN DISSOCIATION CURVE

The majority of O_2 in plasma quickly diffuses into the red blood cells where it chemically binds to the heme groups of the hemoglobin molecule, forming oxyhemoglobin ($HgbO_2$). The chemical binding of O_2 to hemoglobin occurs in the lung and this $HgbO_2$ complex is the major transport mechanism for oxygen. It is also reversible at the tissue level where hemoglobin gives up its oxygen to the tissue. The number of O_2 molecules bound to hemoglobin is dependent on the partial pressure of O_2 in the blood. The *oxyhemoglobin dissociation curve* displays the relationship between the O_2 partial pressure (PO_2) in the blood and the percentage of O_2-binding sites occupied by O_2 molecules (Fig. 8-10). As the partial pressure of O_2 increases, hemoglobin saturation increases. The curve, however, is S-shaped (not linear), reflecting the change in the affinity of Hgb for O_2 with increased binding of O_2 to the heme. The **oxyhemoglobin dissociation curve** demonstrates a number of interesting features. The curve begins to plateau at a PO_2 of about 50 mm Hg and flattens at a PO_2 of 70 mm Hg. At partial pressures below 60 mm Hg, O_2 readily binds to Hgb as the PO_2 increases (linear portion). At a PO_2 of 60 mm Hg, hemoglobin is 90% saturated; increases in PO_2 above this level will have only minor influences on hemoglobin saturation. Specifically, increasing the PO_2 from 60 to 100 mm Hg, will increase hemoglobin saturation

only 7%. The clinical significance of the flat portion of the oxyhemoglobin dissociation curve is that a drop in PO_2 anywhere from 100 mm Hg to 60 mm Hg results in hemoglobin that is more than 90% saturated; this virtually assures adequate O_2 delivery to the tissues. The curve also demonstrates that increasing the PO_2 above 100 mm Hg has little effect on O_2 content in the blood because hemoglobin is already (almost) fully saturated. Along the steep or *linear portion* of the curve, blood O_2 content and thus O_2 delivery to the tissue are significantly compromised when the PO_2 falls below 60 mm Hg. The clinical significance of this portion of the curve is that a large amount of O_2 is released from hemoglobin with only a small change in PO_2; this facilitates the diffusion of O_2 to the tissue. The point on the curve at which 50% of the hemoglobin is saturated with O_2 (two O_2 molecules on one Hgb molecule) is called the P_{50} (Fig. 8-11). In adults at sea level, this occurs at a PO_2 of 27 mm Hg.

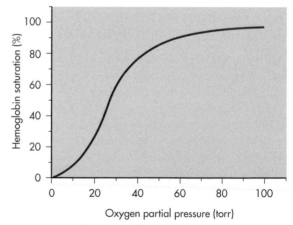

FIGURE 8-10 ■ Oxyhemoglobin dissociation curve showing the relationship between the partial pressure of oxygen in blood and the percentage of the hemoglobin binding sites that are occupied by oxygen molecules (percent saturation). Adult hemoglobin (HgbA) is about 60% saturated at a PO_2 of 30 torr, 90% saturated at 60 torr, and about 75% saturated at 40 torr. *(From Berne RM, Levy ML, Koeppen BM, Stanton BM (eds): Physiology, 5th ed. St. Louis, Mosby, 2004.)*

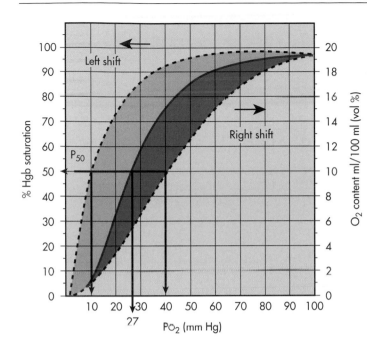

FIGURE 8-11 ■ The P_{50} represents the partial pressure at which hemoglobin is 50% saturated with oxygen. When the oxygen dissociation curve shifts to the right, the P_{50} increases. When the curve shifts to the left, the P_{50} decreases. *(From Berne RM, Levy ML, Koeppen BM, Stanton BM (eds): Physiology, 5th ed. St. Louis, Mosby, 2004.)*

FACTORS ASSOCIATED WITH SHIFTS IN THE OXYHEMOGLOBIN DISSOCIATION CURVE

The oxyhemoglobin dissociation curve can be shifted either to the right or the left as a result of numerous clinical conditions. The curve is shifted to the right when the affinity of hemoglobin for O_2 decreases. This results in decreased hemoglobin binding O_2 at a given Po_2 and is seen as an increase in the P_{50}. The curve is shifted to the left when the affinity of hemoglobin for O_2 increases. This results in a lower P_{50}. A shift in the curve to the right aids in the release of O_2 into tissues and cells, whereas a shift in the curve to the left aids in the uptake/binding of O_2 to hemoglobin in the lung. Processes that shift the oxyhemoglobin dissociation curve are shown in Figure 8-12.

The Bohr Effect

Changes in blood pH will shift the oxyhemoglobin dissociation curve. A decrease in pH shifts the curve to the right (enhancing O_2 dissociation); conversely, an increase in pH shifts the curve to the left (increasing O_2 affinity). During cellular metabolism, CO_2 is produced and released into the blood, resulting in the increased generation of hydrogen ions and a decrease in pH. This results in a shift of the dissociation curve to the right, which has a beneficial effect by aiding in the release (dissociation of O_2 from Hgb) and diffusion of O_2 into the tissue and cells. The shift to the right appears to be not only due to the decrease in pH but also a direct effect of CO_2 on hemoglobin. Conversely, as blood passes through the lungs, CO_2 is exhaled, resulting in a decrease in hydrogen ion content and an increase in pH, which results in a shift to the left in the dissociation curve. The higher hemoglobin affinity for O_2 enhances the binding of O_2 to hemoglobin. This effect of CO_2 on the affinity of hemoglobin for oxygen is known as the **Bohr effect** (named after the Danish physiologist Christian Bohr). The Bohr effect is due in part to the change in pH that occurs as CO_2 increases and in part to the direct effect of CO_2 on hemoglobin. The Bohr effect enhances O_2 delivery to the tissue and O_2 uptake in the lungs (Fig. 8-13).

Temperature

Body temperature increases in muscles during exercise. This increase in temperature shifts the dissociation curve to the right, thus enabling more O_2 to be released in the muscles, where it is needed because of

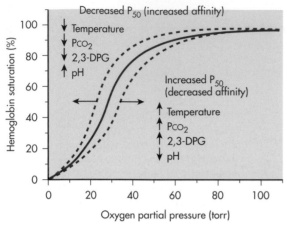

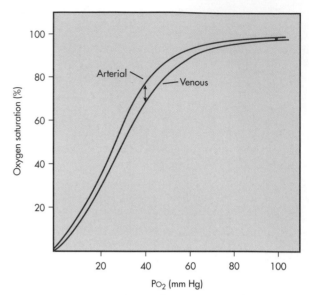

FIGURE 8-12 ■ Factors that shift the oxyhemoglobin dissociation curve. The affinity of hemoglobin for oxygen is expressed as the P_{50}. Increases in P_{CO_2}, temperature, and 2,3-diphosphoglycerate (2,3-DPG) or decreases in pH shift the oxyhemoglobin dissociation curve to the right (increased P_{50} = decreased affinity), whereas opposite changes shift the curve to the left (decreased P_{50} = increased affinity) relative to the standard value of 27 torr. *(From Berne RM, Levy ML, Koeppen BM, Stanton BM (eds): Physiology, 5th ed. St. Louis, Mosby, 2004.)*

FIGURE 8-13 ■ Normal arterial and venous $HgbO_2$ equilibrium curves. In the lung, the effect of the shift to the left caused by a decrease in hydrogen ion concentration enhances oxygen uptake. In the systemic capillaries, significant O_2 unloading begins at about P_{O_2} = 70 mm Hg. The rising hydrogen ion concentration caused by the entry of CO_2 shifts the curve to the right, enhancing oxygen dissociation. The P_{50} of the arterial curve is 27 mm Hg; the P_{50} of the venous curve is 29 mm Hg. *(From Berne RM, Levy ML, Koeppen BM, Stanton BM (eds): Physiology, 5th ed. St. Louis, Mosby, 2004.)*

increased demand. A decrease in body temperature during cold weather, especially in the extremities (lips, fingers, toes, and ears) shifts the curve to the left (higher Hgb affinity). In this instance, the Pa_{O_2} may be normal but the release of O_2 in these extremities is not facilitated. That is why these areas can display a bluish coloration with exposure to cold (known as *acrocyanosis*). Temperature also affects the solubility of O_2 in plasma. At 20° C, 50% more O_2 will be dissolved in plasma.

2,3-Diphosphoglycerate

Mature red blood cells do not have mitochondria and therefore respire via anaerobic glycolysis. During glycolysis, large quantities of the metabolic intermediary 2,3-diphosphoglycerate (2,3-DPG) are formed within the red blood cell. As 2,3-DPG levels increase in the red blood cell, the affinity of hemoglobin for O_2 decreases proportionately, thus shifting the oxyhemoglobin dissociation curve to the right. The affinity of 2,3-DPG for hemoglobin is greater than that for O_2; as a result, 2,3-DPG directly competes with O_2 for Hgb-binding sites. Conditions that increase 2,3-DPG include hypoxia, decreased hemoglobin concentration,

and increased pH. Increases in 2,3-DPG with hypoxia result in greater O_2 release from hemoglobin at any P_{O_2}, mitigating hypoxia's effects on the tissues. Red blood cells with HgbS (sickle cell trait) have increased levels of 2,3-DPG. Decreased levels of 2,3-DPG are observed in stored blood samples; this could theoretically, present a problem due to the greater $HgbO_2$ affinity, which inhibits the unloading of O_2 in tissues.

Fetal Hemoglobin

As discussed previously, fetal hemoglobin has a greater affinity for O_2 than adult hemoglobin. Fetal hemoglobin thus shifts the oxyhemoglobin dissociation curve to the left.

Carbon Monoxide

Carbon monoxide (CO) binds to the heme group of the Hgb molecule at the same site as O_2, forming carboxyhemoglobin (HgbCO). A major difference, however, as illustrated in comparing the oxyhemoglobin and carboxyhemoglobin dissociation curves, is that the affinity of CO for hemoglobin is about 200 times greater than that of O_2 (Fig. 8-14). Thus, small amounts of CO greatly inhibit the binding of O_2 to hemoglobin. In addition, in the presence of CO, the hemoglobin molecules' affinity for O_2 is enhanced, which shifts the dissociation curve to the left, further inhibiting the unloading and delivery of O_2 to tissue. Thus, CO prevents O_2 loading into the blood in the lungs and O_2 unloading in the tissues. As the P_{CO} of blood approaches 1.0 torr, all of the Hgb-binding sites are occupied by CO, and hemoglobin is unable to bind to O_2. This situation is not compatible with life and is the mechanism of death in individuals with CO poisoning. CO is colorless, odorless, and tasteless and does not produce symptoms of breathlessness or difficulty breathing (see Chapter 10 on regulation of respiration for the reason). In healthy individuals, carboxyhemoglobin occupies about 1% to 2% of the Hgb-binding sites; however, in cigarette smokers and in individuals who reside in high-density urban traffic areas, it can be increased to 10%.

Treatment for individuals with high levels of CO, such as after inhaling car exhaust or due to smoke inhalation in a burning building, consists of high concentrations of O_2 to displace CO from hemoglobin. Increasing the barometric pressure above atmospheric, through the use of a barometric chamber, substantially increases the oxygen tension. This increase in barometric pressure promotes the further dissociation of CO from hemoglobin.

Nitric oxide (NO) also has a great affinity (200,000 times greater than O_2) for hemoglobin and binds irreversibly to it at the same site as O_2. Endothelial cells can synthesize NO, which has vasodilatation properties and is used therapeutically as an inhalant in patients with pulmonary hypertension. Although not common, NO poisoning can occur, and one should be cautious when administering NO therapy for long periods.

CLINICAL SIGNIFICANCE OF SHIFTS IN THE OXYHEMOGLOBIN DISSOCIATION CURVE

Shifts of the dissociation curve to the right or left have little effect when they occur at oxygen partial pressures within the normal range (80-100 mm Hg) (plateau part of curve). However, at oxygen partial pressures below 60 mm Hg (steep part of the curve), shifts in the oxyhemoglobin dissociation curve can dramatically influence O_2 transport. For example, in a patient with lung disease who has a Pa_{O_2} equal to 60 mm Hg, the Hbg saturation is 90%, which is still adequate for normal functioning. However, if the patient experiences a decrease in pH, the dissociation curve shifts to the right and the Hgb saturation could drop to less than 70%, which would significantly impair O_2 delivery.

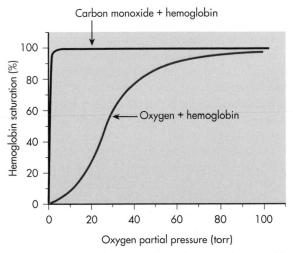

FIGURE 8-14 ■ Oxyhemoglobin and carboxyhemoglobin dissociation curves. Carbon monoxide and oxygen compete for the same binding sites on hemoglobin, but carbon monoxide has an affinity for hemoglobin that is ~200 times greater than O_2. Thus above a blood P_{CO} of about 0.5 torr, all of the hemoglobin-binding sites are occupied by carbon monoxide. *(From Berne RM, Levy ML, Koeppen BM, Stanton BM (eds): Physiology, 5th ed. St. Louis, Mosby, 2004.)*

OXYGEN DELIVERY TO THE TISSUES

As blood circulates from the lungs, it is exposed to tissues with a lower P_{O_2}, and oxygen is released by the hemoglobin. Oxygen delivery from the lungs to the tissue varies with cardiac output (Qt), the hemoglobin content of blood, and the ability of the lung to oxygenate the blood. The total O_2 delivered (DO_2) to the tissue can be calculated by multiplying the cardiac output (Qt) times the O_2 content of arterial blood (CaO_2); that is,

$$DO_2 = Qt \times (CaO_2) \times 10 \text{ (to change the vol\%}$$
$$\text{from mL } O_2/dL \text{ to mL } O_2/L)$$

Under normal conditions, the cardiac output is about 5 L/min and the O_2 content in arterial blood is 20 vol%; thus, in a normal individual,

$$DO_2 = 5 \text{ L/min} \times 20 \text{ vol\%} \times 10$$
$$= 1000 \text{ mL } O_2/min$$

OXYGEN CONSUMPTION

Not all of the O_2 carried in the blood is unloaded at the tissue level. The principle of conservation of mass, also known as the Fick relationship, can be applied to calculate oxygen consumption. The O_2 extracted from the blood by the tissue (that is, the O_2 consumption, or $\dot{V}O_2$) is the difference between the arterial O_2 content (CaO_2) (i.e., the amount of O_2 delivered) and the venous O_2 content (CvO_2) (the O_2 content remaining after release to the tissues) times the cardiac output; that is,

$$\dot{V}O_2 = Qt \, [(CaO_2 - CvO_2) \times 10]$$

Under normal conditions, when the CaO_2 is 20 vol% and the CvO_2 is 15 vol%, the amount of O_2 actually consumed by the tissues is 5 vol% (5 mL of O_2 for each 100/mL of blood or 50 mL of O_2 for each liter of blood). With a cardiac output of 5 L/min, the total amount of O_2 consumed in one minute is 250 mL/min (50 mL O_2/L blood $\times$ 5 L/min).

An interesting but underused approach to understanding O_2 consumption is the **O_2 extraction ratio** (also referred to as the O_2 coefficient ratio), which is the amount of O_2 extracted by the tissue divided by the amount of O_2 delivered:

$$O_2 \text{ extraction ratio} = \frac{CaO_2 - CvO_2}{CaO_2}$$

$$\text{Normal } O_2 \text{ extraction ratio} = \frac{20 \text{ vol\%} - 15 \text{ vol\%}}{20 \text{ vol\%}} = \frac{5 \text{ vol\%}}{20 \text{ vol\%}}$$
$$= 0.25$$

Under normal conditions, only 25% of the O_2 that is delivered to the tissues is actually utilized by the tissues. This significant reserve is one of the reasons why individuals are able to tolerate large changes in O_2 content. It is possible to significantly change the O_2 extraction ratio without a change in the difference between CaO_2 and CvO_2. As shown previously, the normal O_2 extraction ratio is 0.25 with a CaO_2 and CvO_2 difference of 5 vol%. If the CaO_2 decreases to 8 vol% with a CvO_2 of 3 vol%, the O_2 extraction ratio now becomes 0.62 even though the CaO_2 and CvO_2 difference remains 5 vol%; that is,

$$\text{Altered } O_2 \text{ extraction ratio} = \frac{8 \text{ vol\%} - 3 \text{ vol\%}}{8 \text{ vol\%}} = \frac{5 \text{ vol\%}}{8 \text{ vol\%}}$$
$$= 0.62$$

Hypothermia, relaxation of skeletal muscles, and an increase in cardiac output will reduce O_2 consumption and will decrease the O_2 extraction ratio. Conversely, a decrease in cardiac output, anemia, hyperthermia, and exercise increase O_2 consumption and will increase the O_2 extraction ratio.

TISSUE HYPOXIA

Tissue hypoxia occurs when there is insufficient O_2 available to the cells to maintain adequate aerobic metabolism to carry out normal cellular activities. Anaerobic metabolism occurs in association with the generation of increased levels of lactate and hydrogen ions and the subsequent formation of lactic acid. This results in a significant decrease in the blood pH. In severe hypoxia, the body—especially the lips and nailbeds—takes on a blue-gray coloration (cyanosis) due to the lack of O_2 and the increased levels of deoxyhemoglobin. **Hypoxemia** and/or tissue hypoxia can occur (see Chapter 7). Hypoxemia refers to an abnormal PO_2 in arterial blood, which at sea level on room air, is a PaO_2 less than 80 torr. Hypoxia usually less occurs at a lower PO_2 and, although various mitigating circumstances can influence the absolute level at which there is insufficient O_2 for cell function, hypoxia is commonly said to occur when the PaO_2 falls below 60 torr.

As shown in Table 8-1, four major types of tissue hypoxia can occur via different mechanisms. *Hypoxic hypoxia* is the most common and occurs in lung diseases such as chronic obstructive pulmonary disease

				MECHANISM	
				TABLE 8-1	
				Tissue Hypoxia	
Type of Hypoxia	Cause	PaO_2	CaO_2	Amount O_2 Delivered	Amount O_2 Utilized
Hypoxic	Pulmonary disease with ↓ PaO_2 ↓ V/Q ratio	Low	Low	Low	Normal
Circulatory	Vascular disease Arterial-venous shunt (malformation)	Normal	Normal	Low	Normal
Anemic	CO poisoning Anemia	Normal	Low	Normal	Normal
Histologic	Cyanide Sodium azide	Normal	Normal	Normal	Low

(COPD), pulmonary fibrosis, and neuromuscular diseases. As a result of these diseases, there is a decrease in PaO_2 and/or CaO_2 with a subsequent decrease in O_2 delivery to tissue. *Circulatory (stagnate) hypoxia* is the result of diminished blood flow to an organ, usually due to vascular disease or an arterial venous shunt. *Anemic hypoxia* is caused by the inability of the blood to carry O_2 either due to low hemoglobin (anemia) or to its inability to carry O_2, as in the case of CO poisoning. *Histologic hypoxia* results when there is a block in the electron transport system in mitochondrial respiration, thus preventing the utilization of O_2 by the cell. Histologic hypoxia occurs with respiratory chain poisoning, such as with cyanide, sodium azide, and the pesticide rotenone.

Tissue oxygenation is directly dependent on the hemoglobin concentration and thus the number of red blood cells available in the circulation. **Erythropoiesis** (red blood cell production in the bone marrow) is controlled by the hormone *erythropoietin*, which is synthesized in the kidney by cortical interstitial cells. Although under normal conditions hemoglobin levels are very stable, under conditions of decreased O_2 delivery, low hemoglobin concentrations, or low PaO_2 levels, the cortical interstitial cells are stimulated to increase erythropoietin secretion, and this leads to increased production of red blood cells. Chronic renal disease can damage the cortical interstitial cells and result in their inability

to synthesize erythropoietin. Anemia ensues, with decreased hemoglobin concentrations directly related to the lack of erythropoietin production. Erythropoietin replacement therapy has been shown to be effective in this condition.

CARBON DIOXIDE TRANSPORT

Carbon dioxide is carried in the blood in three ways: physically dissolved, as bicarbonate ions (HCO_3^-), and chemically bound to amino acids. By far the predominant transport mechanism of CO_2 is via HCO_3^- in red blood cells (Table 8-2). CO_2 is a byproduct of tissue metabolism; approximately 200 to 250 mL of CO_2 is produced per minute. Under steady state conditions at rest, with a cardiac output of 5 L/min, 4 to 5 mL of CO_2 must be eliminated by the lung for every 100 mL of blood.

CARBON DIOXIDE PRODUCTION, METABOLISM, AND DIFFUSION

CO_2 is critical in the maintenance of physiologic homeostasis and is a major factor in regulating hydrogen ion (H^+) concentrations in blood, cells, and other body tissues. It is also an important chemical stimulus in the regulation of respiration in normal individuals via chemoreceptors in the peripheral circulation and central nervous system (see Chapter 10). The major

TABLE 8-2				
Transport of CO_2 per Liter of Normal Human Blood				
		ARTERIAL	MIXED VENOUS	A–V DIFFERENCE
P_{CO_2}	mm Hg	40	46	6
Dissolved	ml/L	25	29	4
Carbamino	ml/L	24	38	14
HCO_3^-	ml/L	433	455	22
Total	ml/L	482	522	40

sources of CO_2 production are in mitochondria during the aerobic cellular metabolism of glucose and in the conversion of carbohydrates to fats. Carbonic acid (H_2CO_3), is a major product of cellular metabolism and is readily metabolized to CO_2 and H_2O. During the metabolism of one glucose molecule, six CO_2 molecules are produced and six O_2 molecules are consumed (see Table 5-1). CO_2 production which at rest is about 200 mL/min can be increased sixfold during conditions of stress or exercise. The body has enhanced storage capabilities for CO_2 compared with O_2. Whereas Pa_{O_2} is dependent on factors in addition to alveolar ventilation, Pa_{CO_2} is *solely* dependent on alveolar ventilation and CO_2 production. There is an inverse relationship between alveolar ventilation and Pa_{CO_2} (see Fig. 5-3).

The diffusion of CO_2 from the cell to the capillaries occurs through passive diffusion from higher to lower partial pressures of CO_2. When the intracellular concentration of CO_2, or its partial pressure (Pc_{CO_2}), exceeds the tissue concentration (Pt_{CO_2}), CO_2 moves out of the cell and into the surrounding tissue. Subsequently, Pt_{CO_2} is increased; when it exceeds the capillary P_{CO_2}, diffusion of CO_2 occurs from the tissue into the capillaries just before the blood enters the venous system. The CO_2 is then carried in venous blood to the lungs, where it is removed in exhaled gas. Diffusion of CO_2 occurs so readily from the alveolar lumen to the capillaries, and vice versa, that the PA_{CO_2} and Pa_{CO_2} are equal. Under normal conditions, Pt_{CO_2} is 50 mm Hg, venous P_{CO_2} (Pv_{CO_2}) is 46 mm Hg, and Pa_{CO_2} is 40 mm Hg. The blood level of CO_2 is highest on the venous side after the CO_2 has been picked up in the capillaries. Under normal conditions the difference in Pa_{CO_2} and Pv_{CO_2} is about 6 mm Hg. In contrast with the exchange of O_2 from the

arterial side of the circulatory system, CO_2 exchange occurs primarily from the venous side.

BICARBONATE

Once CO_2 diffuses through the tissue and reaches the plasma, it quickly physically dissolves and establishes a partial pressure (Pa_{CO_2}). CO_2 readily diffuses from the plasma to the red blood cells and an equilibrium is established between the red blood cells and plasma. The major pathway for the generation of HCO_3^- is the reaction of CO_2 with H_2O to form carbonic acid (HCO_3^-), which then readily dissociates to form bicarbonate (HCO_3^-) and free H^+ ions (Fig. 8-15); that is,

$$CO_2 + H_2O \xleftrightarrow{\text{ CA }} H_2CO_3 \leftrightarrow H^+ + HCO_3^-$$

This reaction occurs very slowly by chemical reaction standards (seconds) in tissue and plasma and is not thought to be of major significance in these compartments. However, it is catalyzed within red blood cells by the enzyme carbonic anhydrase (CA), which speeds up the reaction time to microseconds and is the major source of HCO_3^- generation. Once formed within the red blood cells, the HCO_3^- diffuses out of the cell in exchange for Cl^-. This Cl^- exchange is referred to as the **chloride shift** (also called the Hamburger phenomenon and the anionic shift to equilibrium). The Cl^- binds to K^+, which was released by hemoglobin during the transfer of O_2 from hemoglobin to the tissue. The chloride shift maintains the electrostatic homeostasis of the cells. In addition, osmotic equilibrium is maintained in the red blood cell, because water also accompanies the Cl^- movement. For this reason, red blood cells are actually slightly

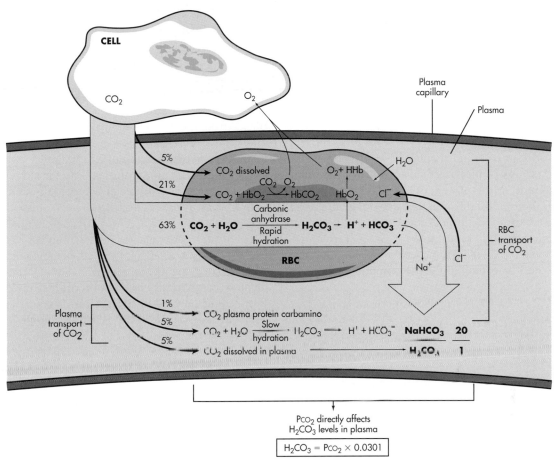

FIGURE 8-15 ■ Mechanisms of CO_2 transport. The predominant mechanism by which CO_2 is transported from the tissue cells to lung is in the form of HCO_3^-. *(From Berne RM, Levy ML, Koeppen BM, Stanton BM (eds): Physiology, 5th ed. St. Louis, Mosby, 2004.)*

swollen in the venous system compared with the arterial system.

This pathway of CO_2 to carbonic acid to bicarbonate is reversible. It is shifted to the right to generate more bicarbonate when CO_2 enters the blood from the tissue, and it is shifted to the left to generate more CO_2 when CO_2 is exhaled in the lungs.

The free H^+ ions are quickly buffered by binding to plasma proteins or, if within the red blood cell, the H^+ ions bind to hemoglobin to form an $H \cdot Hgb$ complex. The H^+ ion buffering is critical to keep the reaction moving toward the synthesis of HCO_3^-; high levels of free H^+ will push the reaction back in the opposite direction. This H^+ source is mainly responsible

for the slightly more acidic nature of venous blood (pH 7.35) compared with arterial blood (pH 7.40).

$$CO_2 + H_2O \leftrightarrow H^+ + HCO_3^-$$
$$\updownarrow$$
$$H^+ + Hgb \leftrightarrow H \cdot Hgb$$

DISSOLVED CARBON DIOXIDE

Although CO_2 is 20 times more soluble than O_2 in water, the dissolved form of CO_2 still remains a small amount of the total transported CO_2. With this said, the dissolved form of CO_2 is much more important in CO_2 transport than is the dissolved form of O_2. Approximately 5% to 10% of the total CO_2 transported by blood is carried in physical solution. Also, one must keep in mind that although CO_2 transport and H^+ regulation occur simultaneously, they occur independently of each other and are controlled by different factors.

CARBAMINO COMPOUNDS

CO_2 can also combine chemically with the terminal amine groups in blood proteins to form carbamino compounds. Most of the CO_2 transported in this way is bound to the amino acids in hemoglobin because most of the protein found in blood is globin. Deoxyhemoglobin binds more CO_2 as carbamino groups than oxyhemoglobin, facilitating loading in the tissues and unloading in the lung. Approximately 5%

to 10% of the CO_2 content in blood consists of carbamino compounds.

CARBON DIOXIDE DISSOCIATION CURVE

In contrast to O_2, the dissociation (removal and uptake) of CO_2 from the blood is almost directly related to the P_{CO_2}, and therefore the dissociation curve for CO_2 is linear (Fig. 8-16). When plotted on similar axes, the CO_2 dissociation curve is steeper than the oxygen dissociation curve. The degree of hemoglobin saturation with O_2 has a major effect on the CO_2 dissociation curve. Although O_2 and CO_2 bind to hemoglobin at different sites, deoxygenated hemoglobin has a greater affinity for CO_2 than oxygenated hemoglobin. The deoxygenated hemoglobin more readily forms carbamino compounds and also more readily binds free H^+ ions released during the formation of HCO_3^-. Thus deoxygenated blood (venous blood) freely takes up and transports more CO_2 than oxygenated arterial blood.

The effect of changes in oxyhemoglobin saturation on the relationship of the CO_2 content to P_{CO_2} is referred to as the **Haldane effect** and is reversed in the lung when O_2 is transported from the alveoli to the red blood cells. As a result of the Haldane effect, the CO_2 dissociation curve for whole blood is shifted to the right at greater levels of oxyhemoglobin and shifted to the left at greater levels of deoxyhemoglobin. Because of the Haldane effect, CO_2 uptake is facilitated in the presence of deoxyhemoglobin, and CO_2 unloading is facilitated in the presence of oxyhemoglobin.

In summary, the red blood cell is ideally constructed to transport O_2 and CO_2. Oxygen unloading along the systemic capillary is enhanced by increases in P_{CO_2} and by decreases in pH (Bohr effect), whereas CO_2 loading into the blood is enhanced by decreases in oxyhemoglobin saturation (Haldane effect). Oxygen is bound to hemoglobin when CO_2 exists in the form of HCO_3^-, which is produced in the red blood cell and transported into the plasma.

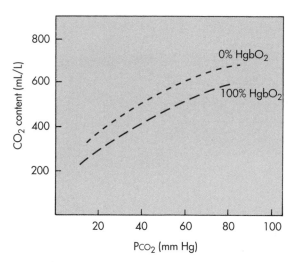

FIGURE 8-16 ■ Blood CO_2 equilibrium curves at different hemoglobin saturations (% $HgbO_2$). Venous blood can transport more CO_2 than arterial blood at any given P_{CO_2}. Compared with the hemoglobin oxygen equilibrium curve, the CO_2 curves are essentially straight lines between a P_{CO_2} of 20 and 80 mm Hg. *(From Berne RM, Levy ML, Koeppen BM, Stanton BM (eds): Physiology, 5th ed. St. Louis, Mosby, 2004.)*

SUMMARY

1. The major source of energy in cells and organs is provided by the intracellular metabolism of oxygen (O_2).

2. O_2 is carried in the blood from the lungs to the tissues in two forms: physically dissolved in the blood and chemically combined to hemoglobin.

3. Carbon dioxide (CO_2) is carried in the blood in three forms: physically dissolved in blood, chemically combined to blood proteins as carbamino compounds, and as bicarbonate.

4. Gases (nitrous oxide [N_2O], ether, helium) with a rapid rate of air-to-blood equilibration are perfusion-limited, and gases (CO) with a slow air-to-blood equilibration rate are diffusion-limited. Under normal conditions, O_2 transport is perfusion-limited but can be diffusion-limited in certain conditions.

5. Fick's law of diffusion states that the diffusion of a gas across a sheet of tissue is *directly* related to the surface area of the tissue, the diffusion constant of the specific gas, and the partial pressure difference of the gas on each side of the tissue and is *inversely* related to tissue thickness.

6. O_2 loading and unloading and CO_2 loading and unloading not only occur simultaneously but also facilitate each other.

7. CO_2 diffuses approximately 20 times more rapidly through the alveolar-capillary membrane than does O_2.

8. O_2 binds quickly and reversibly to the heme groups of the hemoglobin (Hgb) molecule.

9. In its dissolved form, O_2 maintains its molecular structure and gaseous state. It is this form that is measured clinically in an arterial blood gas sample as the PaO_2.

10. The ability of CO_2 to alter the affinity of Hgb for O_2 (the Bohr effect) enhances O_2 delivery to tissue and O_2 uptake in the lungs.

11. Tissue hypoxia occurs when insufficient amounts of O_2 are supplied to the tissue to carry out normal levels of aerobic metabolism.

12. The major source of CO_2 production is in the mitochondria during aerobic cellular metabolism. The reversible reaction of CO_2 with H_2O to form carbonic acid (H_2CO_3) with its subsequent dissociation to HCO_3^- and H^+ is catalyzed by the enzyme carbonic anhydrase within red blood cells and is the major pathway for HCO_3^- generation.

13. The CO_2 dissociation curve from blood is linear and directly related to PCO_2.

14. There are four major types of tissue hypoxia: hypoxic hypoxia, circulatory hypoxia, anemic hypoxia, and histologic hypoxia.

15. The O_2 dissociation curve is S-shaped, not linear. In the plateau area (above 60 mm Hg), increasing the PO_2 has only a minimal effect on Hgb saturation; the same is true if there is a decrease in PO_2 from 100 to 60 mm Hg. This assures adequate Hgb saturation over a large range of PO_2. The steep portion of the curve (20-60 mm Hg) illustrates that during O_2 deprivation (low PO_2) O_2 is readily released from Hgb with only small changes in PO_2, which facilitates O_2 diffusion to the tissue.

KEY WORDS

- 2,3-diphosphoglycerate (2,3-DPG)
- Adenosine triphosphate
- Bicarbonate ions
- Bohr Effect
- Bulk flow
- Carbamino compounds
- Carbon monoxide
- Carbonic anhydrase
- Carboxyhemoglobin (HgbCO)
- Chloride shift
- CO content
- CO_2 dissociation curve
- CO_2 transport
- Conservation of mass
- Deoxyhemoglobin
- Diffusion
- Diffusion constant
- Diffusion-limited gas exchange
- Effective solubility
- Erythropoeisis

- Fetal hemoglobin
- Fick's law of diffusion
- Haldane effect
- Hemoglobin
- Henry's law
- Hypoxemia
- Hypoxia
- Methemoglobinemia
- Myoglobin
- Nitric oxide
- Nitrous oxide
- O_2 content
- O_2 extraction ratio
- O_2 transport
- Oxidative metabolism
- Oxygen saturation (SO_2)
- Oxyhemoglobin
- Oxyhemoglobin dissociation curve
- Perfusion-limited gas exchange
- Sickle cell anemia
- Tissue hypoxia

SELF-STUDY PROBLEMS

1. What are the physiologic parameters that cause the oxyhemoglobin dissociation curve to shift?

2. How do the shifts in the oxyhemoglobin dissociation curve aid in O_2 and CO_2 uptake and delivery?

3. A patient appears to be suffering from hypoxic symptoms. An arterial blood gas reveals an SaO_2 of 98%. Is it possible for this patient to be hypoxic?

4. What are the major forms in which O_2 and CO_2 are transported in the blood?

5. Using the oxyhemoglobin dissociation curve, explain why giving supplemental oxygen to increase the PO_2 has little effect in improving oxygen delivery in most patients and is beneficial only in patients with a PaO_2 of less than 60 mm Hg.

6. What is tissue hypoxia and what are the mechanisms that cause it?

7. Explain why some gases are diffusion-limited and others are perfusion-limited and how under certain circumstances oxygen can be either.

REFERENCES

Hlastala MP, Swenson ER: Blood-gas transport. In Fishman AP, Elias JA, Fishman JA, et al (eds): Pulmonary Diseases and Disorders, 3rd ed. New York, McGraw-Hill, 1998.

Jelkmann W. Erythropoietin: Structure, control of production and function. Physiol Rev 72:449-489, 1992.

Klocke RA: Carbon dioxide transport. In Crystal RG, West JB, Barnes PJ, Weibel ER (eds): The Lung: Scientific Foundations, 2nd ed. New York, Raven Press, 1997.

Leach RM: Treacher DF. Oxygen transport—2. Tissue hypoxia. BMJ 317:1370-1373, 1998.

*Perrella M, Bresciani D, Rossi-Bernardi L: The binding of CO_2 to human hemoglobin. J Biol Chem 250:5413-5418, 1975.

Reeves RB, Park HK: CO uptake kinetics of red cells and CO diffusion capacity. Respir Physiol 88:1, 1992.

Russell JA, Phang PT: The oxygen delivery-consumption controversy. Am J Respir Crit Care Med 149:433-437, 1994.

Treacher, DF, Leach RM: Oxygen transport—1. Basic principles. BMJ 317:1302-1306, 1998.

*Weibel ER: Morphological basis of alveolar-capillary gas exchange. Physiol Rev 1973; 53:257-312.

*West JB: Effect of slope and shape of dissociation curve on pulmonary gas exchange. Respir Physiol 8:66-85, 1969.

_____

*These are the classics.

PULMONARY ASPECTS OF ACID-BASE BALANCE AND ARTERIAL BLOOD GAS INTERPRETATION

OBJECTIVES

1. Explain the nine types of acid-base conditions.
2. Distinguish between acute and chronic acid-base conditions and compensatory mechanisms.
3. Explain respiratory compensatory mechanisms.
4. Explain renal compensatory mechanisms.

5. Describe use of base excess and anion gap in understanding acid-base status.
6. Develop an approach to the interpretation of arterial blood gases.

With an understanding of the transport mechanisms of O_2 and CO_2 throughout the body, we can begin to explore the clinical interpretation of altered Po_2 and Pco_2 levels in blood. The partial pressures of O_2, CO_2 and pH in the blood can be measured readily. Their values show the net effect of lung disease on gas exchange and thus, the arterial blood gas measurement is the best overall test of lung function. Arterial blood gas values cannot be determined by clinical assessment alone even by experienced clinicians. For example, cyanosis does not become apparent until the arterial oxygen falls to less than 50 torr or 80% saturation, and quality of air exchange determined by auscultation is a poor assessment of alveolar ventilation. Thus arterial blood gas measurements are an important and essential tool in caring for critically ill patients, in guiding therapy, and in monitoring the progression of chronic lung disease.

Just as other laboratory tests such as chest radiographs benefit from a careful, systematic approach, so does the interpretation of arterial blood gas values. First, we will present some general principles about

acid-base balance and oxygenation that are important to proper interpretation and then we will examine the major respiratory and metabolic processes associated with changes in arterial blood gas values. Finally, we will describe a systematic approach to arterial blood gas interpretation.

PRINCIPLES OF INTERPRETING ARTERIAL BLOOD GAS VALUES

Arterial blood gases should always be interpreted in light of the patient's history and symptoms. Recall the Irish proverb: *Normal values are normal in normal people.* For example, if a patient's respiratory rate is three times normal and the measured arterial $Paco_2$ is 40 mm Hg ("normal"), it does not necessarily mean that this patient has normal lungs. Rather, this patient is maintaining normal alveolar ventilation (i.e., a normal $Paco_2$) by markedly increasing his or her respiratory rate. As we shall see, a number of different mechanisms (such as an increase in minute ventilation) can compensate for abnormalities in gas exchange and can bring the body back toward homeostasis. Normal values for arterial blood gas measurements are shown in Table 9-1.

TYPES OF ACID-BASE ABNORMALITIES

There are nine fundamental acid-base conditions: normal, acute and chronic respiratory acidosis, acute and chronic respiratory alkalosis, acute and chronic metabolic acidosis, and acute and chronic metabolic alkalosis. Acute conditions occur over a relatively short period of time; chronic conditions occur over longer periods (hours and days) and are associated with compensation, usually by the kidney but occasionally by the lung. **Acidemia** occurs when there is an excess of hydrogen ions in the blood, and **alkalemia** occurs when there are too few hydrogen ions in the blood. Values associated with various blood gas disturbances are listed in Table 9-1.

MEASURING ARTERIAL BLOOD GASES

Obtaining an Arterial Blood Gas Sample

Arterial blood can readily be sampled by needle puncture of a radial artery (Fig. 9-1). Other sites, used occasionally but associated with a greater potential risk of complications, are the brachial and femoral arteries. Blood is collected into a heparinized syringe to prevent clotting. Air bubbles are expelled to prevent equilibration of the sample with ambient air, and the sample is kept on ice until analyzed. Routinely three measurements are obtained: Pao_2, $Paco_2$, and pH. Base excess (or deficit) and HCO_3^- (using the Henderson-Hasselbach equation) can be calculated from the measured values for Pco_2 and pH. (HCO_3^- can also be directly measured as part of serum electrolytes.) When frequent sampling of arterial blood is needed, a catheter can be inserted, usually in the radial artery.

PULSE OXIMETRY

Arterial puncture is uncomfortable for patients and is associated with a small but finite risk. Pulse oximetry is a noninvasive method of assessing arterial oxygenation that is now widely used in hospitalized patients.

TABLE 9-1	
Normal Values and Acid-Base Disturbances*	
pH Normal	7.35 to 7.45
Acidosis	
Mild	7.30 to 7.35
Moderate	7.25 to 7.30
Severe	<7.25
Alkalosis	
Mild	7.45 to 7.50
Moderate	7.50 to 7.55
Severe	>7.55
Pao_2 Normal	>85 mm Hg
Hypoxemia	
Mild	55 to 85 mm Hg
Moderate	40 to 55 mm Hg
Severe	<40 mm Hg
$Paco_2$ Normal	35-45 mm Hg
Hypercapnia	
Mild	45-50 mm Hg
Moderate	50 to 60 mm Hg
Severe	>60 mm Hg
Hypocapnia	
Mild	30 to 45 mm Hg
Moderate	25 to 30 mm Hg
Severe	<25 mm Hg
HCO_3^- Normal	22 to 28 mEq/L
Depression	
Mild	19 to 22 mEq/L
Moderate	17 to 19 mEq/L
Severe	<17 mEq/L
Elevation	
Mild	28 to 31 mEq/L
Moderate	31 to 35 mEq/L
Severe	>35 mEq/L
Base Excess Normal	−3 to +4 mEq/L
Depression	
Mild	−4 to −7 mEq/L
Moderate	−7 to −10 mEq/L
Severe	>−10 mEq/L
Elevation	
Mild	+4 to +8 mEq/L
Moderate	+8 to +12 mEq/L
Severe	>+12 mEq/L
Anion Gap	5 to 11 mEq/L
$AaDo_2$†	10 to 25 mm Hg (on room air)

*For a 25-year-old adult at sea level on room air.
†The alveolar-arterial oxygen difference ($AaDo_2$) widens with age.

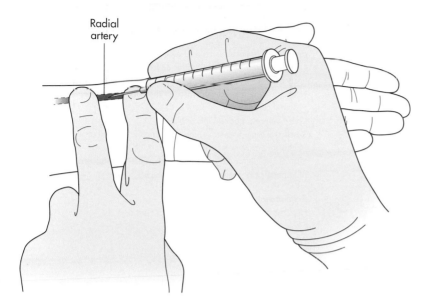

Radial
artery

FIGURE 9-1 ■ Radial artery puncture. Before performing a radial artery puncture, test the efficacy of the ulnar collateral supply by compressing the radial artery and noting that the palm does not blanch. The syringe should be rinsed with sodium heparin to prevent clotting of the sample. *(Redrawn from Waring WW, Jeansonne LO III: Practical Manual of Pediatrics, 2nd ed. St. Louis, Mosby, 1982.)*

The sensor device can be clipped on the patient's finger and oxygen saturation can be displayed continuously on a monitor. Specific wavelengths of light are passed through the finger and the oximeter measures the pulsatile absorption of light by arteriolar blood. Because oxygenated and deoxygenated hemoglobin have different patterns of light absorption, they produce different results. The major advantage of pulse oximetry is that it provides a continuous measurement. However, this method has two major limitations: (1) the oximeter measures O_2 saturation, not P_{O_2}; and (2) it provides no information about P_{CO_2} and pH.

ARTERIAL pH

pH is the negative log of the hydrogen ion concentration. Measurement of arterial pH is the only way to determine if the body is too alkaline or too acid. Low pH values (<7.35) indicate **acidemia** or an increase in hydrogen ions; pH values greater than 7.45 indicate **alkalemia**, a decrease in hydrogen ions. Acid*emia* and alkal*emia* refer to conditions in the *blood*; acid*osis* and alkal*osis* refer to the process that causes the *abnormality*. Maintenance of a normal or near-normal pH in the blood is important because arrhythmias can result when the pH falls below 7.25, and seizures and vascular collapse can occur when the pH rises above 7.55.

The acid-base status of blood can be analyzed using the **Henderson-Hasselbach equation** for the bicarbonate buffer system. This equation states that the pH in blood is equal to a constant (pK) plus the log ratio of bicarbonate to P_{CO_2}. That is,

$$pK + \log \frac{[HCO_3^-]}{0.3 \times P_{CO_2}}$$

The pK is a constant (p$K = 6.1$) that is related to the dissociation of carbonic acid (H_2CO_3). The bicarbonate concentration is determined by the kidney, whereas the lung determines the P_{CO_2}. When the HCO_3^- is constant, increases in P_{CO_2} result in decreases in pH, and decreases in P_{CO_2} result in increases in pH. As long as the ratio of bicarbonate to 0.03 · P_{CO_2} is 20, the pH remains at 7.4. Compensatory mechanisms in the body are responsible for maintaining the ratio of HCO_3^- to 0.03 · P_{CO_2} at 20.

RESPIRATORY ACIDOSIS AND ALKALOSIS

Respiratory effects on acid-base status center around the elimination of CO_2. The two basic respiratory alterations are respiratory acidosis and respiratory alkalosis (Table 9-2). Respiratory acidosis is associated

TABLE 9-2			
Patterns of Acid-Base Disturbances			
	P_{CO_2}	pH	HCO_3^-
Respiratory Acidosis			
No compensation	↑↑	↓↓	NL
Metabolic compensation	↑↑	↓	↑↑
Respiratory Alkalosis			
No compensation	↓↓	↑↑	NL
Metabolic compensation	↓↓	↑	↓↓
Metabolic Acidosis			
No compensation	NL	↓↓	↓↓
Respiratory compensation	↓	↓	↓↓
Metabolic Alkalosis			
No compensation	NL	↑↑	↑↑
Respiratory compensation	↑	↑	↑↑

NL, normal; ↑↑ and ↓↓ represent a greater increase and decrease, respectively, than ↑ and ↓.

TABLE 9-3
Respiratory Causes of Acidosis and Alkalosis

Respiratory Acidosis
Central respiratory control center depression (narcotics, anesthetics, sedatives)
Neuromuscular disorders (muscular dystrophy, myasthenia gravis, spinal cord injury)
Chest wall restriction (kyphoscoliosis)
Restrictive lung disease (pulmonary fibrosis, pneumothorax, pleural effusion, extreme obesity)
Obstructive pulmonary disease (emphysema, chronic bronchitis, upper airway obstruction, cystic fibrosis)

Respiratory Alkalosis
Hyperventilation (anxiety, encephalitis, tumors)
Fever
Acute asthma
Pulmonary embolism
Hypoxia, high altitude
Salicylate ingestion
Progesterone (hyperventilation of pregnancy)

with a decrease in pH secondary to an increase in Pa_{CO_2} and is due to a decrease in the elimination of CO_2 by the lungs. Increases in Pa_{CO_2} can be due to either increased dead-space ventilation or hypoventilation (see Chapter 7). In contrast, respiratory alkalosis is associated with an increase in pH secondary to a decrease in Pa_{CO_2} and is due to an increase in the elimination of CO_2 by the lungs. Excess removal of CO_2 from the blood by the lungs is called **hyperventilation**.

A respiratory acidosis can be either acute or chronic. Imagine a situation in which an individual is given a narcotic, a respiratory depressant. Minute ventilation quickly decreases and arterial P_{CO_2} levels rise. The increase in P_{CO_2} occurs over minutes and is associated with an immediate decrease in pH (see Equation 1). There is not sufficient time for any compensatory mechanism to occur. This is an example of an acute, or uncompensated, respiratory acidosis.

In individuals with chronic lung disease, the changes in gas exchange in the lung occur slowly and, as disease progresses, the arterial CO_2 levels begin to slowly rise. The CO_2 combines with water to form H_2CO_3, which dissociates to form H^+ and HCO_3^-. Prompted by the increase in P_{CO_2} in the renal tubular cells, the kidney conserves HCO_3^- and excretes H^+ ions as H_2PO_4 or NH_4^+. The increase in plasma HCO_3^- shifts the HCO_3^-/ $0.03 \cdot P_{CO_2}$ ratio back toward its normal level. Renal compensation, however, like all other compensatory

mechanism is not "perfect" or complete, and thus although the pH approaches 7.4, it remains slightly less than this value. In this example, although Pa_{CO_2} rises, the change in pH is buffered by an increase in HCO_3^- ion. Examples of diseases associated with respiratory acid-base balance disturbances are listed in Table 9-3.

METABOLIC ACIDOSIS AND ALKALOSIS

Respiratory alterations in acid-base status are related to changes in CO_2, and metabolic abnormalities are associated with either a gain or a loss of fixed acid or bicarbonate in the extracellular fluid. For example, with vomiting there is a loss of stomach acid; this results in a metabolic alkalosis due to loss of fixed acid. The lung is able to quickly compensate for these metabolic abnormalities by changing ventilation, resulting in either increased or decreased elimination of CO_2. Thus a metabolic acidosis stimulates ventilation, CO_2 elimination, and a rise in pH toward normal levels, whereas a metabolic alkalosis suppresses ventilation and CO_2 elimination and the pH decreases toward the normal range. This is then followed by the slower elimination by the kidneys of excess acid or bicarbonate. For example, in individuals with

TABLE 9-4
Metabolic Causes of Acidosis and Alkalosis

Metabolic Acidosis

Drug ingestion (methanol, ethanol, ethylene glycol, ammonium chloride)

Diarrhea

Renal dysfunction

Lactic acidosis (shock, acute respiratory distress syndrome [ARDS], carbon monoxide)

Ketoacidosis (diabetes, starvation, alcoholism)

Metabolic Alkalosis

Vomiting (nasogastric suctioning)

Diuretics

Antacid ingestion

uncontrolled diabetes, the increase in blood sugar is associated with an increase in ketones and the development of ketoacidosis. The pH in the blood decreases. This decrease in pH is buffered, however, by an increase in minute ventilation, resulting in a decrease in PCO_2 followed by ketone elimination in the urine. Common diseases associated with metabolic acid-base balance disorders are listed in Table 9-4.

RESPIRATORY AND RENAL COMPENSATORY MECHANISMS

Homeostasis is a process of control mechanisms that helps to stabilize body systems by returning them to a more normal state. Because cells are unable to function outside of a relatively narrow pH range, homeostatic or compensatory mechanisms are important for cell and organ survival. Compensatory mechanisms are quickly activated to offset disturbances in acid-base balance; as a result, it is unusual to see uncompensated primary acid-base abnormalities. Changes in function in the respiratory and renal systems are the major acid-base compensatory mechanisms. The respiratory system compensates for metabolic acidosis or alkalosis by altering alveolar ventilation. The kidneys compensate for a respiratory acidosis or metabolic acidosis of nonrenal origin by excreting fixed acids and by retaining filtered bicarbonate; they compensate for a respiratory alkalosis and metabolic alkalosis of nonrenal origin by decreasing hydrogen ion excretion and retention of bicarbonate.

Most acid-base disorders are complex, with elements of both acute (uncompensated) and chronic (compensated) changes present. In examining acid-base abnormalities, then, the question frequently arises about what is the primary abnormality and what is the compensatory response. How is it possible to sort out the primary abnormality from the compensatory response? There are two important principles to remember. The first is that *compensation is rarely complete*; the second is that *compensatory acid-base responses rarely overcompensate*.

RESPIRATORY COMPENSATION

The respiratory system compensates for metabolic acid-base balance disorders by altering alveolar ventilation. When CO_2 production is constant, alveolar PCO_2 is inversely proportional to alveolar ventilation (see Fig 5-3). When a metabolic acidosis is present, the increased blood or H^+ concentration stimulates chemoreceptors, which in turn stimulate alveolar ventilation and decrease arterial PCO_2. Respiratory compensation for a metabolic alkalosis is to decrease alveolar ventilation, resulting in an increase in alveolar CO_2.

The relation between arterial levels of CO_2 and pH with and without renal compensation is demonstrated by the following two rules. For each increase of 10 mm Hg in $PaCO_2$, the pH will fall 0.03 units if time is allowed for renal compensation, and 0.08 units if the process is acute and insufficient time for renal compensation has occurred. (Renal compensation takes around 48 hrs to occur.) For example, is the following elevation in $PaCO_2$ acute or chronic?

pH, 7.20; $PaCO_2$, 65 mm Hg

If the increase in $PaCO_2$ is acute, an increase in $PaCO_2$ from 40 to 65 mm Hg will result in a decrease in pH; that is,

$$0.08 \times 25/10 \text{ mm Hg} = 0.20 \text{ units}$$

or

$$7.40 - 0.20 = 7.20$$

If the increase in $PaCO_2$ is *chronic*, an increase in $PaCO_2$ from 40 to 65 mm Hg will result in a decrease in pH; that is,

$$0.03 \times 25/10 \text{ mm Hg} = 0.075 \text{ units}$$

or

$$7.40 - 0.075 = 7.32$$

Therefore, in this patient, the elevation in P_{ACO_2} is entirely acute. Note that if the process had occurred over days, renal compensation would have occurred and the change in pH would have been smaller—that is, closer to 7.32 instead of 7.20.

Although it is useful to think about acid-base changes as either acute or chronic, with few exceptions (such as the acute administration of a respiratory depressant in the example given earlier), compensation for changes in P_{CO_2} begins immediately. Examine now the following pH and P_{CO_2} combination.

$$\text{pH, 72.8; } P_{CO_2}, 70 \text{ mm Hg}$$

If the increase in P_{ACO_2} is *acute*, an increase in P_{ACO_2} from 40 to 70 mm Hg will result in a decrease in pH; that is,

$$0.08 \times 30/10 \text{ mm Hg} = 0.24 \text{ units}$$

or

$$7.40 - 0.24 = 7.16$$

If the increase in P_{ACO_2} is *chronic*, an increase in P_{ACO_2} from 40 to 70 mm Hg will result in a decrease in pH; that is,

$$0.03 \times 30/10 \text{ mm Hg} = 0.09 \text{ units}$$

or

$$7.40 - 0.09 = 7.31$$

Here the decrease is in between 7.31 and 7.16, suggesting that an increase in P_{CO_2} has occurred some time between 24 and 48 hours. Furthermore, this is a respiratory acidosis, because the P_{ACO_2} is increased to more than 40 mm Hg with a reduced pH.

RENAL COMPENSATION

The kidneys compensate for acidosis either of respiratory or non-renal origin by excreting fixed acids and by retaining filtered bicarbonate. An increase in CO_2 inside the renal tubular cells, produced either by the tubular cell or by an increase in dissolved CO_2

in the blood, combines with water to form carbonic acid via the **carbonic anhydrase reaction**:

$$CO_2 + H_2O \xleftrightarrow{CA} H_2CO_3 \leftrightarrow H^+ + HCO_3^-$$

Equation 2

The hydrogen ions generated in this reaction are transported into the tubular lumen, and the bicarbonate is reabsorbed into the peritubular capillary (Fig. 9-2). Electrical neutrality is maintained by the exchange of sodium ions for the hydrogen ions. The hydrogen ions in the tubular lumen are buffered by tubular bicarbonate, phosphate, and other buffers and may be converted to H_2O and CO_2 by the carbonic anhydrase in the brush border of the proximal tubular cells. Approximately 90% of all filtered bicarbonate ions are reabsorbed in the proximal tubule.

The kidneys normally secrete 50 mEq of H^+ and reabsorb about 50 mEq of bicarbonate daily.

In alkalosis, the kidney decreases both hydrogen ion secretion and bicarbonate reabsorption. At plasma bicarbonate levels greater than 28 mEq/L, the kidney excretes bicarbonate.

BASE EXCESS AND ANION GAP

Two other calculated values can also be used to determine the processes responsible for the acid-base status. These are the **base excess** and the **anion gap**. Base excess can be used to determine if a metabolic acidosis is present while the anion gap can help to identify the cause of the metabolic acidosis. Base excess represents the change in buffer base (BB), which is the sum of HCO_3^- and buffer in the blood. It is the number of milliequivalents (mEq) of acid or base needed to titrate 1 liter of blood to pH 7.4 at 37° C *if the P_{ACO_2} is held constant at 40 torr*. Base excess (BE) changes from its normal value of 0 ± 2 to 3 *only* with metabolic acid-base changes.

The reaction shown in Equation 2 determines the base excess:

$$CO_2 + H_2O \xleftrightarrow{CA} H_2CO_3 \leftrightarrow H^+ + HCO_3^-$$ Equation 2

$$\updownarrow$$

$$\text{H Buf} \leftrightarrow H^+ + \text{Buf}$$ Equation 3

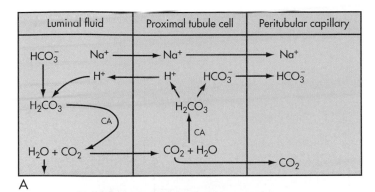

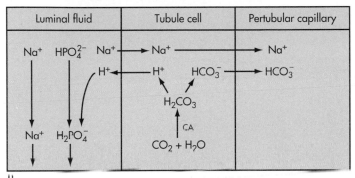

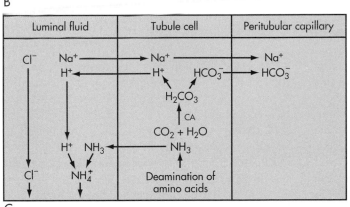

FIGURE 9-2 ■ Renal fixed acid excretion and bicarbonate retention. Approximately 90% of all filtered bicarbonate ions are reabsorbed directly or by the mechanism shown in **A**. The remaining 10% is reabsorbed in the process of titration of tubular phosphate ions (**B**) or by the generation of ammonium ions (**C**). *(Redrawn from Levitzky MG: Pulmonary Physiology, 4th ed. New York, McGraw-Hill, 1995.)*

The sum of HCO_3^- and Buf is called the buffer base (BB):

Base excess (BE) = Change in buffer base (BB)

If carbon dioxide is retained and increases in Equation 2, then H^+, generated by the shift to the right (**Le Chatelier's principle**), moves down to be buffered in Equation 3; HCO_3^- concentration increases; and buffer (Buf) concentration decreases. A respiratory change therefore, results in no change in the sum (BB) of HCO_3^- and Buf; hence BE equals zero. A change in pH of 0.15 units results from a base change of 10 mEq/L.

Changes in base excess can be seen graphically in the **Davenport diagram** (Fig. 9-3). The Davenport pH-HCO_3^- diagram is a graphic representation of the Henderson-Hasselbach equation (Equation 1). Three different buffer lines (slanting down and to the right) define the [HCO_3^-] and pH responses to the

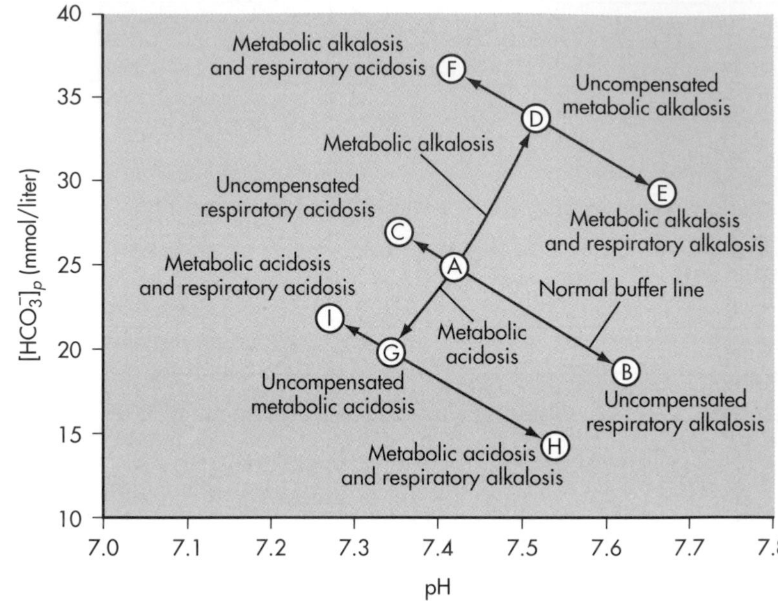

FIGURE 9-3 ■ Acid-base paths in vivo. *(Redrawn from Davenport HW: The ABC of Acid-Base Chemistry, 6th ed. Chicago, University of Chicago Press, 1974.)*

addition of acid or base to plasma. The CO_2 isopleth line (slanting up and to the right) relates pH to $[HCO_3^-]$ and is shown here for a P_{CO_2} level equal to 40 torr. Point A represents the normal situation with pH = 7.40, $[HCO_3^-]$ = 24 mEq/L, and P_{CO_2} = 40 mm Hg. An increase in bicarbonate concentration shifts the buffer line from CAB to DF (see Fig. 9-3). In this case, the base excess, given by the vertical distance between the two buffer lines, is increased. A reduction in bicarbonate concentration displaces the buffer line from CAB to GH and results in a negative base excess, which is also called a **base deficit**.

Once a metabolic acidosis has been identified, the anion gap can be used to identify its cause. The anion gap represents the difference between the concentration of the major plasma cation (Na^+) and the major plasma anions (Cl^- and HCO_3^-); that is,

$$\text{Anion gap} = [Na^+] - ([Cl^-] + [HCO_3^-]) \quad \text{(Equation 4)}$$

The rationale for this is that when acid is added to body fluids the $[H^+]$ increases and the $[HCO_3^-]$ decreases (Equation 2). In addition, the concentration of the anion, which is associated with the acid, will increase. It is important to remember, however, that a real anion gap does not exist. It is just that there are anions that are not being measured. The full, correct Equation 4 should be:

$$[Na^+] + [\text{unmeasured cations}] = [Cl^-] + [HCO_3^-] + [\text{unmeasured anions}]$$

Normally the anion gap ranges from 5 to 11 mEq/L, with most of this gap being made up by the negative charges on plasma proteins; an anion gap greater than 12 mEq/L is abnormal.

A change of 10 mm Hg in Pa_{CO_2} will result in an approximate change of 4 mEq/L in $[HCO_3^-]$ if renal compensation has occurred. If the anion of the acid is Cl^-, the anion gap will be normal (i.e. the decrease in $[HCO_3^-]$ is matched by an increase in $[Cl^-]$). Thus the metabolic acidosis associated with diarrhea or renal tubular acidosis is associated with a normal anion gap. In contrast, if the anion of the nonvolatile acid is not Cl^- (e.g. lactate) the anion gap will increase (i.e., the decrease in $[HCO_3^-]$ is not matched by an increase in the $[Cl^-]$ but rather by an increase in the concentration of the unmeasured anion). Thus the anion gap is increased in the metabolic acidosis associated with renal failure, ketoacidosis, lactic acidosis, or the ingestion of large quantities of aspirin.

ARTERIAL OXYGENATION

The arterial measurement of Po_2 reports the partial pressure of O_2 physically dissolved in blood. It is determined by the gradient for O_2 transport across the alveolar-capillary membrane, which is largely determined by the alveolar O_2. As previously described (see Chapter 5), the ideal alveolar O_2 is given by the alveolar gas equation, and the difference between the ideal alveolar O_2 and the actual arterial O_2 (the alveolar-arterial oxygen difference, or $AaDo_2$) is used to determine whether there is evidence of abnormal arterial oxygenation (see Chapter 7).

In interpreting arterial blood gas values, it is essential to know whether the individual was receiving supplemental O_2 or was on room air. One quick check of this is to add the Pao_2 and the $Paco_2$ together. The sum of the Pao_2 and $Paco_2$ with the patient breathing room air should be less than 130 mm Hg (at sea level). If it is greater than 130 mm Hg, the patient may have been on supplemental oxygen.

The exact quantity of inspired oxygen (Fio_2) that a patient is receiving can also be difficult to determine if he or she is receiving oxygen by nasal cannula. To convert nasal oxygen flow (L/min) to approximate Fio_2, assume a 4% increase in Fio_2 per liter of nasal flow. This is a reasonable approximation, however, only if the patient's minute ventilation (respiratory rate × tidal volume) is nearly normal. Normal values for arterial oxygen tension also decrease with age. One way to estimate the normal Pao_2 with increasing age is:

$$Pao_2 = 105 - \text{patient's age}/2 \qquad \text{Equation 5}$$

Thus the normal arterial oxygen tension of an 80-year-old individual is 65 mm Hg. It is apparent that in elderly individuals there is only a small margin between normal and what could be harmful to various organs and cells in the body

Finally, the arterial Po_2 response to 100% supplemental oxygen can be used to determine the pathophysiologic process responsible for hypoxemia. Persistent hypoxemia despite 100% oxygen or an increasing Fio_2 indicates the presence of an anatomic shunt and is frequently seen in children with cyanotic congenital heart disease.

ANALYZING ARTERIAL BLOOD GAS VALUES

A systematic approach to interpreting arterial blood gas values can help the student have a better understanding of underlying physiologic principles.

Step 1: Is there an acidosis or alkalosis?

The first step in examining the acid-base component of an arterial blood gas is to determine the net disturbance in acid-base balance by examining the pH. If the pH is 7.45 or greater, an alkalosis, respiratory or metabolic or both, is present. Similarly, a pH of 7.35 or less is indicative of an acidosis. A normal pH indicates normal acid-base status or a mixed disturbance that is balanced (e.g., a respiratory acidosis with a metabolic alkalosis).

Step 2: Is the primary disorder of respiratory or metabolic origin?

Next examine the Pco_2 and its relation to the pH. An abnormal Pco_2 is greater than 45 mm Hg or less than 35 mm Hg. If the pH value moves in the appropriate direction of the Pco_2 (i.e., increased pH with decreased Pco_2 or decreased pH with increased Pco_2), a respiratory disorder is the primary disturbance. Similarly, if the pH value does not move in the appropriate direction of the Pco_2, a metabolic disorder is the primary disturbance. Specifically, if there is an acidosis and the Pco_2 is greater than 45 mm Hg, the acidosis is respiratory in nature. If there is an acidosis and the Pco_2 is less than 40 mm Hg, the acidosis is metabolic with respiratory compensation (hyperventilation). In the same way, if there is an alkalosis and the Pco_2 is greater than 40 mm Hg, the alkalosis is metabolic with respiratory compensation (hypoventilation), and if there is an alkalosis and the Pco_2 is less than 40 mm Hg, the alkalosis is respiratory in nature.

Step 3: Is there evidence of respiratory or metabolic compensation?

The final step in analysis of acid-base balance is to determine whether the changes are acute or chronic. For a primary respiratory abnormality, calculate the change in pH that would occur if the change in Pco_2 were acute (0.08/10–mm Hg change

TABLE 9-5			
Compensation Formulas for Acid-Base Disturbances			
PRIMARY DISORDER	PRIMARY RESPONSE	COMPENSATORY RESPONSE	CHRONIC RESPONSE MAGNITUDE
Respiratory Acidosis	P_{CO_2}	HCO_3^-	HCO_3^- increases 3.5 mEq/L for each 10 mm Hg increase in P_{CO_2}
Respiratory Alkalosis	P_{CO_2}	HCO_3^-	HCO_3^- falls 5 mEq/L for each 10 mm Hg increase in P_{CO_2}
Metabolic acidosis	HCO_3^-	P_{CO_2}	$P_{CO_2} = 1.5 \ (HCO_3^-) + 8 \pm 2$
Metabolic alkalosis	HCO_3^-	P_{CO_2}	P_{CO_2} increases 6 mm Hg for each 10 mEq/L increase in HCO_3^-

Adapted from Weinberger SE: Principles of Pulmonary Medicine, 4th ed. Philadelphia, WB Saunders, 1998.

in P_{CO_2}) or chronic (0.03/10–mm Hg change in P_{CO_2}). For a primary metabolic disorder, a rough guide is that the Pa_{CO_2} should approximate the last two digits of the pH value (e.g., 7.25 should be associated with a P_{CO_2} of 25 mm Hg). Equations to calculate respiratory compensation for primary metabolic disorders are available but are not widely used clinically (Table 9-5).

Step 4: What Is the Alveolar-Arterial Oxygen Difference (AaDo$_2$)?

It is important to determine if oxygen exchange is normal. Using the alveolar gas equation, determine the ideal PA_{O_2}. Compare this value with the measured Pa_{O_2}. If the difference is greater than 25 mm Hg with the patient breathing room air, there is a problem with oxygenation.

SUMMARY

1. The arterial blood gas measurement of Pa_{O_2}, Pa_{CO_2}, and pH is the best overall test of lung function.
2. Arterial blood gas values should always be interpreted in light of the patient's history and symptoms.
3. Pulse oximetry measures oxygen saturation continuously.
4. The Henderson-Hasselbach equation for the bicarbonate buffer system states that the pH in blood is equal to a constant (pK) plus the log ratio of bicarbonate (kidneys) to P_{CO_2} (respiratory system).
5. Respiratory effects on acid-base status center around the elimination of carbon dioxide, whereas renal effects center around the excretion of fixed acids and the retention of filtered bicarbonate.
6. A respiratory acidosis is associated with a decrease in pH secondary to an increase in Pa_{CO_2} and is due to a decrease in the elimination of CO_2 by the lungs. A respiratory alkalosis is associated with an increase in pH secondary to a decrease in Pa_{CO_2} and is due an increase in the elimination of CO_2 by the lungs.

7. Compensation for metabolic abnormalities by the respiratory system occurs quickly, whereas renal compensation for respiratory abnormalities occurs over a period of 24 to 48 hours.
8. Compensation by the kidneys or lungs is rarely complete, and responses rarely overcompensate.
9. For each increase of 10 mm Hg in Pa_{CO_2}, the pH will fall 0.03 units if time is allowed for renal compensation, and 0.08 units if the process is acute and insufficient time for renal compensation has occurred.
10. The base excess represents the change in buffer base in the blood and is increased if a metabolic acidosis is present.
11. The anion gap represents the difference between the concentration of the major plasma cation (Na^+) and the major plasma anions (Cl^- and HCO_3^-) and can be used to determine the cause of a metabolic acidosis.
12. There are four steps in interpreting an arterial blood gas: (1) determine if an acidosis or alkalosis

is present; (2) determine whether the primary disorder is of respiratory or metabolic origin; (3) determine if there is respiratory or metabolic compensation; (4) determine the alveolar-arterial oxygen difference (AaDo$_2$).

KEY WORDS

- Alveolar-arterial oxygen difference (AaDo$_2$)
- Acid-base balance
- Alveolar ventilation
- Anion gap
- Arterial pH
- Base deficit
- Base excess
- Bicarbonate
- Buffer base
- Carbonic anhydrase reaction
- Davenport diagram
- Fixed acid
- Henderson-Hasselbach equation
- Homeostasis
- Hyperventilation
- Hypoventilation
- Metabolic acidosis
- Metabolic alkalosis
- Pulse oximetry
- Renal compensation
- Respiratory acidosis
- Respiratory alkalosis
- Respiratory compensation

SELF-STUDY PROBLEMS

1-5. Match the blood gas values and the basic defect or disease. All blood gases were drawn with the individual on room air.

a. pH = 7.40; Paco$_2$ = 40 mm Hg; Pao$_2$ = 110 mm Hg   1. Metabolic acidosis

b. pH = 7.34; Paco$_2$ = 60 mm Hg; Pao$_2$ = 60 mm Hg   2. Metabolic alkalosis

c. pH = 7.25; Paco$_2$ = 25 mm Hg; Pao$_2$ = 110 mm Hg   3. Laboratory error or patient on oxygen

d. pH = 7.50; Paco$_2$ = 30 mm Hg; Pao$_2$ = 50 mm Hg   4. Chronic hypoventilation; normal lung parenchyma

e. pH = 7.47; Paco$_2$ = 45 mm Hg; Pao$_2$ = 80 mm Hg   5. Hypoxemia with hyperventilation

6. A 55 year-old-woman, who is in good health, is upset because she has just learned that her husband is having an affair and has gambled away all their savings. She is brought to the emergency room in an agitated and breathless state. Three possible sets of arterial blood gas measurements are given in the following table. Which set of measurements best fits the patient's condition and history?

	Set A	Set B	Set C
pH	7.20	7.52	7.52
Pao$_2$ (mm Hg)	100	100	120
Paco$_2$ (mm Hg)	20	20	20
HCO$_3^-$ (mEq/L)	0	24	24
BE (mEq/L)	−15	+1	11

7. A 3-month-old infant is admitted to the hospital with wheezing, vomiting and decreased appetite. She is diagnosed with respiratory syncytial virus bronchiolitis and moderate dehydration from vomiting and decreased oral intake. Her arterial blood gas values while breathing room air are: pH = 7.32; Paco$_2$ = 25 mm Hg; Pao$_2$ = 66 mm Hg; BE = −12. mEq/L. The best interpretation of theses blood gas values is:

a. Metabolic acidosis, respiratory alkalosis
b. Metabolic acidosis, respiratory acidosis
c. Metabolic alkalosis, respiratory acidosis
d. Metabolic alkalosis, respiratory alkalosis
e. Respiratory alkalosis

8. A 59-year-old man is admitted to the hospital in acute respiratory distress resulting from emphysema complicated by pneumonia. He is conscious but confused, disoriented, and slow to respond to questions. He uses accessory muscles to breathe and there is decreased chest expansion and motion of the diaphragm. The man is started on oxygen therapy using a 24% Venturi mask (Fio$_2$, 24%). An arterial blood gas analysis reveals the following values: pH = 7.33; Pao$_2$ = 48 mm Hg; Paco$_2$ = 67 mm Hg; HCO$_3^-$ = 34 mEq/L.

The best interpretation of these values is:
  a. Metabolic acidosis, respiratory alkalosis
  b. Metabolic acidosis, respiratory acidosis
  c. Metabolic alkalosis, respiratory acidosis
  d. Metabolic alkalosis, respiratory alkalosis
  e. Respiratory acidosis

REFERENCES

Levitsky MG: Pulmonary Physiology, 4th ed. New York, McGraw-Hill, 1995.

Lim KG, Morgenthale, TI: Pulmonary function tests, part 2: Using pulse oximetry. J Respir Dis 26:85-88, 2005.

Morganroth ML: An analytic approach to diagnosing acid-base disorders. J. Crit Illness 5:138-150, 1990.

Shapiro BA, Peruzzi WT, Kozelowski-Templin R: Clinical Application of Blood Gases. 5th ed. St. Louis, Mosby, 1994.

Weinberger SE: Principles of Pulmonary Medicine, 4th ed. Philadelphia, WB Saunders, 2004.

Williams AJ: ABC of oxygen: Assessing and interpreting arterial blood gases and acid-base balance. BMJ 317:1213-1216, 1998.

CONTROL OF RESPIRATION

OBJECTIVES

1. Provide an overview of the three basic elements of the ventilatory control system.

2. Explain the structure and function of central chemoreceptors and peripheral chemoreceptors and their interrelationship.

3. Describe five chest wall and lung reflexes important in the control of respiration.

4. Describe the anatomy of the central respiratory control center and the relationship between the ventral and dorsal respiratory groups.

5. Describe the role of cerebrospinal fluid hydrogen ion and HCO_3^- in the regulation of respiration.

6. Explain the effects of hypoxemia, increased work of breathing, sleep, and acidosis on the ventilatory response to CO_2.

7. List three diseases associated with abnormal respiratory control.

R espiration demonstrates automaticity as well as self-modulation (voluntary). Although intermittent respiratory movements have been observed in utero, regular, automatic respiration begins at birth. Inspiration and exhalation occur automatically under the control of neurons located in the brainstem. At the same time, however, voluntary hyperventilation is easy, breath-holding is possible within limits, and our breathing pattern is modulated by the need for speech and singing.

Ventilatory control refers to the generation and regulation of rhythmic breathing by the respiratory center in the brainstem and its modification by the input of information from higher brain centers and systemic receptors. From a mechanical perspective, the goal of breathing is to minimize work; from a physiological perspective, the goal is to maintain blood gas levels and specifically to regulate arterial PCO_2. A third goal of breathing is to maintain the acid-base environment of the brain through the effects of ventilation on arterial PCO_2.

OVERVIEW OF VENTILATORY CONTROL

First, we will describe an overview of ventilatory control from a functional perspective. Then, we will examine each of the major areas in greater detail. Finally we will examine ventilatory control's integrated role in maintaining a normal $PaCO_2$.

The ventilatory control system consists of three basic elements (Fig. 10-1):

1. Sensors (peripheral and central chemoreceptors and pulmonary mechanoreceptors) that gather information and feed that information to the central controller.

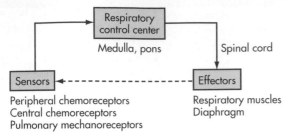

FIGURE 10-1 ■ The three major elements of the respiratory control system. Sensors, including central and peripheral chemoreceptors and pulmonary mechanoreceptors, feed information to the respiratory control center. In turn, the respiratory control center sends signals to the effectors such as the respiratory muscles and the diaphragm. Stimulation of the effectors subsequently reduces sensor activity through negative feedback.

2. The central controller (the respiratory control center) located in the brain that integrates and coordinates the information and sends signals to the effectors.

3. The effectors (respiratory muscles including the diaphragm) that produce changes in the ventilatory pattern.

As previously described in Chapter 5, alveolar ventilation is a function of respiratory rate and tidal volume. The respiratory rate is determined by the signal frequency from the central controller to the effectors, whereas the tidal volume is determined by the activity of the individual nerve fibers in the effectors to their motor units, including the frequency and duration of discharges and the number of units activated.

The **respiratory control center** is located in the reticular formation of the medulla oblongata beneath the floor of the fourth ventricle. This center is not a discrete nucleus but rather a poorly defined collection of different nuclei that generate and modify the basic rhythmic ventilatory pattern. It consists of two main parts—a **ventilatory pattern generator**, where the rhythmic pattern is generated, and an **integrator**, which processes inputs from higher brain centers and chemoreceptors and controls the rate and amplitude of the ventilatory pattern. The integrator controls the pattern generator and determines the appropriate ventilatory drive. Input to the integrator arises from higher brain centers including the cerebral cortex, hypothalamus, amygdala, limbic system, and cerebellum.

Within the central nervous system, **central chemoreceptors** are located just below the ventrolateral surface of the medulla. These chemoreceptors detect changes in the P_{CO_2}/pH of brainstem interstitial fluid and modulate ventilation.

Peripheral structures also provide input to the integrator and control ventilatory drive. Chemosensitive **peripheral chemoreceptors** are located on specialized cells in the aortic arch (**aortic bodies**) and at the bifurcation of the internal and external carotid arteries in the neck (**carotid bodies**). These chemoreceptors respond to changes in their local environment associated with decreases in P_{O_2}, increases in P_{CO_2}, and decreases in the pH of arterial blood and give afferent information to the central respiratory control center through the vagus nerve (aortic bodies) and the carotid sinus nerve, a branch of the glossopharyngeal nerve (carotid bodies), to make adjustments in alveolar ventilation that change whole body P_{CO_2}, pH, and P_{O_2}. And finally, the ventilatory pattern can be modulated by pulmonary **mechanoreceptors** and **irritant receptors** in the lung in response to the degree of lung inflation or the presence of an irritant in the airways.

The collective output of the respiratory control center to the motor neurons controls the muscles of respiration (the effectors) and it is this output that results in automatic, rhythmic respiration. The responsible motor neurons are located in the anterior horn of the spinal column. Intercostal muscles and the accessory muscles of respiration are controlled by motor neurons located in the thoracic region of the spinal column. Diaphragmatic motor neurons are situated in the cervical region of the spine and control diaphragmatic activity through the phrenic nerve.

In contrast to automatic respiration, voluntary respiration bypasses the medullary respiratory control center. It originates in the motor cortex, with information passing directly to the motor neurons in the spine through the corticospinal tracts. The respiratory muscle motor neurons thus act as the final site of integration of voluntary (corticospinal tract) and automatic (ventrolateral tract) control of ventilation. Voluntary control of these muscles competes with automatic influences at the level of the spinal motor neurons and can be demonstrated by breath holding. At the start of a breath hold, voluntary control dominates the spinal motor neurons, but as the breath hold continues, automatic ventilatory control eventually overpowers the voluntary effort and limits the duration of the breath hold.

There are also motor neurons that innervate the muscles of the upper airway. These are located within the medulla near the respiratory control center. They innervate muscles in the upper airways through cranial nerves. When activated, they result in dilation of the pharynx and large airways at the initiation of inspiration.

THE RESPIRATORY CONTROL CENTER

Most of what we know about the control of ventilation comes from studies in animals in which focal areas of the brain have been destroyed (ablation) or in which the brainstem has been surgically cross-cut (Fig. 10-2). When the brain is cross-cut between the medulla and the pons, periodic breathing is maintained even if all other afferents to the area, including the vagus

nerve, are severed, demonstrating that the inherent rhythmicity of breathing originates in the medulla. If the brain is transected below this area, breathing ceases. While no single group of neurons in the medulla has been found to be the breathing "pacemaker," there are two distinct groups of nuclei within the medulla that are involved in respiratory pattern generation (Fig. 10-3).

The first group is the **dorsal respiratory group** (DRG), which is composed of cells in the nucleus tractus solitarius located in the dorsomedial region of the medulla. These cells have the property of intrinsic periodic firing and are primarily responsible for inspiration and for the basic rhythm of ventilation. The tractus solitarius is also the primary projection site of visceral afferent fibers of the 9th cranial nerve (glossopharyngeal) and the 10th cranial nerve (vagus). These nerves provide information about P_{O_2}, P_{CO_2}, and pH from peripheral chemoreceptors and systemic arterial blood pressure. The vagus nerve also carries information from pulmonary mechanoreceptors. The input from the 9th and 10th cranial nerves to the

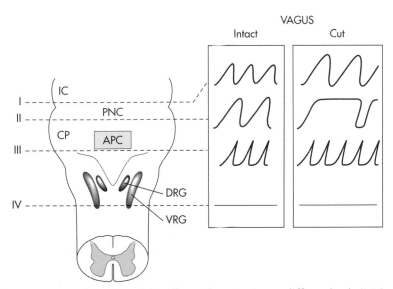

FIGURE 10-2 ■ The respiratory control center and the effects of transection at different levels (I-IV) on the ventilatory pattern. The respiratory control center is located in the medulla (the most primitive portion of the brain). Respiratory control neurons are located in two areas called the nucleus tractus solitarius and the nucleus retroambiguus. Transection at various sites in this area results in different breathing patterns depending upon the location and whether the vagus nerve is intact or has also been transected (cut). APC, apneustic center; CP, cerebellar peduncle; DRG, dorsal respiratory group; IC, inferior colliculus; PNC, pneumotaxic center; VRG, ventral respiratory group. (*Redrawn from Berger AJ, Mitchell RA, Severinghaus JW: Regulation of respiration. N Engl J Med 297:92, 1977. With permission of the New England Journal of Medicine.*)

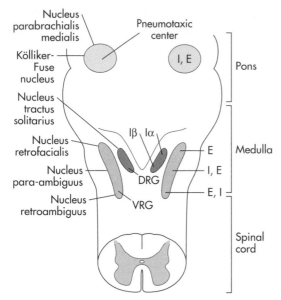

FIGURE 10-3 ■ Dorsal view of the location of the pontine and medullary respiratory neurons. DRG, dorsal respiratory group; E, expiratory; I, inspiratory; Iα and Iβ, two populations of inspiratory neurons in the DRG inhibited and excited, respectively, by lung inflation; VRG, ventral respiratory group. *(Modified from Berger AJ: Control of Breathing. In Murray J, Nadel JA (eds): Textbook of Respiratory Medicine. Philadelphia, WB Saunders, 1988.)*

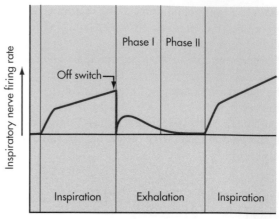

FIGURE 10-4 ■ Neural signaling of inspiratory motor neurons involves one inspiratory and two expiratory phases. Inspiration is abrupt followed by a steady ramp-like increase in neuron firing rate. At the end of inspiration, there is an off switch event resulting in a rapid decline in firing rate. Exhalation begins with a paradoxical increase in inspiratory neuron firing that brakes the expiratory phase. During the second phase of exhalation, this neuron firing becomes absent. *(Redrawn from Leff A, Schumacker P: Respiratory Physiology: Basics and Applications. Philadelphia, WB Saunders, 1993.)*

DRG is thought to constitute the initial intracranial processing station for these afferent inputs. However, even when all afferent stimuli to the DRG have been abolished, the DRG continues to generate repetitive bursts of action potentials. Thus, the DRG represents the breathing "pacemaker." Nuclei in this area project primarily to the contralateral spinal cord, where they serve as the principal initiators of phrenic nerve activity (supplying the diaphragm). The DRG also sends many fibers to the ventral respiratory group.

The second group of cells is the **ventral respiratory group** (VRG). The VRG is located bilaterally in the ventrolateral region of the medulla and is composed of three cell groups (the rostral nucleus retrofacialis, the caudal nucleus retroambiguus, and the nucleus para-ambiguus). The VRG contains both inspiratory and expiratory neurons. The primary function of these neurons is to drive either spinal respiratory neurons innervating the intercostal and abdominal muscles or the upper airway muscles of inspiration. Specifically, inspiratory neurons from the nucleus retroambiguus project to the contralateral external intercostals and to inspiratory and expiratory cells within the medulla, whereas expiratory neurons project to the contralateral spinal cord to drive the internal intercostals and abdominal muscles. The neurons in the nucleus para-ambiguus are primarily vagal motoneurons that innervate the laryngeal and pharyngeal muscles and are active during both inspiration and exhalation. Discharge from the cells in these areas appears to excite some cells and to inhibit other cells. The retrofacialis nucleus consists primarily of expiratory neurons. One group of expiratory cells located most rostrally in the retrofacialis nucleus is called the **Bötzinger complex.** This is the only group of neurons in the VRG that have been demonstrated to inhibit inspiratory cells in the DRG.

Inspiration and exhalation at the level of the respiratory control center involve three phases—one inspiratory phase and two expiratory (exhalation) phases (Fig. 10-4). After a latent period of several seconds during which there is no activity, inspiration begins with an abrupt increase in discharge in a crescendo pattern from cells in the nucleus tractus solitarius, and the nucleus retroambiguus. This steady ramp-like increase in firing rate occurs throughout inspiration, during which respiratory muscle activity becomes stronger. At the end of inspiration, there is an "off-switch" event that results in a marked decrease in neuron firing, at which point inspiratory muscle tone falls to its pre-inspiratory level and exhalation begins. At the start of exhalation (phase I), there is a paradoxical increase in inspiratory neuron firing that slows down or "brakes" the expiratory phase by increasing inspiratory muscle tone as well as expiratory neuron firing. This inspiratory neuron firing decreases and becomes absent during phase II of exhalation.

Although many different neurons in the DRG and VRG are involved in ventilation, each cell type appears to have a specific function. For example, within the DRG there are cell populations called Iα cells, which are inhibited by lung inflation, and Iβ cells, which are excited by lung inflation. These two cell populations may be important in the Hering-Breuer reflex, an inspiratory-inhibitory reflex that arises from afferent stretch receptors located in the smooth muscle of the airways. Increasing lung inflation stimulates these stretch receptors and results in an early exhalation by stimulating neurons associated with the off-switch phase of inspiratory muscle control.

Two other areas located in the brainstem are also important in respiratory control. The **pneumotaxic center** is located in the upper pons in the nucleus parabrachialis medialis and the Kölliker-Fuse nucleus. Impulses from the pneumotaxic center result in premature termination of the inspiratory ramp, resulting in a shortened inspiration. As a result of a shortened inspiration, respiratory rate increases. Thus the pneumotaxic center can regulate tidal volume and respiratory rate. It appears to be important in fine-tuning respiratory rhythm.

The **apneustic center** is located in the lower pons. When the brain is sectioned just above this area (level II), *apneusis*, or prolonged inspiratory gasps, are seen if the vagus nerves are also transected. (Apneusis does not occur if the vagus nerves are intact.) Apneusis is probably caused by a sustained discharge of medullary respiratory neurons. Its role in humans is unclear, but it may be the site of afferent information that terminates inspiration. Apneustic breathing is seen after head trauma that damages the pons, and its presence helps to localize the site of injury.

Thus rhythmic breathing depends on a continuous (tonic) inspiratory drive from the dorsal respiratory group and on intermittent (phasic) expiratory inputs from the cerebrum, thalamus, cranial nerves, and ascending spinal cord sensory tracts. The DRG may drive the VRG, but contrary to early thought, reciprocal inhibition between the two groups is unlikely.

SPINAL PATHWAYS

Axons from the respiratory control center from the cortex and from other supraspinal sites descend in the spinal cord white matter to the diaphragm and to the intercostal and abdominal muscles. These descending axons are coupled with local spinal reflexes in an integrated manner. Descending axons with inspiratory activity excite external intercostal motor neurons and, at the same time, inhibit internal intercostal motor neurons by exciting spinal inhibitory interneurons. Premature infants have uncoordinated respiratory muscle activity, especially during sleep, that can result in paradoxical chest wall and abdominal motion. In addition to contributing to abnormal gas exchange, this paradoxical motion can result in respiratory muscle fatigue and respiratory failure.

CENTRAL CHEMORECEPTORS

Chemoreceptors are receptors that respond to a change in the chemical composition of the blood or other fluid around it. Central chemoreceptors are specialized cells that are located on the ventrolateral surface of the medulla but are anatomically separate from the medullary-located respiratory control center (Fig. 10-5). These chemoreceptors are sensitive to the pH of the extracellular fluid around them. Because this extracellular fluid is in contact with the cerebrospinal fluid (CSF), changes in the pH of the CSF affect ventilation by acting on these chemoreceptors.

CSF is in part an ultrafiltrate of plasma that is secreted continuously by the choroid plexus and reabsorbed by the arachnoid villi. Because it is in contact

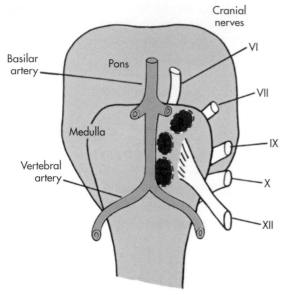

FIGURE 10-5 ■ The locations of the three CO_2 ([H+])-sensitive areas on the ventrolateral medulla. The receptor cells are not actually at the surface but are close to it. R, I, and C refer to the rostral, intermediate, and caudal receptor areas, respectively. *(From Berne RM, Levy ML, Koeppen BM, Stanton BM (eds): Physiology, 5th ed. St. Louis, Mosby, 2004.)*

with the extracellular fluid in the brain, CSF reflects the conditions surrounding the cells in the brain. Although the origin of CSF is the plasma, the composition of CSF is not the same as plasma because there is a barrier to free ion flow between the two sites. This barrier is termed the **blood-brain barrier**, and it separates CSF from the arterial blood. It is composed of endothelial cells, smooth muscle, and pial and arachnoid membranes, and it regulates ion flow. In addition, the choroid plexus also determines the composition of CSF.

The blood-brain barrier is relatively impermeable to hydrogen and HCO_3^- ions, but molecular CO_2 diffuses across it readily (Fig. 10-6). Because of this, alterations in arterial P_{CO_2} are rapidly transmitted to the CSF with a time constant of about 60 seconds. Thus, the P_{CO_2} in the CSF parallels the arterial P_{CO_2} tension. It is not identical, however, because carbon dioxide is also produced by the cells of the brain as a product of metabolism. As a consequence, the P_{CO_2} in the CSF is usually a few torr higher than the P_{CO_2} in

the arterial blood and the pH is slightly more acidic (7.32-7.33) than in plasma.

In addition to being a plasma ultrafiltrate with a slightly lower pH, the P_{CO_2} of CSF is about 10 mm Hg higher than arterial P_{CO_2} and the protein content is considerably lower than plasma (15-45 mg/100 mL, compared with 6.6-8.6 g/100 mL in plasma). As a result of this lower protein concentration, CSF has a lower buffering capacity compared with blood.

Similar to plasma, the **Henderson-Hasselbach equation** relates the pH of CSF to the bicarbonate ion concentration (HCO_3^-):

$$pH = pk + \log \frac{[HCO_3^-]}{0.03 P_{CO_2}}$$

where 0.03 is the solubility coefficient of CO_2 in mmol/liter torr and pK is the negative log of the dissociation constant for carbonic acid (pK = 6.1). The Henderson-Hasselbach equation demonstrates that increases in P_{CO_2} will be associated with decreases in pH at any given bicarbonate concentration. Likewise, increases in CSF bicarbonate will result in an increase in CSF pH at any given P_{CO_2}. As a consequence of this relationship, an increase in arterial P_{CO_2} will result in an increase in CSF P_{CO_2} and a decrease in CSF pH. Compared with blood, the buffer line of CSF is lower and not as steep as the buffer line of blood (because of the reduced buffering capacity). As a result, arterial hypercapnia leads to a greater change in hydrogen ion concentration in CSF compared with arterial blood.

An increase in H^+ ion concentration or P_{CO_2} or both results in a decrease in CSF pH that stimulates the central chemoreceptors, resulting in an increase in ventilation (Fig. 10-7). Ventilation increases almost linearly with changes in H^+ concentration. Thus the CO_2 in blood regulates ventilation by its effect on the pH of CSF. The resulting hyperventilation reduces P_{CO_2} in the blood and, therefore, in CSF. Increased arterial P_{CO_2} is also accompanied by cerebral vasodilation that enhances the diffusion of CO_2 into CSF. Although central chemoreceptors are very sensitive to changes in carbon dioxide, *central chemoreceptors do not respond to hypoxia.*

Changes in arterial pH that are not caused by changes in P_{CO_2} take longer to influence CSF. This is because hydrogen ions cross the blood-brain barrier

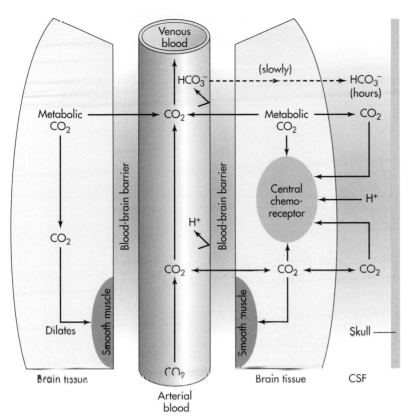

FIGURE 10-6 ■ CO_2 and the blood-brain barrier. Arterial CO_2 crosses the blood-brain barrier and rapidly equilibrates with cerebrospinal fluid (CSF) CO_2. H^+ and HCO_3^- ions cross the barrier only slowly. Arterial CO_2 combines with metabolic CO_2 to dilate smooth muscle. The pH of the CSF is lower and the P_{CO_2} is higher with little protein buffering compared with arterial blood. *(Modified from Levitzky MG: Pulmonary Physiology, 4th ed. New York, McGraw-Hill, 1995.)*

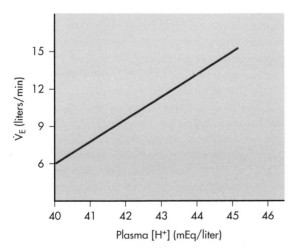

FIGURE 10-7 ■ The effect of H^+ concentration on minute ventilation ($\dot{V}_E$). Note that the relationship is linear. *(Redrawn from Levitzky MG: Pulmonary Physiology, 4th ed. New York, McGraw-Hill, 1995.)*

too slowly to affect the central chemoreceptors. Other receptors, particularly peripheral chemoreceptors, respond to a metabolic acidosis of nonbrain origin. Alveolar ventilation increases secondary to acidotic stimulation of peripheral chemoreceptors and arterial P_{CO_2} falls (Table 10-1). This results in diffusion of CO_2 out of CSF, an increase in CSF pH, and a decrease in central chemoreceptor stimulation. Over hours to days, the HCO_3^- concentration in CSF falls and the pH in the CSF returns toward normal (7.32). How the HCO_3^- concentration in CSF falls in not clear. Mechanisms that have been suggested include diffusion of HCO_3^- across the blood-brain barrier, active transport of HCO_3^- out of the CSF or decreased HCO_3^- formation as a result of carbonic anhydrase activity. That it occurs, however, is unquestioned because the pH of CSF in individuals with chronic obstructive pulmonary disease and a chronic respiratory acidosis

TABLE 10-1

Effects of Metabolic Acidosis (of Nonbrain Origin) on Arterial and Central Chemoreceptor Ventilatory Drive

| | ARTERIAL BLOOD | | | CEREBROSPINAL FLUID | | |
	pH	Pco_2	ARTERIAL CHEMO-RECEPTOR DRIVE	Pco_2	pH	CENTRAL CHEMO-RECEPTOR DRIVE
Initial acidosis	↓↓	Normal	↑↑	Normal	Normal	Normal
Ventilatory compensation for arterial acidosis	↓	↓↓	↑	Normal	Normal	Normal
"Diffusion" of CO_2 from CSF to blood	↓	↓↓	↑	↑	↓	↓

↑↑ and ↓↓ imply a greater increase and decrease, respectively, than ↑ and ↓.

is nearly normal, with a CSF HCO_3^- concentration that is proportional to the increased CO_2 in the blood. Thus, in CSF homeostasis, mechanisms and processes exist that regulate changes in pH and bring the system back to almost normal. The changes in CSF bicarbonate concentration, however, occur slowly over several hours, whereas the changes in Pco_2 in CSF can occur over minutes. Adjustments in ventilation attempt to maintain a normal CSF and arterial pH and Pco_2.

PERIPHERAL CHEMORECEPTORS

The carotid and aortic bodies are peripheral chemoreceptors that respond to decreases in arterial Po_2 (but not to changes in O_2 content), increases in Pco_2, and decreases in pH and transmit afferent information to the central respiratory control center. *The peripheral chemoreceptors are the only chemoreceptors that respond to decreases in Po_2.* Both the central and peripheral chemoreceptors respond to changes in Pco_2, with the peripheral chemoreceptors being responsible for approximately 40% of the ventilatory response to CO_2. Peripheral chemoreceptors respond rapidly; in fact, they are able to respond to breath-to-breath alterations in arterial blood composition. The carotid bodies appear to exert a greater influence on the respiratory control center than the aortic bodies, which appear to have a greater influence on the cardiovascular system.

The peripheral chemoreceptors are small, highly vascularized structures located near the bifurcations of the common carotid arteries (carotid bodies) and

in the arch of the aorta (aortic bodies) (Fig. 10-8). They consist of type I (glomus) cells that are rich in mitochondria and endoplasmic reticulum. They also contain several different types of cytoplasmic granules (synaptic vesicles) that contain different neurotransmitters, including dopamine, acetylcholine, norepinephrine, and neuropeptides. The type I cells are especially rich in dopamine and are the cells primarily responsible for sensing Po_2, Pco_2, and pH. Small increases in chemoreceptor discharge occur even with small decreases in arterial Po_2, but marked increases in chemoreceptor activity occur when arterial Po_2 decreases to less than 75 mm Hg. Increases in ventilation result when the Po_2 falls below 50 to 60 mm Hg. Afferent nerve fibers synapse with type I cells and transmit information to the brainstem through the carotid sinus nerve (carotid body) and vagus nerve (aortic body). It is not known how they respond to arterial changes in Po_2, Pco_2, and pH.

It can be seen from the preceding discussion that ventilation is regulated by changes in arterial and CSF pH and their effects on peripheral and central chemoreceptors. Homeostasis, the return toward normal ventilation, is regulated by changes in HCO_3^- transport in CSF and by renal compensatory mechanisms (Fig. 10-9). Box 10-1 illustrates this relationship.

CHEST WALL AND LUNG REFLEXES

A number of reflexes arise from the chest wall and lung and affect ventilation and ventilatory patterns (Table 10-2). First described in 1868, the **Hering-Breuer**

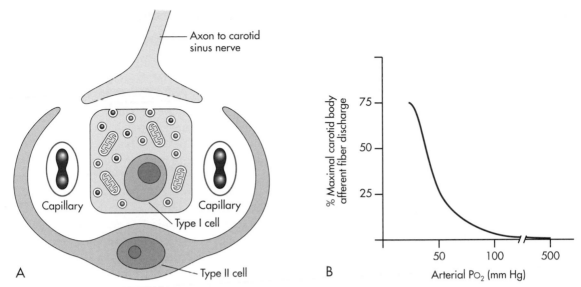

FIGURE 10-8 ■ Structure and function of the carotid body. **A,** The carotid body consists of type I and type II cells and has a rich capillary network. The type II, or glomus, cells contain large numbers of synaptic vesicles that contain neurotransmitters. These neurotransmitters are released in response to increased Pco₂, decreased pH, or decreased Po₂ in the arterial blood. The released neurotransmitters act upon adjacent nerve terminals. Signals from these nerve terminals are transmitted to the medullary respiratory control center through the carotid sinus nerve. **B,** Effect of Po₂ on carotid body afferent fiber discharge. There is a marked increase in activity when the arterial Po₂ falls below 75 mm Hg. When the Po₂ falls below 60 mm Hg, ventilation increases. *(Modified and redrawn from Leff A, Schumacker P: Respiratory Physiology: Basics and Applications. Philadelphia, WB Saunders, 1993.)*

inspiratory-inhibitory reflex is stimulated by increases in lung volume, especially those associated with an increase in both ventilatory rate and tidal volume. It is a stretch reflex mediated by vagal fibers located within the smooth muscle of large and small airways, which when elicited, results in cessation of inspiration by stimulating off-switch neurons in the medulla. This reflex is inactive during quiet breathing and plays a role in ventilatory control only at tidal volumes greater than 1 L in adults. It may help to minimize the work of breathing by inhibiting large tidal volumes and preventing alveolar overdistention. Its importance in humans other than newborns is unclear.

A second described Hering-Breuer reflex is the **Hering-Breuer deflation reflex**. It is associated with an increase in ventilatory rate due to abrupt lung deflation. The mechanism for this reflex is unknown, but decreased stretch receptor activity and stimulation of other receptors such as J receptors have been implicated.

The Hering-Breuer deflation reflex is thought to contribute to the increased ventilation in individuals with a pneumothorax and the periodic deep breaths (sighs) that occur normally; it may be important in preventing atelectasis (lung collapse), particularly in individuals who are being mechanically ventilated.

Stimulation of nasal or facial receptors with cold water initiates the **diving reflex**. When this reflex is elicited, apnea, or cessation of breathing, and bradycardia occur. This reflex protects individuals from aspirating in the initial stages of drowning. Activation of receptors in the nose is also responsible for the **sneeze reflex**.

Receptors are also present in the epipharynx and pharynx. Mechanical stimulation of these receptors produces the aspiration or **sniff reflex**. This is a strong, short-duration inspiratory effort that brings up material from the epipharynx to the pharynx where it can be swallowed or expectorated. These receptors are

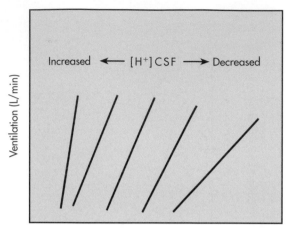

Increased ⟵ [H⁺] C S F ⟶ Decreased

Ventilation (L/min)

PaCO₂ (mm Hg)

FIGURE 10-9 ■ The ventilatory response to P_{CO_2} is affected by the hydrogen ion concentration, [H⁺], of the cerebrospinal fluid (CSF) and brainstem interstitial liquid. When a subject is in chronic metabolic acidosis (e.g., diabetic acidosis), the [H⁺] CSF is increased and the ventilatory response to inspired P_{CO_2} is increased (steeper slope). Conversely, when a subject is in chronic metabolic alkalosis (a relatively uncommon condition), the [H⁺] CSF is decreased and the ventilatory response to inspired P_{CO_2} is decreased (reduced slope). The positions of the response lines are also shifted, indicating altered response thresholds. *(From Berne RM, Levy ML, Koeppen BM, Stanton BM (eds): Physiology, 5th ed. St. Louis, Mosby, 2004.)*

important in swallowing by inhibiting respiration and causing laryngeal closure.

The larynx contains both superficial and deep receptors. Activation of the superficial receptors results in apnea, cough, and expiratory movements that protect the lower respiratory tract from aspirating foreign materials. The deep receptors are located in the skeletal muscles of the larynx. Negative pressure in the upper airway causes reflex constriction of the dilator muscles.

In the tracheobronchial tree, there are three major types of receptors. Inhaled dust, noxious gases, and cigarette smoke stimulate **irritant receptors** in the trachea and large airways, which transmit information through myelinated, vagal afferent fibers. This results in an increase in airway resistance, reflex apnea, and cough. These receptors are also known as **rapidly**

adapting pulmonary stretch receptors because their activity decreases rapidly during a sustained stimulus.

Slowly adapting pulmonary stretch receptors respond to mechanical stimulation and are activated by lung inflation. They also transmit information through myelinated, vagal afferent fibers. The increased lung volume in people with COPD stimulates these pulmonary stretch receptors and delays the onset of the next inspiratory effort. This allows the long, slow expiratory effort in these individuals that is essential to minimize dynamic, expiratory airway compression.

Specialized receptors exist in the lung parenchyma that respond to chemical or mechanical stimulation in the lung interstitium. These receptors are called **juxta-alveolar receptors** or **J receptors**. They transmit their afferent input through unmyelinated, vagal C-fibers. They may be responsible for the sensation of dyspnea (shortness of breath) and the altered ventilatory patterns (rapid, shallow) seen in individuals with interstitial lung edema and in some inflammatory lung states.

There are also **somatic receptors** in the intercostal muscles, rib joints, accessory muscles of respiration, and tendons that respond to changes in the length/tension of the respiratory muscles. Although they do not directly control respiration, they do provide information about lung volume and play a role in terminating inspiration. Somatic receptors are especially important in individuals with increased airway resistance and decreased pulmonary compliance because they can augment muscle force within the same breath. They also help to minimize the chest wall distortion during inspiration in the newborn who has a very compliant rib cage.

NONPULMONARY REFLEXES

The ventilatory pattern is also under voluntary control. Purposeful hyperventilation can result in a decrease in P_{aCO_2} and an increase in pH. The alkalosis that accompanies this hyperventilation can cause **carpopedal spasm**, contraction of the muscles of the hand and foot. An increase in arterial blood pressure stimulates aortic and carotid sinus baroreceptors and can cause reflex hypoventilation or apnea. Pain and temperature receptors can also affect ventilation.

BOX 10-1

In 1968, the summer Olympic games were held in Mexico City, Mexico. Mexico City is 7,240 feet above sea level or 1/2 mile higher than Denver, Colorado. Imagine that you are an athlete who lives in Boston and flies to Mexico City for the competition. The barometric pressure in Boston is ~760 mm Hg, whereas the barometric pressure in Mexico City is 585 mm Hg. At sea level, your Po_2 in arterial blood = ~95 torr. (Using the alveolar air equation in Chapter 5, $Pao_2 = [760 - 47 \text{ mm Hg}] \times 0.21 - 40/0.8 = 100$ torr. Assuming an $AaDo_2$ of 5 torr, your $Pao_2 = 100 - 5 = 95$ torr). In the cerebrospinal fluid (CSF), your pH would be ~7.33, your Pco_2 would be 44 torr ($Paco_2 + CO_2$ produced by metabolism of the brain cells) and your CSF HCO_3^- would be approximately 22 mEq/L.

When you arrive in Mexico City, there is an abrupt decrease in inspired O_2 ($Pio_2 = [585 - 47] \times 0.21 = 113$ torr) and a decrease in alveolar O_2 ($Pao_2 = 113$ torr $- 40$ torr$/0.8 = 63$ torr). If your $AaDo_2$ remained at 5, your Pao_2 would decrease to 58 torr. This decrease in arterial O_2 will result in stimulation of peripheral chemoreceptors and an increase in alveolar ventilation. The increase in ventilation will produce a decrease in $Paco_2$ and an increase in arterial pH. The net result of the increase in ventilation and decrease in $Paco_2$ is to minimize the hypoxemia by increasing your Pao_2 (For example, assume that the $Paco_2$ decreases to 31 torr; then $Pao_2 = [585 - 47$ torr$] \times 0.21 - 31$ torr$/0.8 = 74$ torr, an increase in Pao_2 of 11 torr.) The decrease in arterial Pco_2 also produces a decrease in CSF Pco_2. Because the bicarbonate concentration is unchanged, there is an increase in CSF pH. This increase attenuates the rate of discharge of central chemoreceptors and decreases their contribution to ventilatory drive.

Over the next 12 to 36 hours, the bicarbonate concentration in the CSF decreases as ion pumps or other mechanisms in the blood-brain barrier are activated. The result is that the CSF pH returns toward normal. Central chemoreceptor discharge increases and minute ventilation is further increased. At the same time that the bicarbonate concentration in the CSF is decreasing, there is a gradual excretion of bicarbonate ions from plasma by the kidney. This results in a gradual return of the arterial pH toward normal. Peripheral chemoreceptor stimulation increases further as arterial pH becomes normal (peripheral chemoreceptors are inhibited by elevated arterial pH).

The final result is that within 36 hours of arriving at high altitude, there is a significant increase in minute ventilation that is greater than the immediate effect of the hypoxemia on ventilation. This further increase is due to both central and peripheral chemoreceptor stimulation. Thus, by the end of the weekend, both arterial and CSF pH are approaching normal, minute ventilation is increased, arterial Po_2 is decreased (but less than when you arrived), and arterial Pco_2 is decreased.

You now return home. When you land in Boston, your Pio_2 returns to normal and the hypoxic stimulus to ventilation is removed. Arterial Po_2 returns to normal and the peripheral chemoreceptor stimulation to ventilation decreases. This results in an increase in arterial CO_2 toward normal. CSF CO_2 also increases toward normal. This increase is associated with a decrease in CSF pH, because the bicarbonate concentration in CSF is now reduced and ventilation is augmented.

Over the next 12 to 36 hours, ion pumps in the blood-brain barrier move HCO_3^- ions back into the CSF, with a gradual return of the CSF pH toward normal. Similarly, the pH in the blood decreases as the arterial Pco_2 rises because the arterial bicarbonate concentration is also decreased. This stimulates peripheral chemoreceptors, and minute ventilation remains augmented. Over the next 12 to 36 hours, renal mechanisms increase the blood HCO_3^- concentrations, the arterial pH returns to normal, and minute ventilation returns to normal.

RESPONSE TO CARBON DIOXIDE

Ventilation is regulated by the levels of CO_2, O_2, and pH in the arterial blood. Of these, the arterial Pco_2 is the most important. Both the rate and depth of breathing are controlled to maintain the $Paco_2$ close to 40 mm Hg. Even during periods of activity, rest, and sleep, the arterial Pco_2 is held at 40 ± 2 to 3 mm Hg. The importance of arterial CO_2 in ventilation can be demonstrated by having an individual breathe a low concentration of oxygen to which CO_2 is added to maintain a constant level of CO_2. Hypoxemia is sensed

TABLE 10-2			
Tracheobronchial Receptor Properties			
RECEPTOR TYPE	END-ORGAN LOCATION	STIMULI	REFLEXES
Myelinated Vagal Fibers			
Slowly adapting receptor	Among airway smooth muscle cells	Lung inflation	Hering-Breuer inflation reflex
			Hering-Breuer deflation reflex
			Inspiratory time-shortening
			Bronchodilation
			Tachycardia
			Hyperpnea
Rapidly adapting receptor (irritant receptor)	Among airway epithelial cells	Lung hyperinflation	Hering-Breuer deflation reflex
		Exogenous and endogenous agents	Cough
		Histamine	Mucus secretion
		Prostaglandins	Bronchoconstriction
Unmyelinated Vagal Fibers			
C-fiber ending (J receptors)	Pulmonary interstitial space	Large hyperinflation	Apnea, followed by rapid shallow breathing
	Close to pulmonary circulation	Exogenous and endogenous agents	Bronchoconstriction
	Close to bronchial circulation	Capsaicin	Bradycardia
		Phenyl diguanide	Hypotension
		Histamine	Mucus secretion
		Bradykinin	
		Serotonin	
		Prostaglandins	

by the peripheral chemoreceptors, which increase their rate of firing in response to the decrease in Pa_{O_2}. This stimulation in ventilation, however, does not occur until the Pa_{O_2} has dropped below 60 mm Hg. Below 60 mm Hg, there is marked stimulation of ventilation. However, if arterial Pa_{CO_2} is increased only a small amount (~5 mm Hg), ventilation is increased even in the presence of an increased level of Pa_{O_2} (Fig. 10-10). Only voluntary hyperventilation and the hyperpnea of exercise can surpass the minute ventilation observed with increasing hypercapnia.

The relationship between Pa_{CO_2} and ventilation is best shown in a classic experiment that was first performed many years ago. In this experiment, the alveolar P_{O_2} is maintained at a constant level and the subject rebreathes from a bag so that the inspired P_{CO_2} gradually rises. Ventilation is then plotted against alveolar P_{CO_2}, as shown in Figure 10-11. The central and peripheral chemoreceptors detect the change in Pa_{CO_2} and transmit this information to the medullary respiratory centers. The respiratory control center then regulates minute ventilation in order to control arterial P_{CO_2} within the normal range. Ventilation increases

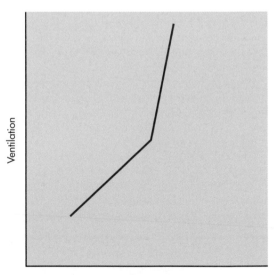

FIGURE 10-10 ■ Relationship between overall ventilation and tidal volume is depicted in awake state when ventilation is increased in response to respiratory stimuli such as hypercapnia. *(Redrawn from Murray JF, Nadel JA (eds): Textbook of Respiratory Medicine, 3rd ed, vol 1. Philadelphia, WB Saunders, 1994.)*

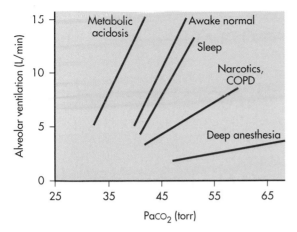

FIGURE 10-11 ■ Relationship between alveolar ventilation and changing P_{CO_2}. Responses to sleep and wakefulness, narcotic ingestion, chronic obstructive pulmonary disease (COPD), deep anesthesia, and metabolic acidosis. Both the slopes and the positions of the response curves are changed, indicating differences in ventilatory responses and response thresholds. *(Redrawn from Levitzky MG: Pulmonary Physiology, 4th ed. New York, McGraw-Hill, 1995.)*

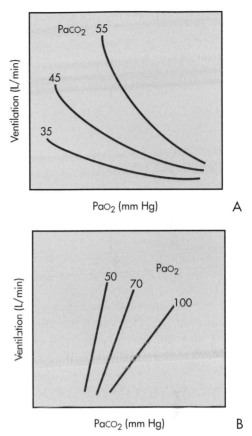

FIGURE 10-12 ■ The effects of hypoxia (**A**) and hypercapnia (**B**) on ventilation as the other respiratory gas partial pressure is varied. **A**, At a given Pa_{CO_2}, ventilation increases more and more as Pa_{O_2} decreases. When Pa_{CO_2} is allowed to decrease (the normal condition) during hypoxia, there is a little stimulation of breathing until P_{O_2} falls below 60 mm Hg. The hypoxic response is mediated through the carotid body chemoreceptors. **B**, The sensitivity of the ventilatory response to CO_2 is enhanced by hypoxia. *(From Berne RM, Levy ML, Koeppen BM, Stanton BM (eds): Physiology, 5th ed. St. Louis, Mosby, 2004.)*

as P_{CO_2} increases. In the presence of a normal Pa_{O_2}, the ventilation increases by about 3 L/min for each millimeter rise in Pa_{CO_2}. In the presence of a low Pa_{O_2}, there is greater ventilation for any given Pa_{CO_2} and the increase in ventilation with increasing Pa_{CO_2} is greater (steeper slope). The relationship between minute ventilation and the inspired CO_2 concentration is used as a test of CO_2 sensitivity. The slope of the response between minute ventilation and inspired CO_2 is termed the **ventilatory response to CO_2**. It is important to recognize that this relationship is amplified by low oxygen levels. This is because separate mechanisms are responsible for sensing P_{O_2} and P_{CO_2} in the peripheral chemoreceptors. Thus the presence of both hypercapnia and hypoxemia (sometimes called asphyxia when hypoxia is present) has an additive effect on chemoreceptor output and the resulting ventilatory stimulation (Fig. 10-12).

The ventilatory response to CO_2 is reduced by sleep, hyperventilation, increasing age, and genetic, racial, and personality factors. Trained athletes and divers, in general, have a lower CO_2 response. Drugs that depress the respiratory center such as morphine, barbiturates,

and anesthetic agents decrease the ventilatory response to both CO_2 and O_2. In these instances, there is an inadequate stimulus to drive the motor neurons that innervate the muscles of respiration. Hypoventilation results, and arterial P_{CO_2} increases.

The ventilatory response to CO_2 is also reduced if the work of breathing is increased. This is primarily because the neural output of the respiratory center, which is (almost) normal, is not as effective in producing ventilation because of the mechanical limitation to ventilation. In addition, in individuals with chronic obstructive pulmonary disease (COPD), there is evidence that the sensitivity of the respiratory control center is reduced. Metabolic acidosis shifts the CO_2 response to the left, demonstrating an increase in ventilation during metabolic acidosis for any particular Pa_{CO_2}.

RESPONSE TO HYPOXIA

The ventilatory response to hypoxia arises solely from stimulation of peripheral chemoreceptors and, most especially, stimulation of the carotid body. If an individual rebreathes air from a bag in which the P_{CO_2} is held constant at 40 mm Hg, there is little change in ventilation until the arterial P_{O_2} falls below 50 to 60 mm Hg. As one might anticipate, the response to arterial P_{O_2} is potentiated at higher arterial P_{CO_2} levels. The response to hypoxia is the response to P_{O_2}, not to O_2 content. This is why neither anemia nor carbon monoxide poisoning stimulates ventilation.

ABNORMALITIES IN CONTROL OF BREATHING

Changes in ventilatory pattern can occur for both primary and secondary reasons. During sleep, the carbon dioxide response curve shifts to the right (increased set point), and the slope of the response decreases slightly. As a result, during slow wave sleep, arterial P_{CO_2} rises as much as 5 to 6 torr. Approximately one third of normal individuals have brief episodes of apnea or hyperventilation during sleep that have no significant effect on arterial P_{O_2} and P_{CO_2}. These apneas usually last less than 10 seconds and occur during the lighter stages of slow-wave and rapid eye movement (REM) sleep. In a small number of individuals, the duration of apnea is abnormally prolonged, resulting in changes in arterial P_{O_2} and P_{CO_2}. These individuals have sleep-disordered breathing.

There are two major categories of **sleep disordered breathing—obstructive sleep apnea** (OSA) and **central sleep apnea.**

OSA (Fig. 10-13) is the most common of the sleep apnea abnormalities and occurs when the upper airway (usually the hypopharynx) closes during inspiration.

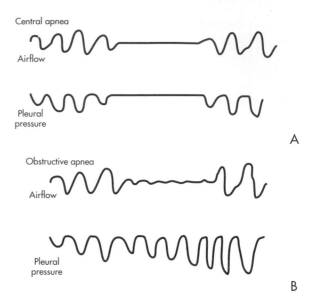

FIGURE 10-13 ■ The two main types of sleep apnea. **A**, Central apnea is characterized by the absence of an attempt to breathe, as demonstrated by no pleural pressure oscillations. **B**, In obstructive sleep apnea, the pleural pressure oscillations increase as CO_2 rises. This indicates that airflow resistance is very high, owing to upper airway obstruction. *(From Berne RM, Levy ML, Koeppen BM, Stanton BM (eds): Physiology, 5th ed. St. Louis, Mosby, 2004.)*

Although the process is similar to what happens during snoring, it has more severe effects, obstructing the airway and causing cessation of airflow.

The histories of individuals with OSA are similar. A spouse usually reports that the individual snores. The snoring becomes louder and louder and then suddenly stops while the individual continues to make vigorous respiratory efforts. The individual is then aroused, goes back to sleep, and begins the same process repetitively throughout the night.

The upper airway is the source of the airway obstruction and the obstruction is due to failure of the pharyngeal muscles to contract properly as a result of excessive fat around the pharynx or airway blockage by the tongue. The arousal occurs when the arterial hypoxemia and hypercarbia stimulate both peripheral and central chemoreceptors. Respiration is restored briefly before the next apneic event occurs. Individuals with OSA can have hundreds of these events each night.

As a consequence, they are sleep-deprived even though they do not awaken fully with each episode.

Other complications of OSA include polycythemia, right-sided cardiac failure (cor pulmonale), and increased risk for aortic dissection and pulmonary hypertension secondary to the recurrent hypoxic events. The most common cause of OSA is obesity. Other causes include excessive compliance of the hypopharynx, upper airway edema, and structural abnormalities of the upper airway. Treatment includes weight loss, oral appliances to pull the tongue forward, and bi-level positive airway pressure (Bi-PAP), which keeps the upper airway distended during inspiration.

Central sleep apnea occurs when there is a decrease in ventilatory drive to the respiratory motor neurons. The individual with central sleep apnea makes no respiratory efforts for abnormally long periods (1-2 minutes). Although the mechanism for this disorder is not clear in all individuals, a depressed response to CO_2 during sleep may be involved.

Central alveolar hypoventilation (CAH) is a rare disease in which voluntary breathing is intact but abnormalities in automaticity exist. It is also called **Ondine's curse**, named after a mythological tale in which the suitor of Neptune's daughter (Ondine) was cursed to lose automatic control over all bodily functions during sleep.

While awake, individuals with CAH have sufficient voluntary control over ventilation to maintain normal blood gas values, but during sleep or during times when ventilation is dependent on automatic ventilatory control (e. g., the individual is distracted by reading, watching TV, or playing a game), marked hypoventilation or apnea may occur. For these individuals, mechanical ventilation or, more recently, bilateral diaphragmatic pacing (similar to a cardiac pacemaker) can be life-saving.

Another problem potentially related to abnormal ventilatory control is **sudden infant death syndrome** (SIDS). SIDS is the most common cause of death in infants in the first year of life outside of the perinatal period. Although the cause of SIDS is not known, abnormalities in ventilatory control and particularly in CO_2 responsiveness have been implicated. Placing infants on their back to sleep (reducing the potential for CO_2 rebreathing) has dramatically decreased (but not eliminated) the death rate from this syndrome.

Cheyne-Stokes ventilation, another abnormality in ventilatory control, is characterized by a varying tidal

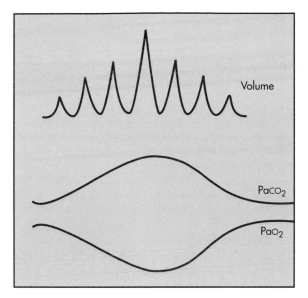

FIGURE 10-14 ■ In Cheyne-Stokes breathing, tidal volume and consequently arterial blood gases wax and wane. Generally, Cheyne Stokes breathing is a sign of vasomotor instability, particularly low cardiac output. *(From Berne RM, Levy ML, Koeppen BM, Stanton BM (eds): Physiology, 5th ed. St. Louis, Mosby, 2004.)*

volume and ventilatory frequency (Fig. 10-14). Following a period of apnea, tidal volume and respiratory frequency increase progressively over several breaths and then progressively decrease until apnea occurs. This irregular breathing pattern is seen in some individuals with central nervous system diseases including head trauma and increases in intracranial pressure. It is also present occasionally in normal individuals during sleep at high altitude. The mechanism for Cheyne-Stokes respiration is unknown. In some individuals, it appears to be due to slow blood flow in the brain associated with periods of overshooting and undershooting ventilatory efforts in response to changes in P_{CO_2}.

Apneustic breathing, another abnormal breathing pattern (Fig. 10-15), is characterized by sustained periods of inspiration separated by brief periods of exhalation. The mechanism for this ventilatory pattern appears to be due to loss of inspiratory-inhibitory activities that results in the augmented inspiratory drive. The pattern is sometimes seen in individuals with central nervous system injury.

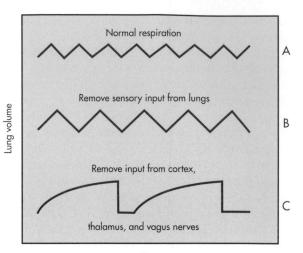

FIGURE 10-15 ■ Some patterns of breathing. **A,** Normal breathing at about 15 breaths/min in humans. **B,** The effect of removing sensory input from various lung receptors (mainly stretch) is to lengthen each breathing cycle and to increase tidal volume so that alveolar ventilation is not significantly affected. **C,** When input from the cerebral cortex and thalamus is also eliminated, together with vagal blockade, the result is prolonged inspiratory activity broken after several seconds by brief expirations (apneusis). *(From Berne RM, Levy ML, Koeppen BM, Stanton BM (eds): Physiology, 5th ed. St. Louis, Mosby, 2004.)*

SUMMARY

1. Respiratory control is both automatic and voluntary.
2. Ventilatory control is composed of sensors (central chemoreceptors, peripheral chemoreceptors, and pulmonary mechanoreceptors), controllers (the respiratory control center), and effectors (respiratory muscles).
3. The arterial P_{CO_2} is the major factor influencing ventilation.
4. The respiratory control center is composed of the dorsal respiratory group and the ventral respiratory group. Rhythmic breathing depends on a continuous (tonic) inspiratory drive from the dorsal respiratory group and on intermittent (phasic) expiratory inputs from the cerebrum, thalamus, cranial nerves, and ascending spinal cord sensory tracts.
5. The peripheral and central chemoreceptors respond to changes in P_{CO_2} and pH. The peripheral chemoreceptors (carotid and aortic bodies) are the only chemoreceptors that response to changes in P_{O_2}.
6. The blood-brain barrier is relatively impermeable to H^+ and HCO_3^- but CO_2 readily diffuses across it. Acute and chronic hypercarbia affect breathing differently because of slow adjustments in cerebrospinal fluid $[H^+]$ and $[HCO_3^-]$, which alter CO_2 sensitivity.

7. Hypoxia enhances CO_2 responsiveness. The ventilatory response to hypoxia alone arises solely from stimulation of peripheral chemoreceptors and in particular the carotid body and occurs in response to decreases in P_{O_2} and not to changes in O_2 content.
8. The pneumotaxic center regulates tidal volume and respiratory rate and is important in fine-tuning respiratory rhythm.
9. Pulmonary stretch receptors respond to mechanical stimulation and are activated by lung inflation.
10. Irritant receptors protect the lower respiratory tract from particles, chemical vapors, and physical factors, primarily by inducing cough.
11. C-fiber juxta-alveolar or J receptors in the terminal respiratory units are stimulated by distortion of the alveolar walls (lung congestion or edema).
12. The two most important clinical abnormalities of breathing are obstructive sleep apnea and central sleep apnea.

KEY WORDS

■ Aortic body
■ Apneustic breathing
■ Apneustic center

- Blood-brain barrier
- Carotid body
- Central alveolar hypoventilation
- Central chemoreceptors
- Central sleep apnea
- Cerebrospinal fluid
- Cheyne-Stokes respiration
- CO_2 ventilatory response curve
- Diving reflex
- Dorsal respiratory group
- Henderson-Hasselbach equation
- Hering-Breuer inspiratory inhibitory reflex
- Hering-Breuer lung deflation reflex
- Integrator
- Irritant receptor
- Juxta-alveolar receptor (J receptor)
- Obstructive sleep apnea
- Peripheral chemoreceptors
- Pneumotaxic center
- Pulmonary mechanoreceptors
- Pulmonary stretch receptors, rapidly adapting
- Pulmonary stretch receptors, slowly adapting
- Respiratory control center
- Sniff reflex
- Somatic receptors
- Sudden infant death syndrome
- Ventilatory control
- Ventilatory pattern generator
- Ventral respiratory group

SELF-STUDY PROBLEMS

1. Underwater swimmers sometimes hyperventilate before they go under water for long periods of time. What then is the impetus for respiration and why is this potentially dangerous?
2. Explain the acute and chronic ventilatory responses to altitude? What regulatory processes take place as a consequence of the change in arterial pH that develops during the first day of exposure to altitude?
3. How does an increase in $Paco_2$ influence the sensitivity of carotid bodies to Pao_2?
4. What is the mechanism of respiratory failure in individuals who have ingested an overdose of sleeping pills?

REFERENCES

Coleridge HM, Coleridge JC: Pulmonary reflexes: Neural mechanisms of pulmonary defense. Annu Rev Physiol 56:69-91, 1994.

Corne S, Webster K, Younes M: Hypoxic respiratory response during acute stable hypocapnia. Am J Resp Crit Care Med 167: 1193-1199, 2003.

de Castro D, Lipski J, Kanjhan R: Electrophysiological study of dorsal respiratory neurons in the medulla oblongata of the rat. Brain Res 639:49-56, 1994.

Funk GD, Feldman JL: Generation of respiratory rhythm and pattern in mammals: insights from developmental studies. Curr Opin Neurobiol 5:778-785, 1995.

Gonzalez C, Dinger B, Fidone SJ: Mechanisms of carotid body chemoreception In Dempsey JA, Pack AI (eds): Regulation of Breathing. New York, Marcel Dekker, 1995.

Jammes Y, Speck DF: Respiratory control by diaphragmatic and respiratory muscle afferents. In Dempsey JA, Pack AI (eds): Regulation of breathing. New York, Marcel Dekker, 1995.

Lee LY, Kou YR, Frazier DT, et al: Stimulation of vagal pulmonary C-fibers by a single breath of cigarette smoke in dogs. J Appl Physiol 66:2032-2038, 1989.

Robin ED, Whaley RD, Crump CH, Travis DM: Alveolar gas tensions, pulmonary ventilation and blood pH during physiologic sleep in normal subjects. J Clin Invest 37:98-989, 1958.

Sampol G, Romero O, Salas A, et al:. Obstructive sleep apnea and thoracic aorta dissection. Am J Resp Crit Care Med 168:1528-1531, 2003.

Sant'Ambrogio G, Tsubone H, Sant'Ambrogio FB: Sensory information from the upper airway: Role in the control of breathing. Respir Physiol 102:1-16, 1995.

Voipio J, Ballanyi K: Interstitial Pco_2 and pH and their role as chemostimulants in the isolated respiratory network of neonatal rats. J Physiol (Lond) 499:527-542, 1997.

Younes M. Contributions of upper airway mechanics and control mechanisms to severity of obstructive apnea. Am J Resp Crit Care Med 168:645-658, 2003.

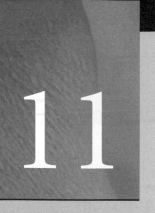

11 NONRESPIRATORY FUNCTIONS OF THE LUNG

OBJECTIVES

1. List the three major mechanisms of particle deposition in the airways.

2. Describe the three major components of mucociliary transport and their interaction in the defense of the lung.

3. Explain how the lung functions as an organ of the mucosal immune system.

4. Explain the roles of phagocytic, dendritic, and natural killer cells in lung defense.

5. Describe the function of the lung in humoral immune mechanisms.

6. Outline the immune response to bacteria in the normal lung.

7. List four pulmonary diseases associated with abnormalities in mucociliary transport and innate and adaptive immunity.

In addition to its primary function of gas exchange, the lung also functions as a major defense organ to protect the inside of the body from the outside world. Just as the respiratory system has developed unique systems to bring in and transport oxygen and simultaneously transport and expel carbon dioxide, it has also developed a unique series of defense systems to cope with environmental exposure and the constant insult of foreign agents.

The respiratory tract is continuously exposed to dust, pollen, ash, and other products of combustion; to microorganisms such as pathogenic viruses and bacteria; to particles or substances such as asbestos and silica; and to hazardous chemicals and toxic gases. In addition, liquids and food particles can be accidentally aspirated (inspired) from the oropharynx or nasopharynx into the airways. The respiratory tract processes and disposes of these foreign substances using three categories of defense mechanisms: (1) mucociliary

clearance that moves inhaled and trapped particles cephalad toward the mouth, (2) phagocytic and inflammatory cells that destroy inhaled material, and (3) a specialized mucosal immune system. The fact that the distal lung parenchyma is normally sterile is testimony to the effectiveness of these three defense systems.

First, we will describe the structural features of the mucociliary clearance system that limit exposure; next we will describe the major phagocytic mechanisms of defense, and finally we will describe the immunologic defense systems in the lung involved with retained particles. Epithelial defense, phagocytic cells, complement, and other blood-derived mediators of inflammation and a variety of cytokines are the principal components of innate immunity, a system of rapid, nonspecific responses to repetitive exposures. In contrast, T-lymphocyte responses, including humoral and cell-mediated responses, are part of the adaptive immune system, a system of specific immune responses to foreign substances known as **antigens**.

AEROSOL DEPOSITION IN THE LUNG

Aerosols are collections of particles that remain airborne for a substantial length of time. Large-particle aerosols tend to settle rapidly down to the floor in a sealed room, whereas fine-particle aerosols remain airborne for longer periods of time. In the respiratory tract, the pattern of aerosol deposition is based mainly on particle size (Fig. 11-1), although distance traveled, mode and pattern of breathing, size and shape of the airways, particle density, and relative humidity also influence patterns of deposition. There are three major mechanisms of particle deposition in the airways: impaction, sedimentation, and diffusion (Fig. 11-2).

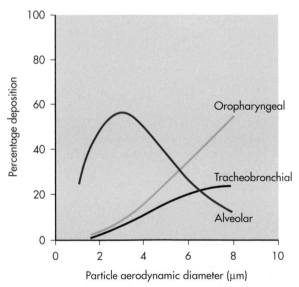

FIGURE 11-1 ■ Inhaled particles are trapped at different locations in the airways, according to their size. Particles with diameters greater than ~5 mm tend to impact into the nasopharynx, oropharynx, or large conducting airways. Smaller particles are more likely to become trapped in the distal airways or in the alveoli. *(Redrawn from Clarke SW, Pavia D: Mucociliary clearance. In Crystal RG, West JB (eds): The Lung: Scientific Foundation. New York, Raven Press, 1991.)*

Impaction

Impaction is the tendency of large particles to land on the posterior nasopharynx as the inspired air stream abruptly changes direction. In general, particles larger than 5 μm in diameter are deposited by impaction in the nasal passages, where airflow is high and changes direction abruptly as a result of the upper airway anatomy. The nose is remarkably efficient at removing these large particles; almost all particles greater than 20 μm in diameter and approximately 95% of particles greater than 5 μm in diameter are filtered by the nose during quiet breathing. The anatomy of the nose is ideally suited for this function (see Fig. 1-1), with ribbons of tissue (turbinates) and nasal hairs (vibrissae) over which air is scrubbed. Smaller particles (2-5 μm in diameter) impact in the lower respiratory tract at points where the air stream changes direction (airway birfucations) and creates eddies that travel perpendicular to the airflow; the inertia of these particles prevents them from changing directions rapidly (**inertial impaction**). This usually occurs in areas with turbulent airflow such as the trachea and bronchi to the first 10 to 12 airway generations.

Sedimentation

In more distal areas, where airflow is slower, smaller particles (0.2-2 μm in diameter) deposit on the surface or on mucus secondary to gravity. This gradual settling of particles based on their weight is called **sedimentation**. Particle deposition by sedimentation occurs extensively in the small airways, including the terminal and respiratory bronchioles, in large measure because these airways are so small that particles have a short distance to fall, and airflow is so slow. (As discussed later, these sedimented particles are important in a number of respiratory diseases.) In addition, most bacteria fall within this size range, making this the most common site for their deposition in the lower respiratory tract.

Diffusion

Random movement of particles (Brownian motion) as a result of their continuous bombardment by gas molecules is called **diffusion** and is the third mechanism of particle deposition. Particle deposition by diffusion occurs with particles less than 0.1 μm in

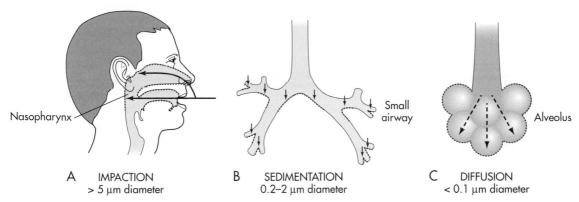

A　IMPACTION
> 5 µm diameter

B　SEDIMENTATION
0.2–2 µm diameter

C　DIFFUSION
< 0.1 µm diameter

FIGURE 11-2 ■ Aerosol deposition in the lung. **A,** Large particles deposit in the nose, mouth and posterior pharynx by impaction. **B,** Smaller particles deposit by gravity and sediment in smaller airways and at the bifurcations of larger airways. **C,** The smallest particles reach the alveoli and deposit on the alveolar surface by diffusion. *(Adapted from West J: Pulmonary Physiology and Pathophysiology. Philadelphia, Lippincott Williams & Wilkins, 2001.)*

diameter and mainly takes place in the smallest airways and alveoli. These particles are cleared by endocytosis by the alveolar macrophages, or they are carried away by lymphatics/lymphoid tissue or transported to the beginning of the mucociliary transport system.

REMOVAL OF DEPOSITED PARTICLES

Not all inhaled particles are deposited in the respiratory tract. Approximately 80% of particles between 0.1 and 0.5 µm in diameter stay suspended as aerosols and are exhaled. Deposited particles are efficiently removed either by **mucociliary transport** or by **phagocytic and inflammatory cells**.

Mucociliary Transport

The mucociliary transport system is one of the lung's structural, primary defense mechanisms. It protects the conducting airways by trapping and removing bacteria, inhaled particles, and cellular debris from the lung. Because new particles and toxic substances are continuously inhaled, even with normal respiration, a continuous system for the clearance of this material is needed. The mucociliary transport system is responsible for this continuous process. In general, the longer inhaled material remains in the airways, the greater the probability that lung damage will occur. Once particles

in the terminal airways have entered the interstitium, clearance is even slower and the likelihood of lung damage is even greater.

There are three major components of mucociliary transport: (1) the **periciliary fluid**, (2) the **mucus layer**, and (3) the **cilia** that beat in a lower layer of nonviscid, serous fluid (periciliary fluid) (Fig. 11-3).

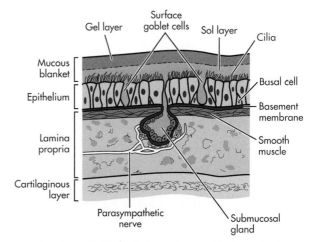

FIGURE 11-3 ■ Epithelial lining of the tracheobronchial tree. The cilia of the epithelial cell reside in the periciliary fluid layer with the mucus on top. Interspersed between the ciliated epithelial cells are surface secretory (goblet) cells and submucosal glands. *(From Berne RM, Levy ML, Koeppen BM, Stanton BM (eds): Physiology, 5th ed. St. Louis, Mosby, 2004.)*

Effective clearance requires both ciliary activity and respiratory tract fluid (periciliary fluid and mucus). Inhaled material is trapped in the relatively tenacious and viscous mucus, whereas the watery periciliary fluid allows the cilia to move freely with only their tips contacting the mucus and propelling it toward the mouth.

Periciliary Fluid

The periciliary fluid layer is produced by the pseudostratified, columnar epithelium that lines the respiratory system and that is joined together by tight junctions (see Fig. 1-9). Airway epithelial cells are ciliated and line the entire respiratory tract to the level of the bronchioles, where they are replaced by a cuboidal, nonciliated epithelium. The only exceptions are parts of the pharynx and the anterior third of the nasal cavity. The respiratory epithelial cells are responsible for maintaining the level of the periciliary

fluid, a layer of water 5 μm in depth, and electrolytes in which the cilia and mucociliary transport system function. The depth of the periciliary fluid is maintained by the movement of ions across the epithelium. Active (i.e., dependent upon energy, as in adenosine triphosphate) chloride secretion into the airway lumen occurs through chloride (Cl^-) channels in the apical membrane. These channels are regulated by intracellular cyclic adenosine monophosphate (cAMP) and calcium. Sodium (Na^+) is absorbed through sodium channels in the apical membrane (Fig. 11-4). Both chloride secretion and sodium absorption translocate water secondarily (osmotic equilibrium) and it is the balance between Cl^- secretion and Na^+ absorption that regulates the depth of the periciliary fluid. A sodium-potassium adenosine triphosphatase (ATPase) (Na^+,K^+-ATPase) pump in the basolateral membrane maintains the sodium gradient, allowing for sodium absorption. An Na^+-Cl^- co-transporter in the basolateral membrane links sodium and chloride flux, leading to a build-up in chloride in the cell above its electrochemical equilibrium and to diffusion down a favorable gradient into the airway lumen. The sodium that accompanies chloride is then transported back across the basolateral membrane by the Na^+,K^+-ATPase pump.

Thus active secretion of Cl^- into the airway lumen produces fluid secretion, whereas active Na^+ absorption accounts for the ability to absorb fluid. It is the balance between chloride secretion and sodium absorption that regulates the depth of the periciliary fluid at 5 to 6 μm (Table 11-1). This depth is important for the normal functioning of the cilia. If it is too deep, cilia splash around, and if it is not deep enough, ciliary function is markedly diminished.

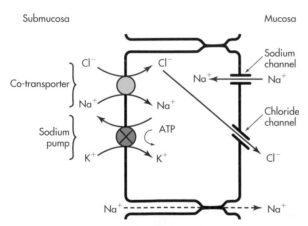

FIGURE 11-4 ■ Mechanisms of ion transport in airway epithelial cells. A co-transporter in the basolateral membrane links sodium and chloride flux, leading to a build-up in chloride above its electrochemical equilibrium. A sodium-potassium ATPase pump in the same membrane transports sodium out of the cell and thus maintains a sodium gradient inside the cell. A sodium channel and a chloride channel in the apical membrane provide for sodium influx into the cell and chloride efflux out of the cell. ATP, adenosine triphosphate. Osmotic equilibrium is maintained by the diffusion of water accompanying net solute flux. *(From Berne RM, Levy ML, Koeppen BM, Stanton BM (eds): Physiology, 5th ed. St. Louis, Mosby, 2004.)*

Mucus Layer

The **mucus layer** or **gel layer** lies on top of the periciliary fluid layer and is propelled by the cilia. Airway mucus is a complex mixture of macromolecules including proteins, glycoproteins, electrolytes, and water. The mucus layer is 5 to 10 μm thick and exists as a discontinuous blanket (i.e., islands of mucus). Three cells produce the mucus layer: surface secretory cells, submucosal tracheobronchial glands, and Clara cells. These cells control both the quantity and composition of macromolecules in the mucus.

TABLE 11-1
Agents that Stimulate Chloride Secretion in Airway Epithelia

AGENT	SURFACE*	cAMP
β-Adrenergic agonist	Submucosal	↑
Prostaglandin E₂	Submucosal	↑
Prostaglandin F₂	Submucosal	—
Vasoactive intestinal peptide	Submucosal	↑
Adenosine	Mucosal	↑
Leukotrienes LTC₄ and LTD₄	Mucosal and submucosal	↑?
Substance P	Mucosal and submucosal	?
Bradykinin	Mucosal and submucosal	↑?

*Surface is the side of the epithelium on which the agents act.
↑, increase; ?, uncertainty; —, no measurable change.
From Welsh MJ: Production and control of airway secretions. In Fishman AP: Pulmonary Diseases and Disorders, 2nd ed. New York, McGraw-Hill, 1988.

links the carbohydrate to the protein), and unlinked proteins form disulfide or peptide bonds. The result is a high molecular weight glycoprotein with low viscosity and high elasticity. It is this elasticity that prevents mucus from backsliding during clearance. Mucus is 95% to 97% water.

Surface secretory cells (also called **goblet cells**) line the respiratory epithelium and are present in approximately every 5 to 6 ciliated cells (see Fig. 1-19). They decrease in number between the 5th and 12th lung divisions and disappear completely beyond the 12th tracheobronchial division. They secrete neutral and acidic glycoproteins rich in sialic acid. In response to a chemical signal, goblet cells discharge their stored material by the process of exocytosis, in which membrane-bound storage granules fuse with the plasma membrane and subsequently open to the airway lumen and release their contents. In the presence of cigarette smoke or in patients with chronic bronchitis, surface secretory cells increase in size and number and extend further down the respiratory tract toward the alveolus. Their output also increases, and

Mucus is composed of glycoproteins and consists of groups of oligosaccharides that are attached to a protein backbone like the bones of a fish to the vertebral column (Fig. 11-5). The oligosaccharides are bound to the amino acids by "O" glycosidic bonds (i.e., oxygen

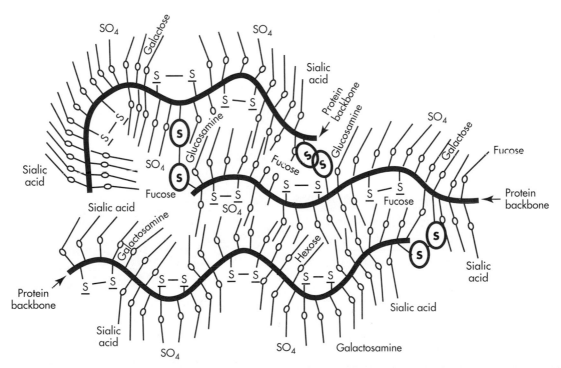

FIGURE 11-5 ■ Schematic drawing of mucus. Note the protein backbone with glycoprotein side chains and the "O" glycosidic and disulfide bonds. *(From Berne RM, Levy ML, Koeppen BM, Stanton BM (eds): Physiology, 5th ed. St. Louis, Mosby, 2004.)*

there is a change in the chemical composition of their secretions.

Submucosal tracheobronchial glands are present normally wherever there is cartilage; they empty into the airway lumen through a ciliated duct. In patients with chronic bronchitis, these glands are increased in number and size and can extend to the bronchioles. The glands' secretory component consists of **mucous cells** near the distal end of the tubule, which is lined by "nonspecified" cells, and of **serous cells** at the most distal end of the tubule (Table 11-2). Mucous cells contain large, often confluent, electron-lucent granules; serous cells contain small, discrete electron-dense secretory granules. The mucous cells of the submucosal tracheobronchial glands secrete acid glycoproteins while the serous cells secrete neutral glycoproteins and contain lysozyme, lactoferrin, and anti-leukoprotease. In disease, the chemical composition of the glycoproteins does not change, but there is an increase in the volume of the secretions and a change in the ratio of neutral glycoproteins to acidic glycoproteins that modifies the physical properties of the mucus. This change in viscosity and elasticity affects the subsequent clearance of the mucus. Gland secretion is under parasympathetic, adrenergic, and peptidergic (vasoactive intestinal peptide) neural control. Local inflammatory mediators such as histamine and arachidonic acid metabolites stimulate mucus production.

Clara cells are located in the bronchioles and contain granules. Although their exact function is not known, they secrete a nonmucinous material containing carbohydrate and protein. They also appear to play a role in bronchial regeneration after injury.

Normal individuals produce approximately 100 mL of mucus each day. Although some people even today refer to the "mucous blanket" in the airways, the mucus layer is actually "spotty" and varies in thickness between 2 and 5 µm. Most of the volume of the mucus is absorbed by the ciliated, columnar, epithelial lining cells, with only 10 mL reaching the glottis per day. This mucus is propelled to the back of the throat, where it is swallowed.

It is perhaps important at this point to distinguish mucus from **sputum**. Sputum is expectorated mucus. In addition to mucus, sputum contains serum proteins, lipids, electrolytes, calcium, and DNA from degenerated white cell nuclei (collectively known as bronchial secretions) and other secretions (e.g., nasal, oral, lingual, pharyngeal, and salivary secretions).

Cilia

Cilia are the microscopic hairlike scrubbers of the respiratory system. It is estimated that there are approximately 200 to 250 cilia per cell (Fig. 11-6). They are 2 to 5 µm in length and have a structure that has

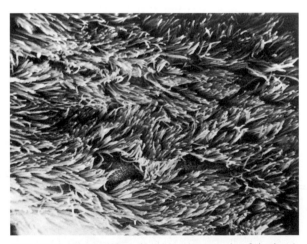

FIGURE 11-6 ■ Scanning electron micrograph of the luminal surface of a bronchiole from a normal man; many cilia are evident surrounding a nonciliated cell (×2000). *(Reprinted by permission from Ebert RV, Terracio MJ: The bronchiolar epithelium in cigarette smokers. Observations with the scanning electron microscope. Am Rev Resp Dis 111:4-11, 1975.)*

	TABLE 11-2	
	Properties of Submucosal Gland Cells	
	SEROUS CELLS	**MUCOUS CELLS**
Granules	Small, electron-dense	Large, electron-lucent
Glycoproteins	Neutral	Acidic
	Lysozyme, lactoferrin	
Hormone	α > β-Adrenergic	β > α-Adrenergic
Receptors	Muscarinic	Muscarinic
Degranulation	α-Adrenergic	β-Adrenergic
	Cholinergic	Cholinergic
	Substance P	

From Welsh MJ: Production and control of airway secretions. In Fishman AP: Pulmonary Diseases and Disorders, 2nd ed. New York, McGraw-Hill, 1988.

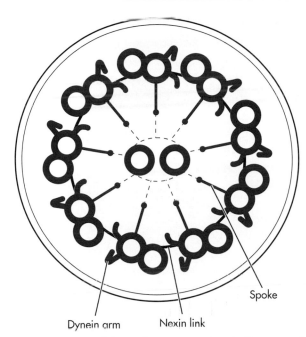

FIGURE 11-7 ■ Schematic cross-sectional diagram of cilium showing its main structural components. *(From Palmbald J et al: Ultrastructural, cellular, and clinical features of the immotile-cilia syndrome. Ann Rev Med 35:481-492, 1984. Reprinted with permission from Annual Reviews Inc.)*

been preserved through evolution from protozoa. Cilia are composed of nine microtubular doublets that surround two central microtubules and are held together by dynein arms, nexin links, and spokes (Fig. 11-7). This structure is ideally suited for their function. The central microtubule doublet contains an ATPase enzyme that is likely responsible for the contractile beat of the cilium. Coordinated ciliary beating can be detected by the 13th week of gestation.

Cilia beat with a coordinated oscillation in a characteristic biphasic, wavelike rhythm called **metachronism** (Fig. 11-8). They beat 900 to 1200 strokes/min with a "power forward" stroke and a slow return or recovery stroke. During their power forward stroke, the tips of the cilia extend upward into the viscous layer, dragging it and entrapped particles. On the reverse beat, the cilia release the mucus and are contained completely in the sol layer. Cilia in the nasopharynx beat in the direction that will propel mucus into the pharynx, whereas cilia in the trachea propel mucus upward toward the pharynx, where it is swallowed.

Ciliary beating is powered by ATP. The bending of the cilia occurs by the sliding of dynein arms interlinking each microtubule pair. This causes a bending to one side. Cilia beat in a coordinated fashion; this coordination occurs by cell-to-cell ion flow, resulting in electrical and metabolic coordination. The mechanism by which cilia and the adjoining cells intercommunicate is unknown. Ciliary function is inhibited or impaired by cigarette smoke, hypoxia, and infection.

Cough, stimulated by irritant receptors that are activated by inhaled or aspirated foreign material, is also an important protective mechanism. Coughing achieves rapid airflow acceleration and extremely high flow rates and when coupled with dynamic airway compression is very effective in squeezing and clearing material and mucus from the airways (see Fig. 3-13).

When functioning normally, the mucociliary transport system is highly effective. Deposited particles can be removed in a matter of minutes to hours. In the trachea and main stem bronchi, the rate of particle clearance is 5 to 20 mm/min, whereas it is slower in the bronchioles (0.5 1 mm/min)

Phagocytic and Inflammatory Cells

Pulmonary **alveolar macrophages** and **dendritic cells** (DCs) are mononuclear phagocytic cells that scavenge particles and bacteria in the airways and in the alveoli. DCs and alveolar macrophages are differentiated cells of the myeloid lineage and are the first nonepithelial cells to contact and respond to foreign substances. They are important components of the innate immune system.

Although B and T lymphocytes are the predominant cells involved in mounting an immune response, DCs are a major cell type for antigen presentation to T cells and are required for a maximum response. DCs are found in the periphery of many tissues and most likely function as sentinels not only to capture antigens but also to bring and process them to lymphocytes in the various lymphoid tissues. They are derived from CD 34+ progenitor cells in the bone marrow developmentally and from the differentiation of blood monocytes in response to the cytokines, GM-CSF and interleukin-4 (IL-4). The major functions of DCs are to capture, process, and present antigen to T cells as well as to either activate or suppress the T-cell response (Table 11-3).

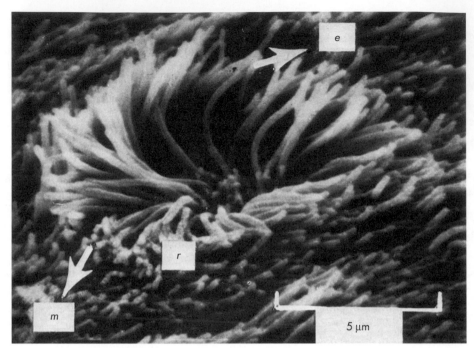

FIGURE 11-8 ■ Scanning electron micrograph of a metachronal wave on rabbit tracheal epithelium. Cilia that move to the left close to the cell surface in their recovery stroke (*r*) swing over toward the right in the more erect effective stroke (*e*). The metachronal wave moves in the direction indicated by arrow (*m*). (Micrograph by MJ Sanderson.) *(From Sanderson MJ, Sleigh MS: Ciliary activity of cultured rabbit tracheal epithelium: Beat pattern and metachrony. J Cell Sci 47:331-347, 1981.)*

Most DCs are present in the peripheral tissues in an immature state. Although they are unable to stimulate lymphocytes at this stage, they are ready to capture and process antigen (Fig. 11-9). The immature DC has several features that optimize its ability to capture antigen; these include phagocytosis, macropinocytosis (large pinocytic vesicles), specialized receptors for endocytosis, and several Fc receptors. After contact with antigen they can mature (increase surface expression of major histocompatibility complex [MHC] and stimulatory molecules) quite rapidly and migrate to

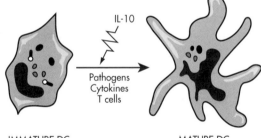

IMMATURE DC	MATURE DC
High intracellular MHCII (MIICs)	High surface MHCII
Endocytosis, including FcR	Low endocytosis and FcR
Low CD54, 58, 80, 86	High CD54, 58, 80, 86
Low CD40, CD25, IL-12	High CD40, CD25, IL-12
Low CD83, p55	High CD83, p55
Low granule antigens	High M342, 2A1,
Actin cables	MIDC-8 antigens
	No actin cables

FIGURE 11-9 ■ Phenotypic and physiologic differences distinguishing immature from mature dendritic cells (DCs). The developmental maturation of immature DCs can be regulated by the cytokine interleukin-10 (IL-10). MHCII, major histocompatibility complex class II. *(From Berne RM, Levy ML, Koeppen BM, Stanton BM (eds): Physiology, 5th ed. St. Louis, Mosby, 2004.)*

TABLE 11-3
Functions of the Dendritic Cell

Capture and process antigen
Migrate to lymphoid tissues
Present antigen to lymphocytes via major histocompatibility complex
Activate lymphocytes and enhance stimulatory response
Express lymphocyte co-stimulatory molecules
Secrete cytokines
Induce tolerance

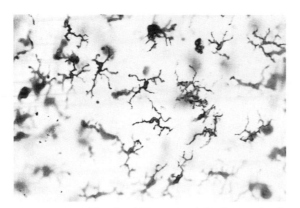

FIGURE 11-10 ■ The dendritic network in the conducting airways. The long, delicate processes of the dendritic cells can be seen throughout the conducting airways. *(Reprinted with permission Lambrecht BN, Prins JB, Hoogsteden HC: Lung dendritic cells and host immunity to infection. Eur Respir J 18:692-704, 2001.)*

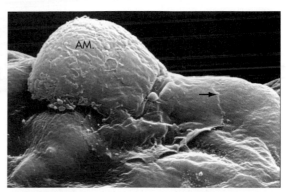

FIGURE 11-11 ■ Scanning electron micrograph of an alveolar macrophage (AM) sitting on an epithelial cell in the lung. *Arrow* points to the advancing edge of the cell. *(From Weibel, 1980. Reproduced with permission.)*

lymphoid tissues to engage lymphocytes, with subsequent initiation of an immune response or, in certain circumstances, the initiation of tolerance. It has been proposed that DCs regulate the immune response via a "cross presentation" mechanism in which the manner (and to which T-lymphocyte type—CD4+ or CD8+ T cells) the DC presents the antigen can either initiate a stimulatory immune response or induce tolerance.

DCs are commonly found from the trachea to the alveoli in the parenchyma of the lung and are usually associated with the epithelium (Fig. 11-10). The upper airways are more densely populated with DCs than the smaller airways in the more peripheral regions of the lung. The anatomic location of these cells correlates well with particle deposition in the airways.

Alveolar macrophages are large, foamy, highly active phagocytic cells derived from myeloid progenitor cells in the bone marrow. Alveolar macrophages have a mean lifespan of 1 to 5 weeks and are derived from blood monocytes, usually as the result of secondary division by other alveolar macrophages. In inflammatory states such as tuberculosis, blood monocytes can, however, migrate into the lung and differentiate into new alveolar macrophages. Alveolar macrophages are found mostly in the alveolus adjacent to the epithelium and less frequently in the terminal airways and interstitial space (Fig. 11-11). They migrate freely throughout the alveolar spaces and serve as a first line

of defense in the lower air spaces. They readily and rapidly (usually within 24 hours) phagocytize foreign particles and substances, as well as cellular debris from dead cells. Once a particle is engulfed, the major mechanisms for killing are typical of phagocytic cells and include oxygen radicals, enzymatic activity, and halogen derivatives within lysosomes. After engulfing a potentially infectious agent, macrophages undergo a burst of metabolic activity and kill the organism. The ability of the alveolar macrophage to kill foreign material rapidly and without mounting an inflammatory response enhances the lung defense system immensely and is a major contributor to the overall defense system. By rapidly phagocytizing particles in the alveolus, the alveolar macrophage inhibits the binding of these substances to the alveolar surface and possible invasion into the interstitial spaces, with potential attendant tissue damage.

Silica dust and **asbestos** are mineral crystals that cannot be dissolved by the macrophage after phagocytosis. The sharp crystals puncture lysosomal membranes, resulting in intracellular lysosomal enzyme release and death of the cell. Chemotactic factors released from the dying macrophage cause fibroblast migration and collagen synthesis in the region. Migration of additional macrophages into the region to ingest the dead macrophages occurs, and these macrophages are also killed by the nondissolved, sharp, mineral crystals. Their death stimulates additional fibroblast migration and additional collagen synthesis (Fig. 11-12). The end

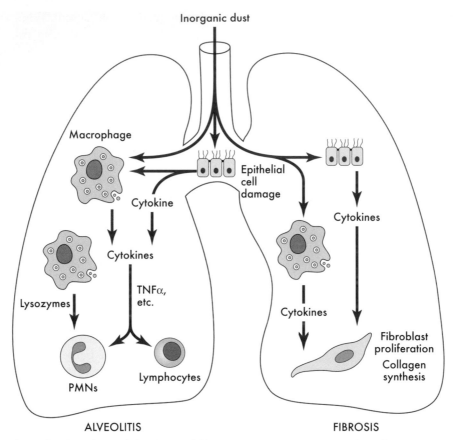

FIGURE 11-12 ■ The pathophysiology of alveolitis and fibrosis in pneumoconiosis. In the inflammatory process *(left side)*, inhaled dust is ingested by alveolar macrophages that are damaged and activated to release cytotoxic O, lysosomal enzymes, and inflammatory cytokines (TNF-α, IL-1). These in turn recruit inflammatory cells (lymphocytes, neutrophils and PMNs) into the alveoli. Epithelial cells are also damaged and they release additional inflammatory cytokines. Alveolar macrophages, lymphocytes, and neutrophils are the cells mainly responsible for the development of alveolitis. In the process of fibrosis *(right side)*, following the inflammatory process, reparation and fibrosis develop. Growth factors (e.g., TNF, IL-1) stimulate the recruitment and proliferation of type II pneumocytes and fibroblasts and induce overproduction of fibronectin and collagen. IL-1, interleukin-1; TNF, tumor necrosis factor. *(Adapted from Fujimura N: Pathology and pathophysiology of pneumoconiosis. Curr Opin Pulm Med 6:140-144, 2000.)*

result is that the alveolar macrophage now has localized and concentrated silica or asbestos particles in a region of the lung in association with the development of **pulmonary fibrosis**, a disease associated with reduced lung compliance, impaired gas exchange, and increased work of breathing.

The alveolar macrophage also has the capability of suppressing an adaptive immune response via T-cell mechanisms. It can suppress T-cell activity via direct contact with the T cell or via the secretion of soluble factors such as nitric oxide, prostaglandin E_2, and the immunosuppressive cytokines IL-10 and transforming growth factor-β (TGFβ). Interestingly, the proinflammatory cytokines, GM-CSF and tumor necrosis factor-α (TNFα), inhibit the suppressive activity of the alveolar macrophage.

The fate of the alveolar macrophage is varied. It can be taken up into the mucociliary clearance system, it can die within the alveolus and get phagocytized by other alveolar macrophages, or it can migrate into lymphoid tissue or the lung interstitium.

Polymorphonuclear leukocytes (PMNs) are important cells in lung defense against established bacterial infection of the lower respiratory tract. While rarely found in normal small airways and alveoli, PMNs are a prominent, histologic feature of a bacterial pneumonia. These cells are recruited to the lung by a variety of stimuli, including chemotactic factors released by alveolar macrophages and by products of complement activation. Movement into the lung from the pulmonary vasculature is orchestrated by many factors that mediate the process of adhesion including integrins on the PMN surface and adhesion molecules on the vascular endothelial cells. PMNs phagocytose and kill invading bacteria by generating products of oxidative metabolism toxic to microbes.

A number of surface enzymes and factors in serum and airway secretions assist in destroying or detoxifying particles and deserve mention. These include *lysozymes* found primarily in PMNs and known to have bactericidal properties; *interferon* (IFN), a potent antiviral compound produced by macrophages and lymphocytes; *complement*, an important co-factor in antigen-antibody reactions; and the bacteriostatic *lactoferrin*, produced by PMNs and glandular mucosal cells. **Antiproteases** found in normal lungs are especially important in inactivating the elastase enzymes released by macrophages and PMNs during phagocytosis. The most important of the antiproteases is α1-antitrypsin. Individuals with α1-antitrypsin deficiency lack the ability to synthesize this enzyme and are predisposed to the development of emphysema in their 30s and 40s. Some individuals who smoke produce increased levels of these proteases beyond the capacity of the antiprotease systems and result in pulmonary inflammation that leads to degradation of the alveolar septal walls and emphysema.

The transition between the conducting airways and their mucociliary transport system and the terminal respiratory units where alveolar mechanisms are important is the "Achilles heel" in what is otherwise a highly effective defense system because the risk of particle retention at this location is high. In the occupational lung disease called **pneumoconiosis** (the "black lung" disease of coal miners) or **silicosis** (the lung disease caused by inhalation of silica during quarrying, mining, or sandblasting), particle sedimentation occurs in the region of the terminal and respiratory bronchioles. The relatively slow rate of particle clearance in this area provides an opportunity for particles to invoke toxic reactions (in the case of silica) or to leave the airway space and enter the interstitial spaces and invoke less intense fibrotic responses. *The terminal respiratory unit is the most common location of airway damage in all types of occupational lung disease.* It is also likely that deposition of atmospheric particles such as tobacco smoke in this area causes some of the earliest changes in chronic bronchitis.

THE LUNG AS A SECONDARY LYMPHOID ORGAN

The lymphatic system and lymphoid tissues in the lung include organized lymphoid structures such as lymph nodes, lymph nodules, and lymph aggregates, in addition to a diffuse submucosal network of scattered lymphocytes and dendritic cells. These lymphoid structures are found throughout the respiratory tract in different anatomic locations. Because there is regional variation in inhaled particle deposition, each lymphoid tissue plays an important and unique role in the overall defense of the lung.

Regional Lymph Nodes of the Lung

The lymph nodes draining the lung are part of the mediastinal network, which drains the head and neck, the lungs, and the esophagus. The peribronchial and hilar lymph nodes are the prominent nodes in the local lung region; less prominent are the intrapulmonary nodes in the pleura and interlobar septal areas. Lymph nodes in these areas have the encapsulated organization typical of lymph nodes in other areas of the body, including the cortex, paracortex, and medulla. When activated, a germinal center is apparent in B cells and plasma cells in the cortical follicles and medullary cords, and in T cells in the paracortical areas between the follicles.

In addition to being the site of antigen presentation via lymph drainage, regional lymph nodes are the sites to receive cancer cells. Thus these mediastinal nodes have significant diagnostic importance for lung cancer.

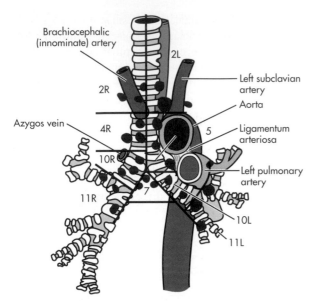

FIGURE 11-13 ■ American Thoracic Society map of regional pulmonary nodes. See Table 11-4 for explanation. *(From Tisi GM, Friedman PJ, Peters RM, et al: American Thoracic Society. Medical section of the American Lung Association. Clinical staging of primary lung cancer. Am Rev Respir Dis 127: 659, 1983.)*

The American Thoracic Society has established a lymph node map and nomenclature for these nodes (Fig. 11-13 and Table 11-4).

Mucosal-Associated Lymphoid Tissue (MALT)

The lymphoid tissue of the mucosal areas in the gastrointestinal, respiratory, and urinary systems consist of loosely organized aggregates of cells known as MALT, which somewhat resemble actual lymph nodes with a similar repertoire of immune cells; however, they are highly specialized. In contrast to lymph nodes, these tissues are not encapsulated and are composed mainly of aggregates or clusters of lymphocytes residing in submucosal regions. In addition to aggregates of cells, MALT contains a substantial number of solitary B and T lymphocytes, which are scattered regularly throughout the connective tissue of the lamina propria (lamina propria lymphocytes) and the epithelial layer (intraepithelial lymphocytes). The B cells found in MALT can selectively differentiate into IgA-secreting plasma cells when stimulated by antigen. MALT in the

	TABLE 11-4
	American Thoracic Society Definitions of Regional Nodal Stations

X	Supraclavicular nodes
2R	**Right upper paratracheal nodes:** nodes to the right of the midline of the trachea, between the intersection of the caudal margin of the innominate artery with the trachea and the apex of the lung
2L	**Left upper paratracheal nodes:** nodes to the left of the midline of the trachea, between the top of the aortic arch and the apex of the lung
4R	**Right lower paratracheal nodes:** nodes to the right of the midline of the trachea, between the cephalic border of the azygos vein and the intersection of the caudal margin of the brachiocephalic artery with the right side of the trachea
4L	**Left lower paratracheal nodes:** nodes to the right of the midline of the trachea, between the top of the aortic arch and the level of the carina, medial to the ligamentum arteriosum
5	**Aortopulmonary nodes:** subaortic and paraaortic nodes, lateral to the ligamentum arteriosum or the aorta or left pulmonary artery, proximal to the first branch of the left pulmonary artery
6	**Anterior mediastinal nodes:** nodes anterior to the ascending aorta or the innominate artery
7	**Subcarinal nodes:** nodes arising caudal to the carina of the trachea but not associated with the lower lobe bronchi or arteries within the lung.
8	**Paraesophageal nodes:** nodes dorsal to the posterior wall of the trachea and to the right or left of the midline of the esophagus
9	**Right or left pulmonary ligament nodes:** nodes within the right or left pulmonary artery
10R	**Right tracheobronchial nodes:** nodes to the right of the midline of the trachea, from the level of the cephalic border of the azygos vein to the origin of the right upper lobe bronchus
10L	**Left peribronchial nodes:** nodes to the left of the midline of the trachea, between the carina and the left upper lobe bronchus, medial to the ligamentum arteriosum
11	**Intrapulmonary nodes:** nodes removed in the right or left lung specimen plus those distal to the mainstem bronchi or carina

Modified from Tisi GM, Friedman PJ, Peters RM, et al: Am Rev Respir Dis 127:659, 1983.

lung is called **BALT** (**bronchus-associated lymphoid tissue**) and provides a first line of defense for this highly exposed mucosal surface. In the upper airways of the respiratory tract, BALT is present in adenoids and tonsils. Unlike lymph nodes, MALT (including BALT) does not have an afferent or efferent lymphatic drainage pattern. This limits systemic sensitization only to mucosal tissues and may be an important part of the defense mechanism.

The anatomic structures of lymphoid tissue in the lung become less organized as one transcends the lung from the most upper airways (hilum) to the periphery (alveoli). Mature lymph nodes with germinal centers and nodules predominate in the hilar region around the main-stem bronchi, whereas lymph aggregates predominate as one approaches the alveoli. There are no organized lymphoid structures in the alveolar spaces. BALT predominates throughout the conducting airways, with aggregates of lymph nodules or solitary lymph nodules found sporadically. Although these lymph nodules are not true lymph nodes, they are still a major processing center for antigens. They reside in the upper airways around major airway branches and blood vessels.

The epithelium associated with areas of BALT is specialized and is called **lymphoepithelium**. It is composed of a mix of epithelial cells and lymphocytes. Lymphoepithelium lacks ciliated epithelial cells, which results in a break in the mucociliary clearance system. This enhances fluid and particulate flow into the BALT area (Fig. 11-14). These epithelial cells secrete cytokines (e.g., IL-6, which favors induction of IgA synthesis), express adhesion molecules essential for antigen-presenting cell (APC) contact with T cells, and themselves have been shown to have APC capabilities. BALT is observed in humans, but only in the presence of pathologic conditions such as upper respiratory tract infections.

HUMORAL IMMUNE MECHANISMS

Immunoglobulin IgA and IgG

Humoral immunity in the respiratory system consists of two major immunoglobulins: IgA and IgG. IgA, and particularly a form of IgA known as **secretory IgA,** is especially important in the nasopharynx and upper airways. Secretory IgA is composed of two IgA

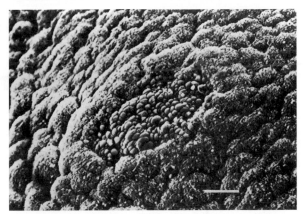

FIGURE 11-14 ■ Scanning electron micrograph of rabbit bronchial epithelium showing island of lymphoepithelium surrounded by ciliated epithelium. Bar = 1 mm. *(Reprinted by permission from Bienenstock J, Johnston N: A morphologic study of rabbit bronchial lymphoid aggregates and lymphoepithelium. Lab Invest 35:343-348, 1976, Williams & Wilkins, Baltimore.)*

molecules (a dimer) joined by a polypeptide that contains an extra glycoprotein called the **secretory component.** Secretory IgA is synthesized locally in submucosal areas by plasma cells and secreted in a dimer form linked by a J-chain. The antibody-dimer migrates to the submucosal surface of epithelial cells where it binds to a surface protein receptor called **poly-Ig** (Fig. 11-15). The poly-Ig receptor aids in the pinocytosis of the dimer into the epithelial cell and its eventual secretion into the airway lumen. During exocytosis of the IgA complex, the poly-Ig is enzymatically cleaved, leaving a portion of it (the secretory component) still associated with the complex. The secretory piece stays attached to the IgA complex in the airway and aids in its protection from proteolytic cleavage in the lumen. Secretory IgA binds to antigens including viruses and bacteria and prevents their attachment to epithelial cells. The IgA also agglutinates microorganisms, which makes them more easily cleared by mucociliary transport.

Unlike IgA, IgG is abundant in the lower respiratory tract. Synthesized locally, IgG neutralizes viruses, is an **opsonin** (a macromolecular coat around bacteria) for macrophage handling of bacteria, agglutinates particles, activates complement, and in the presence of complement causes lysis of Gram-negative bacteria.

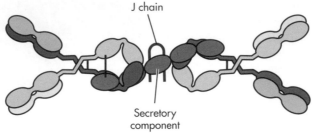

A   Structure of secretory IgA

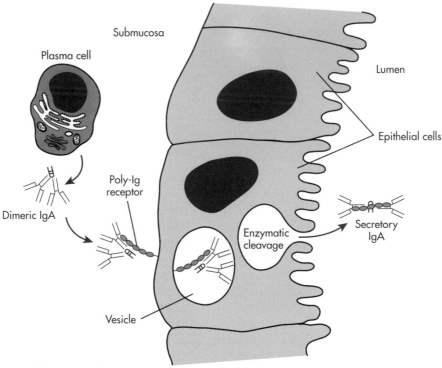

B   Formation of secretory IgA

FIGURE 11-15 ■ Structure and formation of secretory immunoglobin A (IgA). **A,** Secretory IgA consists of at least two IgA molecules that are covalently linked via a J chain and covalently associated with the secretory component. The secretory component contains five Ig-like domains and is linked to dimeric IgA (*thick black line*) between its fifth domain and one of the IgA heavy chains. **B,** Secretory IgA is formed during transport through mucous membrane epithelial cells. Dimeric IgA binds to a poly-Ig receptor on the basolateral membrane of an epithelial cell and is internalized by receptor-mediated endocytosis. After transport of the receptor-IgA complex to the luminal surface, the poly-Ig receptor is enzymatically cleaved, releasing the secretory component bound to the dimeric IgA. *(From Berne RM, Levy ML, Koeppen BM, Stanton BM (eds): Physiology, 5th ed. St. Louis, Mosby, 2004.)*

Natural Killer Cells

Natural killer (NK) cells are derived developmentally from a lymphoid lineage in the bone marrow and require a bone marrow stroma product, IL-15, for differentiation. They are a major component of the body's innate immune defense system against invading pathogens such as herpes viruses and various bacterial infections. Although they share many functional activities similar to those of lymphocytes, they lack surface marker characteristics of either the T or the B lymphocyte. NK cells are named for their ability to kill target cells without prior sensitization. The mechanism of killing is through the release of granular enzymes, perforins, and serine esterases. These enzymes create holes or pores within the target cell membranes, leading to cell death. In addition to their cytotoxic activity, they produce cytokines similar to those of lymphocytes, including IL-4, IL-5, IL-13, IFN-γ, TNF-α, as well as others. The mechanism of antigen or target cell recognition is not known. However, NK cells have many surface receptors that display inhibitory activity in response to MHC class I molecules. Cells that lack or have low expression of MHC class I molecules are targets for NK cells. The inhibitory activity of the NK cell receptors may help distinguish MHC class I molecule self-recognition.

NORMAL ADAPTIVE IMMUNE RESPONSE AND THE RESPONSE TO BACTERIA

The adaptive immune system in the respiratory tract is summoned only after the insulting agent has avoided the unique defense systems established in the respiratory tract. Once triggered, however, it is similar to the response in any other systemic organ.

Under normal circumstances, bacteria such as *Streptococcus pneumoniae* that commonly come into contact with the upper respiratory system (i.e. bronchus to nasopharynx) are expelled by the mucociliary clearance system or are handled by BALT via an IgA response. However, if the bacteria elude these first-line defenses, an inflammatory response develops (e.g., bacterial pneumonia), which is followed by a classic adaptive immune response with T-cell activation and antibody synthesis (Fig. 11-16). These responses take 1 to 2 weeks to develop fully before a resolution of the pneumonia occurs. A typical inflammatory response to a bacterial or viral pneumonia is initially dominated by polymorphonuclear leukocytes and if it persists, a more mononuclear cell infiltrate. As with other organ systems, a transient population of blood-borne phagocytic cells (polymorphonuclear leukocytes and macrophages) resides in local vessels and is on the ready to emigrate into sites of injury. The first inflammatory cells to respond to the injury via chemotactic mechanisms, usually within 4 to 12 hours, are the polymorphonuclear leukocytes and if the injury persists, they are followed by macrophages within 24 to 72 hours.

Under circumstances in which the bacteria or other inciting agent persists and is hard to phagocytize, a **granulomatous response** occurs. The body's reaction to *Mycobacterium tuberculosis* is a classic example of a granulomatous response; that is, a rim of mononuclear cells (lymphocytes and macrophages) forms around the agent in an attempt to wall it off and prevent it from infiltrating into other tissues. This is a T-cell response dominated by CD4+ T cells and T-helper (TH-1) cytokines such as IFN-γ. A granulomatous response is associated with diseases such as silicosis, sarcoidosis, and the hypersensitivity lung diseases (e.g., farmer's lung). Whereas the sequela of many acute bacterial and viral pneumonias is resolution to normal tissue, a common sequela of the chronic granulomatous type of response is scar formation (e.g., pulmonary fibrosis). Extensive injury and cell death (necrosis) occur during the granulomatous response; as a result, the body lays down collagen to form scar tissue, which in essence "sews" up the hole left by the necrotic tissue. Scar formation for the most part is nonreversible. It replaces normal functioning tissue and therefore imparts a dysfunctional state in affected areas. Thus if 10% of the lung scars, technically speaking it may lose 10% of its functional capacity, not taking into account compensatory mechanisms.

In considering lung repair, resolution to normal tissue is always the preferred response; however, in certain circumstances lung scarring occurs, and in those instances, it can be life-saving. Because in many pathologic conditions resolution to normal tissue is not always possible, lung repair can be viewed as a balance in which the body minimizes scar formation and maximizes resolution to normal tissue.

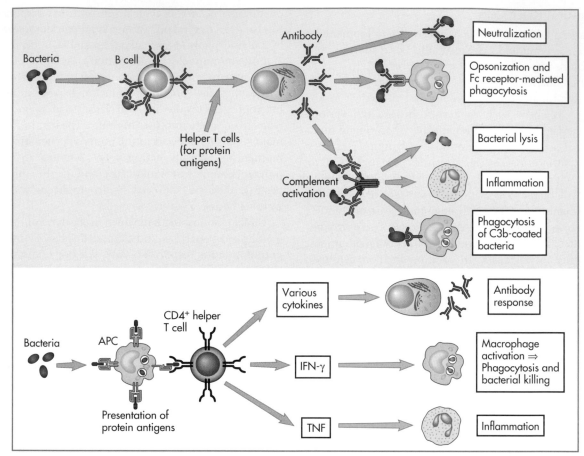

FIGURE 11-16 ■ The adaptive immune response to inhaled bacteria consists of antibody production *(upper panel)* and T cell activation *(lower panel)*. Antibodies neutralize and eliminate bacteria by several mechanisms, whereas T-cell responses stimulate B-cell antibody responses, macrophage activation, and inflammation. APC, antigen-presenting cell; IFN-γ, interferon-γ; TNF, tumor necrosis factor. *(Modified from Abbas AK, Lichtman AH: Cellular and Molecular Immunology, 4th ed. Philadelphia, WB Saunders, 2000.)*

CLINICAL MANIFESTATIONS OF ALTERED PULMONARY DEFENSE

Today's urban industrial environment coupled with occupations in which airborne particles are inhaled can produce a significant burden even on a normal mucociliary transport system. Chronic lung injury often develops after many years of exposure to these foreign materials. Excessive mucus production stresses the mucociliary transport system and stimulates the cough reflex that helps to remove these secretions.

Numerous diseases involving the lung have their origin in abnormalities of lung defense. **Cystic fibrosis** is an autosomal recessive disease characterized by thick, tenacious, dehydrated airway secretions. In this disease, the airway epithelium demonstrates decreased permeability to Cl⁻ because of failure of the chloride ion channel in the apical cell membrane to open even under stimulation by cAMP. The result is a thick mucus with a water content lower than normal. In addition, in cystic fibrosis there is proliferation of goblet cells and hypertrophy of submucosal glands secondary to irritation and/or abnormalities in surface liquid.

Bronchial secretions in normal individuals owe their viscoelastic properties to the size, length, coiling, and cross-linking of the mucus glycoproteins, resulting in flexible elastic fibers. Normal secretions have low viscosity and long relaxation times (highly elastic). In **asthma**—a disease associated with bronchospasm, airway inflammation and airway edema—mucus viscosity instead of elasticity becomes the major physical property, and a glycoprotein gel is formed. Secretions from individuals with asthma have the highest viscosity of mucus in any disease; on occasion, entire mucus casts of a lobe have been expectorated.

Many processes can result in abnormal ciliary beating and thus in abnormal clearance. Ciliary beating is decreased by hypoxia, repeated exposure to the gas phases of tobacco smoke, very dry air, inflammation, and pollution, particularly of ozone. Cilia are also destroyed by infection. **Immotile cilia syndrome** is associated with abnormal ciliary microstructure throughout the body and consequently cilia that do not beat. The triad of situs inversus associated with bronchiectasis and sinusitis associated with immotile cilia is termed **Kartagener's syndrome**.

DISEASES ASSOCIATED WITH ABNORMALITIES IN INNATE AND ADAPTIVE IMMUNITY

By far the most common pathologic conditions associated with mucosal tissues are *allergic diseases* (e.g., allergic asthma, allergic rhinitis, and food and skin allergies). In an allergic response, an antibody synthesis switchover response occurs and IgE, instead of IgA, becomes the predominant antibody synthesized to the allergen. Sensitized T cells and the cytokine IL-4 are required for this to occur. The IgE binds to the surface of tissue mast cells and upon antigen stimulation leads to the degranulation of mast cells (Fig. 11-17). The released granules contain many factors, including eosinophil chemotactic factor and leukotrienes with bronchoconstrictor activity. Symptoms of wheezing, cough, and shortness of breath occur within minutes, and locally there is intense eosinophilia and airway edema. Resolution of the inflammatory response can occur spontaneously or in response to therapy

(anti-inflammatory drugs). Low-grade inflammation may, however, persist and can result in permanent changes in airway structure referred to as *airway remodeling*. The mechanisms for airway remodeling in allergic diseases are not known, but TGF-β may be important.

An interesting group of difficult-to-diagnose lung diseases, first described in the 1930s, are caused by nonpathologic organisms and dusts. These diseases are known as **hypersensitivity lung diseases** and are associated with an altered immune response to the inciting agent. Only a small percentage of equally exposed individuals contract the disease, which is caused by the immune response to the agent and not by the agent itself. It is not a typical allergic response because the symptoms usually occur 4 to 6 hours following exposure, as contrasted with the immediate type of response to allergens; however, some individuals can also have an allergic response. Also, the lesion is not dominated by eosinophils, as occurs in an allergic response. The lung pathology can consist of a polymorphonuclear cell response or a granulomatous-type response followed by pulmonary fibrosis.

Pulmonary complications are common in chronic systemic diseases with possible autoimmune etiologies, including rheumatoid arthritis, systemic lupus erythematosis, and inflammatory bowel diseases (e.g., Crohn's disease, ulcerative colitis). It is not clear why this association exists, but it may be due to a dysregulation of immune responses that initiates a local pulmonary type of autoimmune disease. **Goodpasture's syndrome** is the classic autoimmune response in the lung. It is a pulmonary hemorrhagic disease due to an autoimmune IgG antibody response to type IV collagen in the basement membrane of the lung. Cell injury and death occur through complement activation via an antibody-antigen complex. It is also associated with an intense glomerulonephritis where the disease is thought to have been initiated. The type IV collagen antigen in the kidney basement membrane cross-reacts with the lung basement membrane.

The most common inherited immunoglobulin deficiency is **selective IgA deficiency**, with a prevalence of 1 in 800 births. Although the deficiency is not associated with any specific disease, individuals with the deficiency have a high rate of chronic lung disease, illustrating the importance of this antibody in host defense in the respiratory tract.

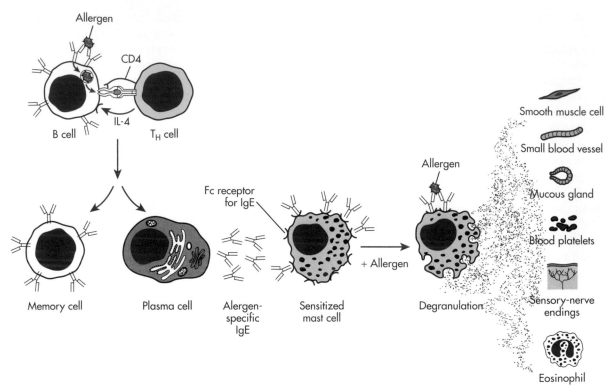

FIGURE 11-17 ■ The general mechanism underlying an allergic reaction. Exposure to an allergen activates B cells to form IgE-secreting plasma cells. The secreted IgE molecules bind to IgE-specific Fc receptors on mast cells and blood basophils. Upon a second exposure to the allergen, the bound IgE is cross-linked, triggering the release of pharmacologically active mediators (*red*) from mast cells and basophils. The mediators cause smooth-muscle contraction, increased vascular permeability, and vasodilation. IgE, immunoglobin E. *(From Berne RM, Levy ML, Koeppen BM, Stanton BM (eds): Physiology, 5th ed. St. Louis, Mosby, 2004.)*

S U M M A R Y

1. The three major components of lung defense against inhaled particles and other inhaled materials are mucociliary transport in the larger airways, phagocytic and inflammatory cells, and a specialized mucosal immune system.

2. Sedimented particles (0.2-2 μm in diameter) deposit in small airways at the junction of the end of the mucociliary transport system and the terminal respiratory units where alveolar mechanisms are important. This is the "Achilles heel" of the respiratory system and plays a significant role in many respiratory diseases.

3. The three components of mucociliary transport are periciliary fluid, mucus, and the cilia.

4. The depth of the periciliary fluid layer is maintained by the balance between chloride secretion and sodium absorption and is essential to normal ciliary beating.

5. Mucus is a complex macromolecule composed of glycoproteins, proteins, electrolytes, and water. The viscoelastic properties of mucus are due to the size, length, coiling, and cross-linking of the mucus glycoproteins. Normal mucus has low viscosity and high elasticity.

6. Three cell types produce mucus: surface secretory cells, tracheobronchial glands, and Clara cells.

7. Pulmonary alveolar macrophages and dendritic cells are mononuclear phagocytic cells that scavenge particles and bacteria in the airways and alveoli. Polymorphonuclear leukocytes are important in lung defense against established bacterial infection.

8. BALT (bronchus-associated lymphoid tissue) is part of the mucosa-associated lymphoid tissue (MALT) system and is mainly composed of aggregates of lymph nodules throughout the conducting airways.

9. Important components of the lung's innate immunity are phagocytic cells (polymorphonuclear leukocytes and macrophages), natural killer cells, the complement system, and cytokines.

10. Lymphocytes and their products (B lymphocytes and humoral immunity; T lymphocytes and cell mediated immunity) are the important components of adaptive immunity.

11. IgA is the predominant antibody produced by plasma cells in BALT, IgG is the predominant antibody in the lower respiratory tract.

12. Allergic diseases are characterized by a switchover response (IgE instead of IgA).

KEY WORDS

- Aerosol
- Alveolar macrophages
- Asthma
- Bronchus-associated lymphoid tissue (BALT)
- Cilia
- Clara cells
- Cystic fibrosis
- Dendritic cells
- Diffusion
- Goblet cells (surface secretory cells)
- Goodpasture's syndrome
- Granulomatous response
- Hypersensitivity lung disease
- IgA deficiency
- Immotile cilia syndrome
- Impaction
- Kartagener's syndrome
- Mucociliary transport
- Mucosa-associated lymphoid tissue (MALT)
- Mucus
- Natural killer cell
- Periciliary fluid
- Polymorphonuclear leukocytes (neutrophils)
- Secretory IgA
- Secretory component
- Sedimentation
- Silica dust
- Sputum
- Tracheobronchial glands

SELF-STUDY PROBLEMS

1. Describe the pathology of the lung in individuals with chronic bronchitis secondary to smoking.

2. What would be the effect on the periciliary fluid layer and mucociliary transport of a drug that blocks sodium absorption and increases intracellular levels of cAMP?

3. Describe the synthesis, structure, and transport mechanisms of IgA.

4. What role do NK cells play in host defense in mucosal tissues and how are they implicated in allergic airway disease?

5. Describe the function of dendritic cells in the lung.

6. How does macrophage phagocytosis of asbestos differ from the usual macrophage processing of microorganisms?

7. Explain how mucosa-associated lymphoid tissues differ from the systemic immune system and lymph nodes.

REFERENCES

Banchereau J, Steinman RM: Dendritic cells and the control of immunity. Nature 392:245-252, 1998.

Chakraborty A, Li L, Chakraborty NG, Mukherji B: Stimulatory and inhibitory differentiation of human myeloid dendritic cells. Clin Immunol 94:88-98, 2000.

Daniele RP: Immunoglobulin secretion in the airways. Annu Rev Physiol 52:177, 1990.

Oberdorster G: Lung clearance of inhaled insoluble and soluble particles. J Aerosol Med 1:289-330, 1988.

Gashi AA, Nadel JA, Basbaum CB: Tracheal gland mucous cells stimulated in vitro with adrenergic and cholinergic drugs. Tissue Cell 21:59, 1989.

Holt PG: Regulation of antigen presenting cell function(s) in lung and airway tissues. Eur Respir J 6:120-129, 1993.

Jiang C, Finkbeiner WE, Widdicombe JH, et al: Altered fluid transport across airway epithelium in cystic fibrosis. Science 262:424-427, 1993.

Kerr A: The structure and function of human IgA. Biochem J 271:285, 1990.

Martonen TB: Deposition patterns of cigarette smoke in human airways. Am Ind Hyg Assoc 53:6-18, 1992.

Salathe M, O'Riordan TG, Wanner A: Treatment of mucociliary dysfunction. Chest 110:1048-1057, 1996.

Sheehan JK, Thornton DJ, Somerville M, et al: The structure and heterogeneity of respiratory mucus glycoproteins. Am Rev Respir Dis 144:S4-S9, 1991.

Sheppard DN, Welsh MJ: Structure and function of the CFTR chloride channel. Physiol Rev 79:S23-S45, 1999.

Sommerhoff CP, Finkbeiner WE: Human tracheobronchial submucosal gland cells in culture. Am J Respir Cell Mol Biol 2:41-50, 1990.

Verdugo P: Goblet cell secretion and mucogenesis. Annu Rev Physiol 52:157-176, 1990.

Wanner A, Salathe M, O'Riordan TG: Mucociliary clearance in the airways. Am J Respir Crit Care Med 154:1868-1902, 1996.

Welsh MJ: Electrolyte transport by airway epithelia. Physiol Rev 67:1143-1184, 1987.

12

THE LUNG UNDER SPECIAL CIRCUMSTANCES

■　■　■　■　■　■　■　■　■　■　■　■　■　■

OBJECTIVES

1. Explain the circulatory and ventilatory changes associated with exercise.

2. Outline three ways that exercise testing can be performed.

3. Describe the five stages of fetal lung development.

4. Explain fetal circulation and the changes that occur during and immediately after birth.

5. Explain the circulatory and ventilatory changes associated with altitude.

6. Describe the physiologic components of acclimatization.

The lung has the reserve and capacity to adapt to a number of special environments. In this chapter, we briefly discuss the respiratory adaptation to exercise and to high altitude as well as in utero respiration and lung development.

EXERCISE

Many books and articles have been written about the cardiorespiratory changes that occur during exercise. The ability to exercise depends on the capacity of the cardiac and respiratory systems to increase oxygen delivery to the tissues and to remove carbon dioxide from the body (Fig. 12-1). Central to this ability is the musculoskeletal system, which facilitates muscle contraction and the conversion of glucose to chemical energy, and the central nervous system (CNS), which delivers coordinated signals to the musculoskeletal system. Also involved in exercise is the autonomic nervous system, which redistributes blood flow among various organs to meet the demands of exercise.

Both tidal volume and respiratory rate increase with exercise, resulting in an increase in minute ventilation (Fig. 12-2). At rest, the minute ventilation in a normal adult is 5 to 6 L/min. The increase in minute ventilation with exercise is linearly related to both CO_2 production and O_2 consumption at low to moderate levels (Fig. 12-3). With maximal exercise, a fit young man can achieve an oxygen consumption of 4 L/min with a minute volume of 120 L/min, almost 15 times resting levels, and a cardiac output that increases only 4 to 6 times above resting level. As a result, in normal individuals it is the cardiovascular system and not the respiratory system that is the rate-limiting factor in exercise.

Exercise is a form of stress to the respiratory system, and, as such, abnormalities in pulmonary mechanics due to airway obstruction or to changes in lung compliance or in oxygenation can become limiting. Work of breathing increases secondary to increases in both lung and chest wall elastic recoil and increases in airway resistance. The larger tidal volumes result in higher lung volumes. Both the lung and the chest wall

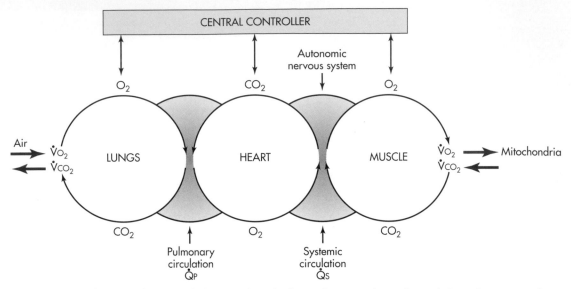

FIGURE 12-1 ■ Physiologic mechanisms during exercise. The lungs, heart, and muscles and the pulmonary and systemic circulations are interrelated and regulated by the central controller and the autonomic nervous system and result in processes commensurate with oxygen consumption ($\dot{V}O_2$) and carbon dioxide production ($\dot{V}CO_2$). *(Modified and redrawn from Murray J: The Normal Lung, 2nd ed. Philadelphia, WB Saunders, 1985.)*

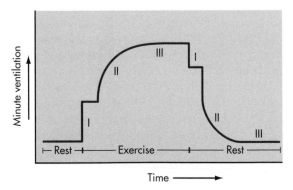

FIGURE 12-2 ■ Ventilation before, during, and after exercise. In phase I there is an abrupt increase in ventilation during the transition between rest and exercise. Phase II occurs after approximately 15 seconds and involves a gradual (exponential) rise in ventilation to reach a new steady state (phase III). Phase III is reached approximately 4 minutes after the onset of exercise. At the end of exercise, there is an abrupt decrease in ventilation (I) followed by a gradual return (II) to the former resting ventilation (III). *(Modified from Berne RM, Levy ML, Koeppen BM, Stanton BM: Physiology, 5th ed. St. Louis, Mosby, 2004.)*

become less compliant at these higher lung volumes, resulting in increased work to overcome the lung and chest wall elastic recoil. In addition, the airway resistance component of work of breathing increases with the higher flow rates generated during exercise (Table 12-1).

Lung Volume Changes with Exercise

With exercise, the increase in tidal volume occurs mainly at the expense of the inspiratory reserve capacity. Total lung capacity decreases slightly as the central blood volume increases (secondary to increased venous return). Residual volume (RV) and functional residual capacity (FRC) are unchanged or increase slightly. Anatomic dead space increases slightly as a result of airway distention at higher lung volumes. This is associated with a decrease in alveolar dead space as cardiac output increases with exercise. The net effect is no change in physiologic dead space. The ratio of dead space volume to tidal volume (V_{DS}/V_T), however, decreases as V_T increases.

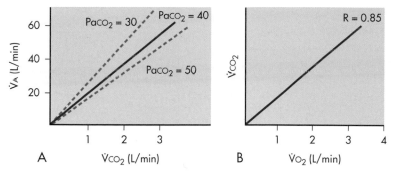

FIGURE 12-3 ■ Relationship between ventilation, O_2 consumption, and CO_2 production. **A,** CO_2 production increases linearly with increased minute ventilation ($\dot{V}A$) during exercise to maintain the $PaCO_2$ at 40 mm Hg. Levels of ventilation at a moderate level of exercise ($\dot{V}CO_2 = 2$ L/min) change with different levels of $PaCO_2$. **B,** CO_2 production and O_2 consumption are linearly related. *(Modified and redrawn from Leff A, Schumacker P: Respiratory Physiology: Basics and Applications. Philadelphia, WB Saunders, 1993.)*

TABLE 12-1

Response of the Respiratory System to Exercise

VARIABLE	MODERATE EXERCISE	SEVERE EXERCISE
Mechanics of breathing		
Elastic work of breathing	↑	↑↑
Resistance work of breathing	↑	↑↑
Alveolar ventilation		
Tidal volume	↑↑	↑↑
Frequency	↑	↑↑
Anatomic dead space	↑	↑
Alveolar dead space (if present)	↓	↓
V_D/V_r	↓	↓↓
Pulmonary blood flow	↑	↑↑
Perfusion of upper lung	↑	↑↑
Pulmonary vascular resistance	↓	↓↓
Linear velocity of blood flow	↑	↑↑
Ventilation-perfusion matching	↑	↑
Diffusion through the alveolar-capillary barrier	↑	↑↑
Surface area	↑	↑↑
Perfusion limitation	↓	↓↓
Partial pressure gradients	↑	↑↑
Oxygen unloading at the tissues	↑	↑↑
Carbon dioxide loading at the tissues	↑	↑↑
PAO_2	↔	↑
PaO_2	↔	↑, ↔, or ↓
$PaCO_2$	↔	↓
pH	↔	↓
O_2 extraction ratio	↑	↑↑

↑, increase; ↓, decrease; ↔, no change; ↑↑, greater increase than ↑; ↓↓, greater decrease than ↓.

Pulmonary Blood Flow during Exercise

Cardiac output increases linearly with oxygen consumption during exercise (Fig. 12-4). The increase in cardiac output is secondary to an increase in heart rate and increased venous return due to deeper inspiratory efforts. Mean pulmonary artery and mean left atrial pressures increase out of proportion to changes in pulmonary blood flow. As a result, there is a decrease in pulmonary vascular resistance. Recruitment of pulmonary blood vessels occurs, especially in upper regions of the lung, and this is associated with a decrease in the regional inhomogeneity observed at rest.

Exercise results in a more uniform ventilation-perfusion ratio ($\dot{V}/\dot{Q}$) throughout the lung, with regional ratios close to 1.0 (Fig. 12-5). Increased pulmonary blood flow during exercise increases the diffusion capacity as oxygen uptake increases. The surface area for diffusion increases as pulmonary blood flow to the upper lung regions increases. Increased velocity of blood flow occurs, and this maintains the partial pressure gradient for diffusion. At maximum levels of exercise associated with great blood velocities, diffusion limitation of gas transfer can occur even in healthy individuals.

Exercise is most remarkable for the lack of significant changes in blood gas values. Except at maximal levels, in general, arterial PCO_2 ($PaCO_2$) decreases slightly and arterial PO_2 (PaO_2) increases slightly during exercise. Arterial pH remains normal at moderate exercise. During heavy exercise, arterial pH begins to fall as lactic acid is liberated during anaerobic metabolism.

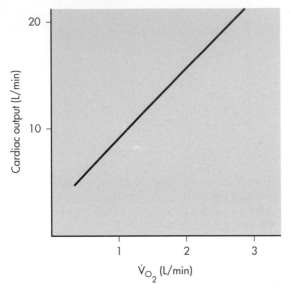

FIGURE 12-4 ■ Cardiac output is linearly related to oxygen consumption. *(Modified and redrawn from Chernick V, Kendig EL: Kendig's Disorders of the Respiratory Tract in Children, 5th ed. Philadelphia, WB Saunders, 1990.)*

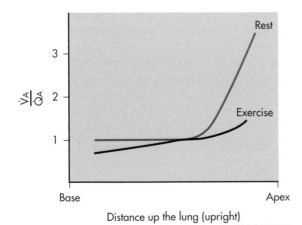

FIGURE 12-5 ■ Regional ventilation/perfusion ratios ($\dot{V}_A/\dot{Q}_A$) in the lung at rest and during exercise. During exercise the $\dot{V}_A/\dot{Q}_A$ is more homogeneous than at rest. *(Modified and redrawn from Levitzky MG: Pulmonary Physiology, 4th ed. New York, McGraw-Hill, 1995.)*

This decrease in arterial pH stimulates ventilation out of proportion to the level of exercise intensity and results in a fall in Pa_{CO_2}. The level of exercise at which a sustained metabolic acidosis begins is called the **anaerobic threshold** (Fig. 12-6). This level is different

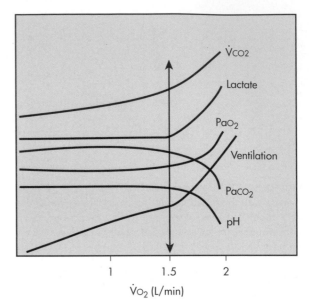

FIGURE 12-6 ■ Some important metabolic changes that occur during exercise. The anaerobic threshold *(arrow)* is marked by a sudden change in the measured variables, which is due mainly to the developing lactic acidosis as anaerobic glycolysis takes over more and more of the muscle energy supply, which is caused by the relative failure of the body to supply sufficient oxygen to the muscles at the rate demanded by the level of exercise. *(Modified from Berne RM, Levy ML, Koeppen BM, Stanton BM: Physiology, 5th ed. St. Louis, Mosby, 2004.)*

in fit compared with unfit individuals. The Aa_{DO_2} also increases during exercise as a result of a number of factors, including diffusion limitation of gas transfer, decreased mixed venous P_{O_2} ($P\bar{v}_{O_2}$), increased alveolar P_{O_2} (PA_{O_2}), and shifts in the oxyhemoglobin dissociation curve.

With activity, CO_2 production increases, and as a result, ventilation must increase. At low levels of exercise (CO_2 production of 1 L/min) there are only small differences in the alveolar ventilation needed to maintain the Pa_{CO_2} over a wide range of values (see Fig. 12-3). As CO_2 production increases with increasing exercise, greater increases in alveolar ventilation are required to maintain the Pa_{CO_2} within this range of values. Although this is not difficult for the individual with normal pulmonary mechanics, CO_2 elimination can be a significant problem for individuals with altered pulmonary mechanics.

The actual cause of the increased ventilation during exercise remains largely unknown. No single mediator or mechanism has been identified to explain why ventilation remains so closely matched to carbon dioxide production. Hypoxic or hypercarbic mechanisms do not play a role, because neither occurs during most exercise. Mechanisms believed to contribute include neural inputs from the motor cortex to the medullary respiratory control center, afferents from muscle and joint mechanoreceptors, and unknown mediators released from working muscles.

EXERCISE TESTING

Exercise testing provides a quantitative assessment of an individual's exercise capacity. A variety of simple and sophisticated tests can be performed to assess exercise capacity. Many of the simpler tests can be performed in the office; more sophisticated tests are usually performed in a hospital's pulmonary function laboratory.

The simplest of all exercise tests is exercise **oximetry**. Oxygen saturation by pulse oximetry is measured at rest; the subject then exercises until becoming short of breath, and the oxygen saturation is recorded. Two types of tests are commonly done—walking and stair climbing.

In the **6- and 12-minute walk test**, the subject is instructed to walk back and forth over a 100-ft distance and the number of laps is counted. The distance walked over a 6- or 12-minute time period is recorded, and the average rate of walking in miles per hour is calculated. This test is particularly useful for titrating oxygen therapy to ensure adequate oxygenation and enhanced exercise capacity.

In the **stair-climbing test**, the number of steps climbed is counted until the subject's symptoms become limiting. On average, the ability to climb 83 steps is equivalent to a maximal oxygen consumption of 20 mL/kg/min. This value is associated with fewer complications after thoracotomy; thus this is a useful test for individuals with chronic obstructive pulmonary disease (COPD) who are undergoing thoracic surgical procedures.

Formal cardiorespiratory exercise testing requires sophisticated equipment and experienced physiologic direction and medical supervision. Such testing is useful in distinguishing between cardiac and pulmonary causes of dyspnea, determining whether symptoms are the result of deconditioning, conducting disability evaluations, assessing work/job capacity, and identifying the malingering patient.

TRAINING EFFECTS

Training increases the ability to perform exercise. Most of the training effect occurs in skeletal muscles and in the cardiovascular system. Maximum oxygen uptake increases with exercise in large part because of an increase in maximal cardiac output. Training lowers the resting heart rate and increases the resting stroke volume without affecting the maximum heart rate. Physical training increases the oxidative capacity of skeletal muscle, improves the strength and endurance of respiratory muscles, induces mitochondrial proliferation, and increases the concentration of oxidative enzymes and the synthesis of glycogen and triglyceride. This results in increased aerobic energy production capacity and lower blood lactate levels in trained subjects. The lower lactate levels in turn result in decreases in ventilation during submaximal exercise.

FETAL LUNG DEVELOPMENT

Fetal lung development can be divided into five stages (Fig. 12-7):

1. Embryonic (day 26 to day 52)
2. Pseudoglandular (day 52 to week 16)
3. Canalicular (week 16 to week 28)
4. Saccular (week 28 to week 36)
5. Alveolar (week 36 to term).

In the **embryonic** stage, the cells of the conducting airways and alveoli develop from endodermally derived epithelium as a ventral outpouching of the primitive gut during the embryonic stage. The primary bronchi then elongate into the mesenchyme and divide into two main bronchi and then undergo dichotomous branching to form the conducting airways. About 23-27 generations of conducting airways are formed, each lined by a columnar epithelium (Fig. 12-8). At the same time, the mesenchyme differentiates around the airways into cartilage, smooth muscle, and connective tissue. By the end of the pseudoglandular stage, all of the conducting airways, including the terminal respiratory bronchioles, are full developed.

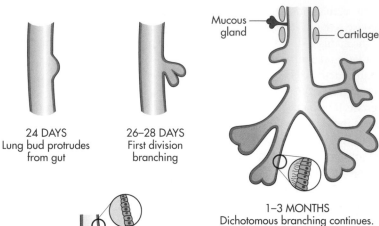

24 DAYS
Lung bud protrudes
from gut

26–28 DAYS
First division
branching

1–3 MONTHS
Dichotomous branching continues.
Lung is glandular: ciliated columnar
epithelium lines airway.

FIGURE 12-7 ■ Stages of lung fetal development. *(Redrawn from Avery ME: The Lung and Its Disorders in the Newborn Infant, 3rd ed. Philadelphia, WB Saunders, 1974.)*

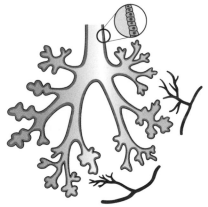

5 MONTHS
Canalized airways lined by
cuboidal epithelium.
Capillaries arise from vascular
structures in mesenchyme.

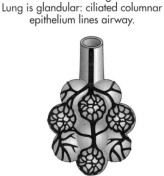

6.5–7 MONTHS
Alveoli appear from alveolar ducts;
epithelium attenuates; capillaries
proliferate around terminal airspaces.

FIGURE 12-8 ■ Development of the tracheobronchial tree in utero. *Line A* represents the number of bronchial generations; *line A′* represents the number of respiratory bronchioles and alveolar ducts; *line B* is the extension of cartilage along the bronchial tree; and *line C* is the extension of mucous glands. *(Redrawn from Bucher U, Reid L: Development of the intrasegmental bronchial tree: The pattern of branching and development of cartilage at various stages of intra-uterine life. Thorax 16:207-218, 1961.)*

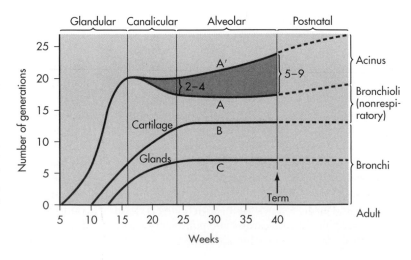

In the **canalicular** stage, respiratory bronchioles with terminal air sacs—the first primitive alveoli—develop. There is also marked proliferation of blood vessels in close proximity to the air sacs with a marked decrease in the amount of connective tissue. Type I and type II epithelial cells appear, and lamellar bodies, the storage place for surfactant, become apparent. Toward the end of the canalicular stage, gas exchange becomes possible as the capillaries rapidly proliferate and the epithelial surface thins.

During the **saccular** stage, there is a marked increase in lung growth; the lung grows to fill the thoracic cavity, and increasing numbers of gas exchanging units develop. Acinar development is complete and is the major site of gas exchange, as there are relatively few true alveoli at birth. **Alveolar** development occurs rapidly following birth, with marked growth in the first 2 years of life; by 8 years of age when alveolar numbers are no longer increasing, there are approximately 300 million alveoli.

FETAL RESPIRATION DEVELOPMENT

Respiratory movements have been observed in utero, but regular, automatic respiration begins at birth. The fetus is well suited to its environment in which the lung is not the gas exchange unit. In utero, the placenta is the organ of gas exchange for the fetus. Its microvilli interdigitate with the maternal uterine circulation and O_2 transport and CO_2 removal from the fetus occur by passive diffusion across the maternal circulation. Blood travels through the umbilical artery to the placenta and returns to the fetus through the umbilical vein (Fig. 12-9). Maternal and fetal circulations are separate and the blood of the fetus and mother do not mix. Compared to adult arterial partial pressures, the Po_2 being delivered to the fetus is low because the uterus extracts its oxygen prior to delivery to the fetus (Fig. 12-10). Thus, the Po_2 in the umbilical vein is only 30 torr and in the umbilical artery is only 20 torr. The fetus, however, is able to thrive in this environment because of the presence of fetal hemoglobin, which has a substantially greater affinity for oxygen than does adult hemoglobin. Fetal hemoglobin is discussed in Chapter 8.

The fetal lung has no respiratory function in utero and, in fact, very little blood actually circulates through the fetal lung. Venous return from the fetus bypasses the lung, instead passing through a **patent foramen ovale**, an opening in the atrial septum of the fetal heart. The foramen ovale remains open because of the high pulmonary vascular resistance in the fetal lung (due to pulmonary hypoxic vasoconstriction), which results in increased pressure in the right atrium. Most of the venous blood that reaches the right ventricle is diverted into the systemic circulation through a **patent ductus arteriosus**, a connection between the pulmonary artery and the aorta. Again, it is the high pulmonary vascular resistance in the lung that produces a pressure gradient favoring blood flow from the pulmonary artery to the aorta.

Birth marks the end of the placenta and the beginning of respiration. With the first breath, there is an increase in oxygen in the lungs. This results in a rapid and marked (one fifth of the systemic circulation) decrease in pulmonary vascular resistance and an increase in blood flow through the lung. The foramen ovale now closes, and over the first several days of life the ductus arteriosus also closes, favored by the change in pressure gradients secondary to further decreases in pulmonary vascular resistance. Recent research suggests that, unlike other vascular tissue, the ductus arteriosus closes in response to the *increased* oxygen content in the systemic circulation. In some individuals, the ductus arteriosus does not close, and surgical closure is required.

POSTNATAL DEVELOPMENT

In the first several months of life many changes occur in the respiratory system. Newborn infants show a strong preference for nasal breathing ("obligate nose breathers"). This adaptation allows newborn infants to breathe and swallow at the same time—a feat lost in the first year of life. It also results in high airway resistance that can be made worse by any nasal congestion. Pulmonary vascular resistance falls and the relatively thick-walled smooth muscle of the pulmonary arterial system thins to adult levels. Airways grow in

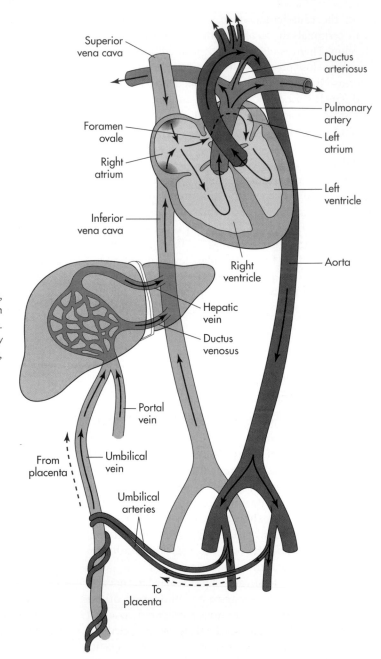

FIGURE 12-9 ■ Fetal circulation. In utero, blood is diverted away from the lungs through the foramen ovale and the ductus arteriosus. *(Redrawn from Leff A, Schumacker P: Respiratory Physiology: Basics and Applications. Philadelphia, WB Saunders, 1993.)*

length and diameter but do not change in number. Alveoli increase in number from approximately 50 million at birth to 300 million in adulthood. Although it is unclear at what age alveolarization is completed, it is known that it occurs early, perhaps by 2 to 3 years of age and certainly no later than 8 years of age. Following completion of alveolarization, alveolar surface area increases in relation to increasing O_2 requirements, because alveoli become more complex in shape as they grow.

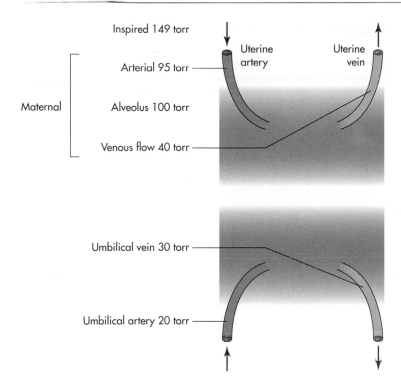

Inspired 149 torr

Uterine artery

Uterine vein

Maternal
Arterial 95 torr
Alveolus 100 torr
Venous flow 40 torr

Umbilical vein 30 torr

Umbilical artery 20 torr

FIGURE 12-10 ■ Blood gas values in the maternal and fetal circulations. *(Redrawn from Leff A, Schumacker P: Respiratory Physiology: Basics and Applications. Philadelphia, WB Saunders, 1993.)*

HIGH ALTITUDE AND ACCLIMATIZATION

At high altitude, ambient air still contains 21% oxygen, but the barometric pressure is lower and the inspired Po_2 and alveolar Po_2 are decreased. Alveolar and thus arterial Pco_2 are also lower because the decreased Po_2 stimulates peripheral chemoreceptors. The result of hyperventilation is an increase in arterial Po_2 (recall the alveolar air equation) (Table 12-2).

Individuals who ascend from sea level to high altitude (unacclimatized) can experience sudden decreases in arterial oxygen and the rapid onset of signs and symptoms of hypoxia with altered function of the CNS. These same symptoms are seen in people on airplanes when there is a sudden loss of cabin pressure. Some individuals who ascend quickly to moderate altitudes develop a syndrome called **acute mountain sickness**. Symptoms include headache, sleeplessness, nausea, vision and hearing diminution, weakness, breathlessness, and dypsnea on exertion. The symptoms are secondary to hypoxia and hypocapnia and require immediate descent. In most individuals, symptoms disappear 1 to 3 days after descent.

Another problem in some individuals who go to high altitude is **high-altitude pulmonary edema**. Symptoms include severe dyspnea, orthopnea, cough, and copious crackles, sometimes to the point of coughing up pink, frothy fluid. High-altitude pulmonary edema is a life-threatening illness. Individuals with this problem should be advised against returning to high altitude, as the problem is likely to recur. A similar problem, known as **high-altitude cerebral edema**, associated with the CNS symptoms of confusion, ataxia, hallucinations, and loss of consciousness, can also occur and requires immediate descent.

Some individuals who reside in high-altitude areas develop a syndrome known as **chronic mountain sickness**, characterized by cyanosis, fatigue, marked polycythemia, and profound hypoxemia. These individuals need to descend to lower altitudes.

Long-term **acclimatization** to high altitude, however, occurs in most individuals and begins within

TABLE 12-2

Physiological Responses to High Altitude—Compared with Sea Level Control Values

	IMMEDIATE	EARLY ADAPTIVE (72H)	LATE ADAPTIVE (2 TO 6 WEEKS)
Ventilation			
Minute ventilation	↑	↑	↑
Respiratory rate	Variable	Variable	Variable
Tidal volume	↑	↑	↑
Arterial P_{O_2}	↓	↓	↓
Arterial P_{CO_2}	↓	↓	↓
Arterial pH	↑	↑ ↔	↑ ↔
Arterial HCO_3^-	↔	↓	↓
Lung Function			
Vital capacity	↔	↔	↔
Maximum airflow rates	↑	↑	↑
Functional residual capacity	↔	↔	↔
Ventilatory response to inhaled CO_2	↔	↑	↑
Ventilatory response to hypoxia	↔	↔	↔
Pulmonary vascular resistance	↑	↑	↑
Oxygen Transport			
Hemoglobin	↔	↑	↑
Erythropoietin	↑	↔	↔
P_{10}	↓	↑	↑
2,3-DPG	↔	↑	↑
Cardiac output	↑	↔	↔ ↓

2,3-DPG, 2,3-diphosphoglycerate; ↑, increased; ↓, decreased; ↔, no change.
Source: Adapted with permission from Guenter CA, Weich MH, Hogg JC: Clinical Aspects of Respiratory Physiology. Philadelphia, Lippincott. 1976 p 3–37.

hours of ascent to high altitude. Hyperventilation is one of the most important features of acclimatization. Renal compensation for the respiratory alkalosis begins within hours, characterized by bicarbonate excretion and hydrogen ion conservation. Hypoxia stimulates erythropoiesis, increasing the hematocrit and oxygen-carrying capacity. As a result, oxygen content (not Pa_{O_2}) increases. Although the polycythemia (increased hematocrit) increases oxygen content, it also increases blood viscosity, which increases ventricular workload. Oxygen release at the tissues is enhanced through increased production of 2,3-diphosphoglycerate secondary to respiratory alkalosis and a rightward shift of the oxyhemoglobin dissociation curve.

Hypoxic stimulation of the peripheral chemoreceptors continues at high altitude, but the ventilatory response curve to CO_2 shifts to the left. Thus at any level of arterial CO_2, the ventilatory response is greater after several days at high altitude. Coincident with this shift, cerebrospinal fluid pH returns toward normal and CNS symptoms abate.

Cardiac output, heart rate, and systemic blood pressure increase with ascent to high altitude. After a month or so, these changes return to normal as a result of a decrease in sympathetic activity. However, pulmonary hypoxic vasoconstriction and pulmonary hypertension persist, leading to right ventricular hypertrophy and cor pulmonale.

Persons born at high altitude have a diminished ventilatory response to hypoxia, whereas those who are born at sea level and subsequently move to high altitude have a normal ventilatory response to hypoxia even after residing at high altitude for a long time. Thus it appears that the ventilatory response to hypoxia is determined at a very young age.

SUMMARY

1. With moderate levels of exercise, the increase in minute ventilation is linearly related to both CO_2 production and O_2 consumption.
2. In normal individuals, the cardiovascular system and not the respiratory system is the rate-limiting factor in exercise.
3. Cardiac output increases linearly with oxygen consumption during exercise.
4. In general, arterial blood gases change little during exercise.
5. The anaerobic threshold occurs when a sustained metabolic acidosis develops during exercise. Training shifts the location of the anaerobic threshold to the right but does not change the maximum heart rate that is achievable.

6. Fetal lung development is divided into five stages: embryonic, pseudoglandular, canalicular, saccular, and alveolar.

7. Airways are fully formed by the 16th week of gestation. Alveoli at birth are relatively few in number and increase dramatically in the first 2 to 3 years of life.

8. Primitive alveoli develop during the latter stages of the canalicular phase of growth and mark the earliest stage of gas exchange and possible extrauterine life.

9. The fetal lung has no respiratory function in utero. Pulmonary hypoxic vasoconstriction is responsible for the maintenance of the patency of the foramen ovale and the ductus arteriosus.

10. High altitude is associated with a decrease in barometric pressure and decreases in PaO_2 and $PaCO_2$.

11. Various syndromes are associated with high altitude, including acute and chronic mountain sickness, high-altitude pulmonary edema, and high-altitude cerebral edema.

12. Hyperventilation is a major feature of acclimatization and results in renal, CNS, and hematologic compensatory mechanisms. Hypoxia stimulates red blood cell production, resulting in polycythemia and an increase in oxygen-carrying capacity.

KEY WORDS

- Acclimatization
- Acute mountain sickness
- Anaerobic threshold
- Canalicular
- Chronic mountain sickness
- Embryonic
- High-altitude cerebral edema
- High-altitude pulmonary edema
- Oximetry
- Patent ductus arteriosus
- Patent foramen ovale
- Pseudoglandular
- Saccular

- 6- and 12-minute walk test
- Stair-climbing test
- Training

SELF-STUDY PROBLEMS

1. What factors limit maximal exercise?

2. What happens to minute ventilation before and after the anaerobic threshold? Why?

3. What is the effect of training on maximum heart rate and cardiac output, respiratory muscle strength, and endurance and ventilation?

4. In congenital diaphragmatic hernia (CDH), the diaphragm fails to close between the thoracic and abdominal cavity. This normally occurs by the 16th week of gestation. As a result abdominal cavity contents fill the space and prevent normal lung development. What components of the respiratory tract (airways, blood vessels, interstitium, and alveoli) will be involved in individuals with CDH?

5. Describe fetal circulation and the circulatory changes that occur at birth.

6. What are the effects of high altitude on arterial oxygenation, lung fluid balance, and the central nervous system?

REFERENCES

Adamson IY. Development of lung structure. In: Crystal RG, West JB, Barnes PJ (eds): The Lung: Scientific Foundation. New York: Raven Press, 1997.

Bangsbo, J: Quantification of anaerobic energy production during intense exercise. Med Sci Sports Exerc 30:47-52, 1998.

Cibella F, Cuttitta G, Romano S, et al: Respiratory energetics during exercise at high altitude. J Appl Physiol 86:1785-1792, 1999.

Harding R, Hooper SB: Regulation of lung expansion and lung growth before birth J. Appl Physiol 81:209-224, 1996.

Kotecha S: Lung growth: Implications for the newborn infant. Arch Dis Child Fetal Neonatal Ed 82:F69-F74, 2000.

Shoene RB: Limits of human lung function at high altitude. J Exp Biol 204:3121-3127, 2001.

*West J, Hackett P, Maret K, et al: Pulmonary gas exchange on the summit of Mt Everest. J Appl Physiol 55: 678-687, 1983.

*A classic.

APPENDIX A
ANSWERS TO SELF-STUDY PROBLEMS

CHAPTER 1

1. The principal muscle of inspiration is the diaphragm. Other muscles of inspiration include the external intercostal muscles, and the accessory muscles of inspiration—the scalene muscles, the alae nasi, and the small muscles of the neck and head.
2. Exhalation is usually passive, but when active, the important muscles are the muscles of the abdominal wall (the rectus abdominus, the internal and external obliques and the transversus abdominus) and the internal intercostals.
3. The pulmonary circulation is a low-pressure, high-compliance system. At rest, many of the vessels are either compressed or not open. Increases in pulmonary flow either universally, as would occur during exercise, or locally, as would occur if one of the main pulmonary arteries were occluded, are associated with maintenance of low pressure, as compressed or occluded vessels open and open vessels distend. Thus transient occlusion of the left main pulmonary artery would double the blood flow through the right pulmonary artery, but this increase in flow would produce only a small change in the pressure in the right pulmonary artery and would certainly not double it.
4. The barrier between gas in the alveolus and the red blood cell consists of the type I alveolar epithelial cell, the capillary endothelial cell, and their respective basement membranes. The distance of the barrier is approximately 1 to 2 μm.
5. The principal function of the lung is gas exchange. The anatomic features that make the lung ideally suited for this function include the large surface area for gas exchange, with millions of alveoli and capillaries; the close proximity between gas in the alveolus and the red blood cell; the dual circulation of the lung, resulting in the entire cardiac output going through the lung; the structure of the type I cell, with its thin, elongated cytoplasm that reduces the distance between alveolar gas and the pulmonary capillary; and the highly distensible, low-pressure pulmonary circulation that allows for accommodation over a wide range of cardiac outputs without a significant change in pressure.

CHAPTER 2

1. Factors that determine total lung capacity (TLC) include lung elastic recoil and the properties of the muscles of the chest wall. TLC occurs when the forces of inspiration decrease because of chest wall muscle lengthening and are insufficient to overcome the lung's elastic recoil.
2. Residual volume occurs when the forces exerted by expiratory muscle shortening decrease and are insufficient to overcome the outward recoil of the chest wall.
3. Acute hypersensitivity pneumonitis is an example of a restrictive lung disease. Thus lung volumes will be reduced. Specifically, TLC and to a lesser extent functional residual capacity (FRC) and residual volume (RV) are decreased, resulting in an increase in the RV/TLC ratio.

CHAPTER 3

1. Increasing lung volume increases the length and diameter of the airways. As a result, resistance to airflow decreases with increases in lung volume, but the relationship is curvilinear. At lung volumes greater than FRC, there is little effect on resistance. Below FRC, resistance increases rapidly and approaches infinity at RV.
2. The cross-sectional area of a conducting airway is determined by the forces of contraction (i.e., the

elastic forces in the airways and the tension of the smooth muscle surrounding the airways) and the forces of dilation or outward traction (i.e., a positive transpulmonary pressure or the interdependence of alveoli and terminal bronchioles).

3. A reduction in elastic recoil pressure, which is present in individuals with emphysema, will result in a decrease in the driving pressure for expiratory gas flow, and in premature airway closure in association with movement of the equal pressure point closer to the alveoli.

4. Airway resistance is determined by flow rate (the more laminar the airflow, the lower the resistance) and airflow velocity becomes very low as the effective cross-sectional area increases. Furthermore, the airways exist in parallel, and as a result the many small airways contribute very little to the resistance.

CHAPTER 4

1A-D.

A. The test appears to be performed in a satisfactory way with a rapid rise to peak flow and a gradual, smooth decline to residual volume. Compared with the normal curve (dotted line), peak flow and expiratory flow rates are decreased. Forced vital capacity (FVC) is normal, with a decreased forced expiratory volume after 1 second (FEV_1); this would result in a decrease in the FEV_1/FVC ratio. These changes are consistent with chronic obstructive pulmonary disease (COPD); the magnitude is approximately 50%, and thus this is moderate COPD.

B. The test demonstrates a rapid rise and a smooth decline to the baseline compatible with acceptable quality. The FVC and FEV_1 are reduced, with a normal FEV_1/FVC ratio. Expiratory flow rates are normal. These changes are consistent with restrictive pulmonary disease; the magnitude is reduced 25% to 50%; thus this is mild-to-moderate restrictive lung disease.

C. The test demonstrates a rapid rise to peak flow, a saw-toothed decline, and an abrupt drop in flow to the baseline. The effort as demonstrated by the initial rise is good, but the subject either coughed (saw-tooth) or periodically closed the

glottis when exhaling. In addition, the subject did not exhale to residual volume (abrupt drop in flow). Thus this flow volume curve is uninterpretable.

D. There is a rapid rise to peak flow followed by a gradual, smooth decline to zero flow or baseline. This is an acceptable test. The FVC and FEV_1 are normal and have a normal ratio. Expiratory flow rates at high lung volume (i.e., early in the maneuver or close to TLC) are normal; flow rates at low lung volume (i.e., late in the maneuver or close to RV) are reduced. This is an example of mild obstructive pulmonary disease (OPD) involving the small airways. It is what you might find in an asymptomatic 20-year smoker.

2. Early in COPD, the spirogram and flow volume curve are normal, but evidence of air trapping (i.e., an elevated RV/TLC ratio) may be present. As the disease progresses, there is further air trapping in association with decreased expiratory flow rates, particularly involving the small airways (see Answer 1D, above). With further progression, peak flow and airway resistance (R_{AW}) are affected, and FEV_1 becomes decreased. When the FVC begins to decrease, the individual has moderate-to-severe obstructive pulmonary disease; when the FVC is below 50% of predicted, the individual has severe obstructive pulmonary disease. Emphysema and chronic bronchitis can both produce pulmonary function abnormalities as described previously. The two diseases can be distinguished by the diffusion capacity for carbon monoxide (D_{LCO}). The D_{LCO} is normal in chronic bronchitis, whereas it is decreased in emphysema.

3. In individuals with restrictive pulmonary disease, both the FVC and the FEV_1 decrease proportionately. This occurs in association with normal (and even supernormal) expiratory flow rates (See Answer 1B, above) and with decreases in TLC, and less so in RV (resulting in an elevated RV/TLC ratio due to a decrease in TLC). Compliance is also reduced in many restrictive lung diseases (but not all). Disease progresses with further reduction in these pulmonary function tests with eventual decreases in expiratory flow rates.

4. A normal D_{LCO} requires a normal surface area for gas diffusion. This is the major requirement.

However, decreased perfusion secondary to emboli or decreased cardiac output or decreased capillary blood volume such as anemia also contributes to an abnormal D_{LCO}.

CHAPTER 5

1. As tidal volume (V_T) increases, there is a decrease in dead space ventilation (V_{DS}) for the same minute ventilation (V_E):

$V_T = 500$ mL	$V_T = 600$ mL
$V_{DS} = 150$ mL $\cdot$ V_E	$V_{DS} = 150$ mL $\cdot$ V_E
500 mL $= 0.30 \cdot V_E$	600 mL $= 0.25 \cdot V_E$

2. Using Fowler's method, the dead space is equal to the volume of the anatomic dead space that contains 100% oxygen and 0% nitrogen plus $\frac{1}{2}$ of the rising nitrogen volume, or:

$$V_{DS} = 130 + \frac{1}{2}(170 - 130)$$
$$= 150 \text{ mL}$$

3. At Pike's peak, the partial pressure of inspired air is:

$$P_{IO_2} \text{ dry} = (445 \text{ mm Hg}) \times 0.21 = 93 \text{ mm Hg}.$$

The air in the conducting airways is:

$$P_{IO_2} = (445 \text{ mm Hg} - 47 \text{ mm Hg}) \times 0.21$$
$$= 83.6 \text{ mm Hg}.$$

4. From the alveolar air equation, it can be seen that an increase in Pa_{CO_2} will result in a decrease in alveolar O_2. This has significant implications in the face of a decrease in oxygen in inspired air. One of the ways that we can increase alveolar O_2 is by changing alveolar CO_2. At high altitude we hyperventilate and decrease alveolar CO_2; this results in an increase in alveolar O_2.

5. If alveolar ventilation is constant, but CO_2 production increases, there will be an increase in alveolar (arterial) CO_2. As a result, using the alveolar air equation, alveolar O_2 will decrease. This is most commonly seen in individuals who are being mechanically ventilated under significant sedation or in patients who are paralyzed, who are on mechanical ventilators, and who develop fever. These individuals will develop an increase in P_{CO_2} in association with a decrease in P_{O_2} as a result of the increase in CO_2 production that is due to the fever.

6. In the upright position, the pleural pressure gradient is most negative at the apex and decreases (becomes less negative) in the dependent regions of the lung. As a result, alveoli at the apex of the lung are bigger, and because of where they are located on the pressure volume curve of the lung, they are less compliant. Thus, with tidal volume breathing most of the ventilation goes to the alveoli at the bases or dependent region. The vertical pressure gradient is maintained when you are standing on your head, but it is now reversed. Namely, the apex of the lung is the dependent portion; its surrounding pleural pressure is less negative; as a result, the alveoli in the apex are now smaller than alveoli at the base of the lung and are positioned at the steeper portion of the pressure volume curve; thus these now dependent alveoli receive a greater portion of the tidal volume.

CHAPTER 6

1. The relationship between total pulmonary vascular resistance and lung volume in the *entire lung* is described by a U-shaped curve. Total pulmonary vascular resistance (PVR) is lowest near FRC and increases at both high and low lung volumes. The pulmonary vascular resistance in *alveolar vessels* increases with increasing lung volume and distention of the air-filled alveoli. Pulmonary vascular resistance in *extra-alveolar vessels* decreases with increasing lung volume due to stretching and an increase in vessel diameter caused by radial traction.

2. Pulmonary blood flow is dramatically affected by gravity. In the absence of gravity, pulmonary blood flow throughout the lung would be equal.

3. A decrease in pulmonary artery pressure, if sufficient, would result in the appearance of Zone 1 regions in the uppermost areas of the lung. A decrease in pulmonary venous pressure could also convert Zone II regions into Zone III regions.

4. Exposure to high altitude results in a decrease in alveolar oxygen tension. This can cause hypoxic vasoconstriction throughout the lung, resulting in an increase in pulmonary arterial pressures.

5. Oxygen is a potent vasodilator. During cardiac catheterization, oxygen is administered to determine whether the pulmonary vasculature is responsive to oxygen. Responsiveness to oxygen is measured by a decrease in pulmonary artery pressure with oxygen administration.

CHAPTER 7

1. An anatomic shunt does not respond to breathing 100% oxygen. In contrast, low $\dot{V}/\dot{Q}$ will respond to increasing the ambient oxygen concentration, and to a lesser extent so will a physiologic shunt. Hypoventilation with hypoxemia will have a normal $AaDO_2$.

2. At the level of a single alveolus, the PO_2 is equal to the alveolar ventilation divided by the capillary flow.

3. With $\dot{V}/\dot{Q}$ inequality, blood from normally ventilated alveoli mixes with blood from lung regions with low ventilation. Because the relationship between oxygen content and partial pressure is sigmoidal, ventilation of normally ventilated alveoli cannot significantly increase the oxygen content in the blood leaving them. This same relationship for CO_2 is more linear; thus excessive ventilation of some alveoli can effectively compensate for under-ventilation of other alveoli in terms of CO_2 exchange. This difference results in a low arterial PO_2 with a normal PCO_2 in many lung diseases until the process is very advanced and compensation can no longer occur for CO_2.

CHAPTER 8

1. The oxyhemoglobin dissociation curve is shifted to the right (increased P_{50}, decreased O_2 affinity) with increases in temperature, PCO_2, and levels of 2.3-diphosphoglycerate (2,3-DPG) and decreases in pH. The curve is shifted to the left (decreased P_{50}, increased O_2 affinity) with decreases in temperature, PCO_2, and 2,3-DPG and increases in pH.

2. The shifts in the oxyhemoglobin dissociation curve aid in the uptake of O_2 and unloading of CO_2 in the lung and in the uptake of O_2 and unloading of CO_2 by the tissues.

3. Yes. Oxygen content and oxygen saturation do not mean the same thing. The oxygen content could be low due to anemia, but in this case the saturation could be normal. Other causes include poor circulation and poisoning of the mitochondrial transport systems.

4. O_2 is primarily transported in two forms: dissolved and chemically bound to hemoglobin. CO_2 is transported in three forms: physically dissolved, as carbamino compounds, and as bicarbonate ions.

5. When hemoglobin is fully saturated, supplemental oxygen will not appreciably affect the Hgb O_2 content. When hemoglobin is not fully saturated, such as in individuals with a PaO_2 less than 60 mm Hg, supplemental oxygen will markedly increase oxygen saturation and thus increase Hgb O_2 content.

6. Tissue hypoxia occurs when the cells or tissues in the body do not receive adequate oxygen to carry out their metabolic functions and switch from oxidative metabolism to anaerobic metabolism. There are four mechanisms of tissue hypoxia: hypoxic hypoxia due to lung disease, anemic hypoxia secondary to inadequate numbers of red blood cells, circulatory hypoxia when there is a marked decrease in cardiac output, and histologic hypoxia due to mitochondrial function poisons.

7. A gas leaving the capillary that has reached equilibrium with alveolar gas is perfusion-limited, whereas a gas leaving the capillary that has not reached equilibrium with alveolar gas is diffusion-limited. The major factors determining whether a gas is perfusion- or diffusion-limited are its solubility in the membrane, its solubility in the blood, and its ability to bind chemically to hemoglobin. Under normal conditions, both O_2 and CO_2 are perfusion-limited; however, they can become diffusion-limited, with very rapid red cell transit in the pulmonary circulation.

CHAPTER 9

1-5. Correct matches are in boldface type.

    a–3. Using the alveolar air equation, the $AaDO_2$ is $[0.21 \times (760 - 47) - 40/0.8] - 110 = -10$ mm Hg; thus this is an impossible gas value on room air. Looked at another way, the sum of the PaO_2 and $PaCO_2$ on room air at sea level should not be greater than 130 mm Hg.

b-4. The pH is less than 7.4, suggesting that there is an acidosis. In order for the elevated $PaCO_2$ to account for the change in pH of 0.06 units, the increase must be chronic ($0.03 \times 20/10$ mm Hg = 0.06 units). Using the alveolar air equation, the $AaDO_2$ is $[0.21 \times (760 - 47) - 60/0.8] - 60 = 15$ mm Hg; this is a normal alveolar-arterial difference demonstrating normal lung parenchyma. Therefore this individual has chronic hypoventilation with normal lung parenchyma.

c-1. The pH is less than 7.4, suggesting that there is an acidosis. In this case the $PaCO_2$ is also low—a compensation for the acidosis. Therefore this must be a metabolic acidosis. What would you predict the base excess to be in this individual? The answer is -10 (0.15 change in pH is associated with a 10 mEq/L change in base excess.) Using the alveolar air equation, the $AaDO_2 = (0.21 \times 760 - 47) - 25/0.8] - 110 = 9$ mm Hg, which is normal, demonstrating no pulmonary parenchymal disease. Thus this individual has a metabolic acidosis (with respiratory compensation).

d-5. This individual has an abnormal $AaDO_2$. ($AaDO_2 = PAO_2 - PaO_2 = [0.21 \times (760 - 47) - 30/0.8] - 50$ mm Hg = 62 mm Hg). The hyperventilation (low $PaCO_2$) appears acute in nature (pH increases 0.08 units for a 10–mm Hg decrease in $PaCO_2$). Why is this individual hyperventilating? In the presence of hypoxia, hyperventilation will increase the PaO_2. The PaO_2 in this individual would be approximately 10 mm Hg lower if this individual did not hyperventilate (if the partial pressure of one gas increases, the other must decrease). The actual amount can be calculated again using the alveolar air equation: $0.21 \times (760 - 47) - 40/0.8 = 100$; in the presence of an $AaDO_2 = 62$ mm Hg, the PaO_2 is $100 - 62 = 38$ mm Hg. Thus, by hyperventilating and decreasing the $PaCO_2$ by 10 mm Hg, this individual achieved a 12 mm Hg increase in PaO_2.

e-2. This individual has an elevated pH and a mildly elevated $PaCO_2$. Because it is unusual to overcompensate, the underlying process is most likely a metabolic alkalosis with respiratory compensation. Is there evidence of underlying lung disease in this arterial blood gas? Using the alveolar air equation, the $AaDO_2 = 0.21 \times (760 - 47) - 45/0.8] - 80 = 14$ mm Hg. This is within the normal range, so this individual does not have pulmonary parenchymal disease. What would the HCO_3^- be in this individual? (Ans.: >24 mEq/L).

6. This woman has no history of lung (or other) disease and is most likely hyperventilating due to an anxiety reaction. Hyperventilation would produce a decrease in $PaCO_2$ and a concomitant increase in PaO_2. Therefore the most appropriate blood gas would be either **b** or **c**. How can you choose between these two? Use the alveolar air equation. In **b**, $AaDO_2 = [0.21 \times (760 - 47) - 20/0.8] - 100 = 25$ mm Hg. In **c**, $AaDO_2 = [0.21 \times (760 - 47) - 20/0.8] - 120 = 5$ mm Hg. Because the $AaDO_2$ increases with age, it would be very unlikely that a person this age would have an $AaDO_2 = 5$ mm Hg. Thus the best answer is **b**. You could have also predicted this individual's $PaO_2 = 102 - 55/3 = {\sim}84$ mm Hg if the $PaCO_2$ were normal (that is, if she had not been hyperventilating). In the face of hyperventilation, the 20 mm Hg decrease in $PaCO_2$ would result in an approximate increase in PaO_2 from 84 mm Hg (predicted) to 104 mm Hg, which is ${\sim}100$ mm Hg (**b**).

7. The correct answer is **a**. The pH is below 7.35, and therefore, the infant has an acidosis. The base excess of -12 mEq/L is indicative of a metabolic acidosis probably secondary to dehydration. This acidosis should be associated with a 0.15 unit decrease in pH. The pH, however, is decreased only 0.08 units. This is because there is a 15 mm Hg decrease in $PaCO_2$, a compensatory respiratory alkalosis (expected pH increase of between 0.12 units with a 15 mm decrease in $PaCO_2$ if acute and 0.045 units if chronic). In addition, there is mild hypoxemia ($PaO_2 = 0.21 \times (760 - 47) - 25/0.8 = 119$;

$AaD_{O_2} = 119 - 66 = 53$. The hypoxemia is due to the bronchiolitis.

8. The correct answer is **e**. The pH is below 7.35, and therefore this individual has an acidosis. Because of his underlying lung disease you suspect that the increase in Pa_{CO_2} is at least partially chronic. An increase of 27 mm Hg, if chronic, should be associated with a decrease in pH of ~0.08 units. Thus all of the change in pH is due to chronic respiratory disease. Despite oxygen therapy, this individual remains hypoxemic.

CHAPTER 10

1. Hyperventilation will reduce the arterial Pa_{CO_2} and will cause an increase in CSF and arterial pH and a reduction in respiratory drive. When an individual is swimming, O_2 will be consumed (CO_2 will begin to rise) but the major stimulus to breathe—a fall in Pa_{O_2}—will not occur until the Pa_{O_2} is reduced to 50 to 60 torr. The swimmer is thus at risk for hypoxemia before the hypercarbic stimulus to breathe is activated.

2. The decrease in $P_{I_{O_2}}$ results in a decrease in Pa_{O_2} and Pa_{O_2} according to the alveolar air equation. The reduced Pa_{O_2} stimulates the carotid bodies, and ventilation increases in response to this hypoxic stimulus. This results in a decrease in Pa_{CO_2} and a respiratory alkalosis. CO_2 also diffuses freely out of the CSF, whereas H^+ and HCO_3^- diffuse very slowly. This results in a marked increase in CSF pH and a decrease in the respiratory stimulus to the central respiratory center. The increased arterial pH may be brought back to normal by renal compensation that occurs over 24 to 48 hours. At the same time, through ion transport in the brain, the CSF pH approaches the pH of arterial blood, and the central respiratory center is again stimulated by a near normal $[H^+]$, so that the hypoxic stimulus on the carotid bodies becomes fully effective.

3. The sensitivity of the carotid bodies to low Pa_{O_2} is elevated when Pa_{CO_2} is elevated.

4. Barbiturates and other centrally active anesthetics are known to depress the respiratory center. Central respiratory depression occurs as a result of overdosage of these drugs and results in life-threatening hypercapnia and hypoxia.

CHAPTER 11

1. Smoking can result in emphysema, chronic bronchitis, and lung cancer. In individuals with chronic bronchitis, the lung pathology consists of goblet cell hyperplasia and hypertrophy with extension into smaller airways beyond the 12th tracheobronchial division, where they normally disappear. In addition, there is mucus gland hypertrophy, with a change in mucus viscosity and elasticity. The airway lumen contains increased mucus, including mucous plugs. Cilia are affected by the smoke, with decreased activity. The combination of decreased ciliary activity and increased and abnormal mucus production results in decreased mucociliary transport. Carbon from the smoke is deposited at bifurcations in small airways, due to impaction and sedimentation of particles in the smoke.

2. The presence of a drug that inhibits sodium absorption from the airway lumen (such as amiloride) would result in an increase in periciliary fluid. Increased cAMP levels in the airway epithelial cell would open chloride channels and result in increased chloride and secondary water in the airway lumen. Both of these would increase the depth of the periciliary fluid and could result in cilia splashing around in the fluid and a decrease in effective mucociliary transport. This is an example of too much of a good thing. Fortunately, most drugs either inhibit sodium absorption or increase chloride secretion but don't do both.

3. Plasma cells in the submucosa of the lung in response to IL-6 synthesize and secrete IgA in a dimer form linked by a J-chain. The dimer migrates to the submucosal surface of epithelial cells where it binds to the protein receptor poly-Ig, which aids in its pinocytosis and secretion into the airway lumen. During exocytosis of the IgA complex, the poly-Ig is enzymatically cleaved, leaving a portion, the secretory piece, still associated with the complex. The secretory piece stays attached to the dimer and aids in its protection from proteolytic cleavage in the lumen.

4. Natural killer (NK) cells kill invading pathogens through the release of granular enzymes, perforins, and serine esterases. These enzymes create holes or pores within the target cell membranes, leading to cell death. In addition to their cytotoxic activity, NK cells produce various pro-inflammatory cytokines similar to lymphocytes. This is an example of how an innate immune response modulates an adaptive immune response. The ability of the NK cell to produce high levels of IL-4 may also be the initiating event in starting the switchover mechanism for IgE synthesis and the eventual development of an allergic response.

5. Dendritic cells (DCs) are derived from the myeloid lineage of monocytes and macrophages and are a major cell type for antigen presentation to T cells. DCs have been found in the periphery of many tissues and function most likely as sentinels, not only to capture antigens but also to bring and process them to lymphocytes in the various lymphoid tissues. There are two known sources of DCs, the first being developmentally from CD 34+ progenitor cells in the bone marrow. The other source is the differentiation of blood monocytes in response to the cytokines GM-CSF and IL-4. DCs are commonly found throughout the respiratory tract in the parenchyma of the lung, from the trachea to the alveolus, and are usually associated with the epithelium. The upper airways are more densely populated with DCs than the smaller airways in the more peripheral regions of the lung. The anatomic location of these cells correlates well with particle deposition in the airways. Immature DCs capture and process antigen, and mature DCs have a more immunoregulatory role.

6. Macrophages phagocytize particles and digest them to amino acids in lysosomes. After ingesting an organism or particle, macrophages undergo a burst of metabolic activity and kill the organism or dissolve the particle. Ingestion is rapid and is not associated with an inflammatory response. The alveolar macrophage, however, is unable to dissolve asbestos; the sharp crystal punctures lysosomes that release their product intracellularly. The macrophage dies and in the process of dying releases chemotactic factors that cause fibroblast migration and collagen synthesis, which attracts other macrophages into the area. These macrophages ingest the asbestos and the process recurs. As a result, the alveolar macrophage localizes asbestos in the airways, and this process results in pulmonary fibrosis.

7. The lymphoid tissues of the mucosal areas (MALT) somewhat resemble actual lymph nodes with a similar repertoire of immune cells. In contrast to lymph nodes, these tissues are not encapsulated and are composed mainly of aggregates or clusters of lymphocytes residing in submucosal regions. In addition to aggregates of cells, MALT contains a substantial number of solitary B and T lymphocytes, which are scattered regularly throughout the tissue within the connective tissue of the lamina propria (lamina propria lymphocytes) and the epithelial layer (intraepithelial lymphocytes). The B cells found in MALT have a selectivity for differentiation into IgA-secreting plasma cells when stimulated by antigen.

CHAPTER 12

1. In healthy individuals, maximal exercise is cardiac-limited—specifically, limited by the heart rate and stroke volume. These factors determine the amount of oxygen delivery to the muscles during maximal activity. In normal, healthy individuals, exercise is never pulmonary-limited.

2. At the beginning of exercise, both tidal volume and respiratory rate increase, resulting in an increase in minute ventilation. This increase is linearly related to both CO_2 production and O_2 consumption. At high to maximal levels of exercise, arterial pH begins to fall as lactic acid is liberated during anaerobic metabolism. The fall in pH stimulates ventilation out of proportion to the level of exercise intensity, and this results in a fall in arterial P_{CO_2}.

3. Maximum heart rate does not change with training. Rather, training lowers the resting heart rate and increases the resting stroke volume. Training increases the oxidative capacity of skeletal muscles and improves strength and endurance of respiratory muscles. As a result, there is increased aerobic capacity with greater exercise, as well as lower lactic acid levels, which results in a decrease in ventilation

during submaximal exercise (compared with the untrained individual).

4. By the 16th week of gestation, all conducting airways, terminal bronchioles, and the primitive acini have formed. Neither rudimentary alveoli nor intra-acinar capillaries have formed. Thus, congenital diaphragmatic hernia (CDH) affects the development of the alveolar capillary barrier and airway growth, but the number of airway divisions is not affected.

5. Before birth, blood flow in the fetus bypasses the lung and is diverted by the foramen ovale and the ductus arteriosus. The circulation is distributed to the developing organs through the systemic circulation, returns to the right side of the heart, passes through the foramen ovale into the left side, and returns to the systemic circulation. Any blood that enters the right ventricle leaves the heart and is diverted across the ductus arteriosus into the descending aorta. After birth, with the first breath, pulmonary vascular resistance decreases, the pressure in the left side of the heart becomes greater than the pressure on the right, and thus the foramen ovale closes. As the pressure in the right side of the heart decreases, oxygenated blood in the aorta passes through the ductus arteriosus and causes it to close, establishing the adult circulation.

6. High altitude results in hypoxemia with hyperventilation. High-altitude pulmonary edema and high-altitude cerebral edema can occur in susceptible individuals.

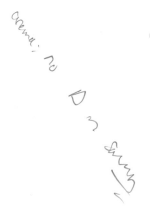

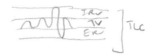

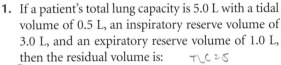

1. If a patient's total lung capacity is 5.0 L with a tidal volume of 0.5 L, an inspiratory reserve volume of 3.0 L, and an expiratory reserve volume of 1.0 L, then the residual volume is:
   a. 0.5 L
   b. 1.0 L
   c. 1.5 L
   d. 2.0 L
   e. 2.5 L

2. The minute ventilation of an individual with a tidal volume of 500 mL and a respiratory rate of 12 breaths per minute is.
   a. 42 mL
   b. 500 mL
   c. 42 L/min
   d. 5 L/min
   e. 6 L/min

3-9. Match the arterial blood gas values (**a to g**) with the most likely condition (**3 to 9**). A condition can be used more than once.

	Pao_2 mm Hg	$Paco_2$ mm Hg	Cao_2 Vol %	Sao_2%
a.	100	40	20	97
b.	100	40	10	98
c.	100	40	10	50
d.	120	20	20	99
e.	650	40	22	100
f.	60	60	17	85
g.	45	48	20	80

3. A person with normal lungs breathing 100% oxygen

4. Anemia

5. Hypoventilation

6. Carbon monoxide poisoning

7. Severe chronic bronchitis

8. Normal

9. Hyperventilation

10. Flow resistance across a set of airways is lowest under the following conditions:
    a. Airway radius is large, airways are in series, gas is of low viscosity
    b. Airway radius is large, airways are in parallel, gas is of high viscosity
    c. Airway radius is small, airways are in series, gas is of low viscosity
    d. Airway radius is small, airways are in parallel, gas is of high viscosity
    e. Airway radius is large, airways are in parallel, gas is of low viscosity

11. The airways most responsible for the resistance of the respiratory system during nasal breathing are:
    a. The nose to the larynx
    b. The trachea to segmental bronchi
    c. The subsegmental airways
    d. The terminal bronchioles
    e. The alveoli and alveolar ducts

12. Which of the following factors does not contribute to lung resistance?
    a. Lung volume
    b. Number and length of conducting airways
    c. Airway smooth muscle tone
    d. Elastic recoil
    e. Static lung compliance

13. Expiratory flow limitation occurs when:
    a. Pleural (intrathoracic) pressure exceeds elastic recoil pressure
    b. The pressure outside an airway is greater than the pressure inside the airway
    c. Dynamic lung compliance is greater than static lung compliance
    d. Lung volume is increased
    e. Expiratory flow rates are high

14. A person's respiratory rate at rest is determined by:
    a. The compliance and resistance of their respiratory system
    b. The minimal oxygen cost of breathing
    c. The metabolic demands of the body
    d. The work of breathing
    e. All of the above

15. Which of the following statements about the measurement of lung volumes is correct?
    a. FRC by helium dilution technique is the same as FRC measured by body plethysmography in individuals with obstructive and restrictive pulmonary disease.
    b. TLC is determined by expiratory muscle strength and lung elastic recoil.
    c. The FVC is greater than the SVC in individuals with obstructive pulmonary disease.
    d. The functional residual capacity is increased in individuals with muscle weakness.
    e. One of the hallmarks of obstructive lung disease is an RV/TLC ratio less than 25%.

16. Which of the following pulmonary function test results best describes an individual with moderate chronic bronchitis?
    a. Normal vital capacity, normal FEV_1, normal FEV_1/FVC, reduced expiratory flow rates, decreased D_{LCO}
    b. Normal vital capacity, reduced FEV_1, decreased FEV_1/FVC, reduced expiratory flow rates, decreased D_{LCO}
    c. Normal vital capacity, normal FEV_1, normal FEV_1/FVC, reduced expiratory flow rates, normal D_{LCO}
    d. Normal vital capacity, reduced FEV_1, decreased FEV_1/FVC, reduced expiratory flow rates, normal D_{LCO}
    e. Reduced vital capacity, reduced FEV_1, normal FEV_1/FVC, reduced expiratory flow rates, normal D_{LCO}

17. A 55-year-old woman, a former smoker, complains of shortness of breath. She has an FVC of 2.4 L and an SVC of 2.9 L. These findings suggest:
    a. Restrictive lung disease
    b. Obstructive lung disease
    c. Muscle weakness
    d. Anemia
    e. Upper airway obstruction

18. Pulmonary function tests might be indicated in all of the following *except*:
    a. Smokers older than 20 years of age
    b. Evaluation of the severity of pulmonary hypertension
    c. Assessment of the risk of lung resection
    d. Congestive heart failure
    e. Children with asthma

19. Factors affecting normal values for pulmonary function tests include all *except*:
    a. Age
    b. Gender
    c. Ethnicity
    d. Barometric pressure
    e. Height

20. Which of the following statements about the effort-independent part of the expiratory flow volume curve is correct?
    a. It occurs in the first 20% of the expiratory maneuver
    b. It depends on expiratory muscle force
    c. It is a measure of small airway function
    d. Abnormalities are indicative of severe airway obstruction
    e. Abnormalities occur early in restrictive lung disease

21. The D_{LCO} is frequently abnormal in all *except* which of the following conditions?
    a. Lung resection
    b. Chemotherapy-induced pulmonary toxicity
    c. Pulmonary hypertension
    d. Multiple pulmonary emboli
    e. Idiopathic pulmonary fibrosis

22. A 40-year-old mountain climber has the following blood gas values at sea level (760 mm Hg): $Pa_{O_2} = 96$ torr, $Pa_{CO_2} = 40$ torr, pH = 7.40, and $F_{IO_2} = 0.21$. He climbs to the top of Pike's Peak (barometric pressure, 445 mm Hg). What is his Pa_{O_2} at the top of Pike's peak (assume that his Pa_{CO_2} and R are unchanged)?
    a. 25 mm Hg
    b. 34 mm Hg
    c. 44 mm Hg
    d. 55 mm Hg
    e. 60 mm Hg

23. An increase in dead space ventilation without a change in tidal volume will result in:
    a. An increase in alveolar PCO_2 without significant change in alveolar PO_2
    b. An increase in alveolar PCO_2 with a decrease in alveolar PO_2
    c. A decrease in alveolar PCO_2 without significant change in alveolar PO_2
    d. A decrease in alveolar PCO_2 without significant change in alveolar PO_2
    e. No change in alveolar PCO_2 or alveolar PO_2

24. The inspired oxygen tension at the level of the trachea when an individual is at the summit of Mt. Everest (barometric pressure, 250 torr) is:
    a. 25 mm Hg
    b. 43 mm Hg
    c. 62 mm Hg
    d. 75 mm Hg
    e. 100 mm Hg

25. Anatomic dead space is determined by:
    a. The size and number of the airways
    b. The number of alveoli that are ventilated but not perfused
    c. The mechanical properties of the chest and chest muscles
    d. The characteristics of inspired gas
    e. Physiologic dead space

26. If the alveolar ventilation is 4 L/min and the CO_2 production is 200 mL/min, what is the $PACO_2$ (assume barometric pressure is 760 torr)?
    a. 31 torr
    b. 36 torr
    c. 38 torr
    d. 50 torr
    e. 55 torr

27. How many milliliters of O_2 does 100 mL of blood contain at a PaO_2 of 40 mm Hg?
    a. 5 mL
    b. 10 mL
    c. 15 mL
    d. 20 mL
    e. 25 mL

28. A patient has a hemoglobin level of 10 g/100 mL of blood. What is his O_2-carrying capacity?
    a. 10 mL O_2/100 mL blood
    b. 13 mL O_2/100 mL blood
    c. 15 mL O_2/100 mL blood
    d. 20 mL O_2/100 mL blood
    e. 25 mL O_2/100 mL blood

29. If the arterial-venous difference is 5 mL O_2/100 mL blood in the question above, what is the O_2 content of the venous blood?
    a. 5 mL O_2/100 mL blood
    b. 8 mL O_2/100 mL blood
    c. 10 mL O_2/100 mL blood
    d. 15 mL O_2/100 mL blood
    e. 18 mL O_2/100 mL blood

30. A sample of blood has a PO_2 of 100 mm Hg and is 98% saturated. The hemoglobin is 15 g/100 mL. The O_2 content of this blood is:
    a. 10 mL/100 mL blood
    b. 15 mL/100 mL blood
    c. 20 mL/100 mL blood
    d. 23 mL/100 mL blood
    e. 25 mL/100 mL blood

31. Investigators are studying a recently discovered gas. This gas has a high solubility in the alveolar capillary membrane and a low solubility in the plasma. It does not appear to bind chemically to blood. Which of the following statements is true about this gas?
    a. The amount of gas absorbed into the blood is inversely proportional to the partial pressure gradient across the alveolar capillary membrane
    b. Diffusion across the capillary-tissue interface will be greater than diffusion across the alveolar-capillary interface
    c. Diffusion will be directly related to the thickness of the membrane
    d. The higher the molecular weight, the greater the diffusion
    e. Diffusion will be perfusion-limited

32. Which of the following factors is associated with enhanced O_2 release to the tissues?
    a. Decreased temperature
    b. Increased PCO_2
    c. Decreased 2,3-DPG
    d. Increased pH
    e. Tissue bicarbonate levels

$Av = (Tv - Ds) \cdot rr$

33. What of the following statements about the Bohr effect is correct?
  a. It is primarily due to the effect of CO_2 on pH and on hemoglobin
  b. It shifts the oxyhemoglobin dissociation curve to the left in the tissues
  c. It enhances CO_2 uptake from the tissues and CO_2 unloading in the lung
  d. It increases the levels of 2,3-DPG in red blood cells
  e. It is related to chloride exchange processes in the red blood cell

34-37. Match the the blood gas values in **a to e** with the acid-base disorders shown in **34 to 37**.

	pH	HCO_3^-	$PaCO_2$
a.	7.23	10	25
b.	7.34	26	50
c.	7.37	28	50
d.	7.46	30	44
e.	7.66	22	20

34. Metabolic acidosis with respiratory compensation $HCO_3 < 24 \quad pCO_2 > 40 \quad A$

35. Respiratory acidosis with renal compensation C

36. Metabolic alkalosis with respiratory compensation $HCO_3 > 24 \quad PCO_2 < 40 \quad D$

37. Respiratory alkalosis with renal compensation E

38. A 65-year-old retired man has been homebound for 5 years because of shortness of breath. He has increased sputum production after a cold and complains of dyspnea so severe that it interferes with his smoking cigarettes. His chest is hyperinflated, with distant breath sounds and loud rhonchi on auscultation. Of the three possible sets of arterial blood gas values shown (**A, B, C**), which best fits the patient's condition and history?

	A	B	C
pH	7.30	7.18	7.45
PaO_2	45	28	65
$PaCO_2$	70	70	70
HCO_3^-	35	24	50
BE	+10	0	+20

39. Which of the following would increase the ventilatory response to CO_2?
  a. Barbiturates
  b. Hypoxia
  c. Sleep
  d. Chronic obstructive pulmonary disease
  e. Anesthesia

40. Breath-holding for 90 seconds will:
  a. Increase PCO_2
  b. Decrease PO_2
  c. Stimulate central chemoreceptors
  d. Stimulate peripheral chemoreceptors
  e. Result in all of the above

41. Which of the following statements is _not_ true about peripheral chemoreceptors?
  a. They respond to decreases in PO_2 and O_2 content
  b. They respond to changes in arterial pH
  c. They respond to increases in PCO_2
  d. They account for ~40% of the ventilatory response to CO_2.
  e. They are rich in dopamine

42. Which of the following responses would be expected in a normal individual after 1 week of residence at an altitude of 12,500 ft?
  a. Increased alveolar ventilation (relative to sea level)
  b. Normal $PaCO_2$
  c. Normal pulmonary artery pressure
  d. Normal PaO_2
  e. Normal plasma bicarbonate

$PAO_2 = FiO_2 (PB - PaO_2)$

43. An 80-year-old man in congestive heart failure has a respiratory rate of 26 breaths/min, arterial pH of 7.08, PO_2 of 60 torr, and PCO_2 of 31 torr. He is treated with diuretics, oxygen, and digitalis and is given bicarbonate intravenously. The following day, his respiratory rate remains elevated and he has an arterial pH of 7.49, PO_2 of 102 torr on 28% O_2, and PCO_2 of 31 torr. The best explanation for his current respiratory alkalosis is:
  a. Excessive bicarbonate administration
  b. CSF central acidosis
  c. Compensatory metabolic acidosis
  d. Peripheral chemoreceptor stimulation
  e. Hypoxia-induced hyperventilation

44. An individual with pneumonia is receiving 30% supplemental O_2 by a facemask. Arterial blood gas values are pH = 7.40, $PaCO_2$ = 44 mm Hg, and a PaO_2 = 70 mm Hg. (assume that the individual is at sea level and his respiratory quotient is 0.8). What is his $AaDO_2$?
    a. 15 mm Hg
    b. 35 mm Hg
    c. 55 mm Hg
    d. 89 mm Hg
    e. 94 mm Hg

45. Moderate levels of exercise result in:
    a. An increase in total lung capacity
    b. An increase in pulmonary vascular resistance
    c. A decrease in the diffusion capacity for carbon monoxide
    d. A lack of significant changes in arterial blood gases
    e. A decrease in CO_2 production

46. The effects of training on the ability to perform exercise can be described as:
    a. A lowering of the resting heart rate
    b. An increase in the maximum heart rate
    c. No change in resting stroke volume
    d. Decreases in glycogen synthesis
    e. Increases in blood lactate levels

47. The first time that extrauterine life can exist is:
    a. When the airways are fully developed.
    b. When acinar development is complete
    c. At the end of the canalicular stage
    d. At the end of the saccular stage
    e. At birth

48. The *most important* change in the pulmonary circulation at birth is:
    a. The decrease in pulmonary vascular resistance
    b. Stimulation of respiration by progesterone
    c. Delivery of the placenta
    d. Pulmonary vasoconstriction
    e. All of the above

49. Ascent to high altitude is associated with:
    a. Hyperventilation
    b. A decrease in inspired oxygen
    c. A respiratory alkalosis
    d. A rightward shift of the oxyhemoglobin dissociation curve
    e. All of the above

50. The respiratory control center is located in the:
    a. Cerebral cortex
    b. Pons
    c. Medulla oblongata
    d. Cerebellum
    e. Spinal motor tract

51. The carotid body responds to:
    a. Hypoxia
    b. Hypercarbia
    c. Change in pH
    d. All of the above
    e. None of the above

52. The response to increases in PCO_2 is characterized by:
    a. A curvilinear increase in minute ventilation
    b. A linear increase in alveolar ventilation
    c. Decreased carotid sinus nerve firing
    d. Inhibition by low levels of O_2
    e. Inhibition by low pH

53. Central chemoreceptors respond to:
    a. Low PO_2
    b. Changes in blood bicarbonate levels
    c. Changes in H^+ ion concentrations
    d. Changes in molecular CO_2
    e. All of the above

54. The Hering-Breuer reflex is stimulated by:
    a. Spinal motor neurons
    b. Nasal or facial receptors
    c. Increases in lung volume
    d. Irritant receptors
    e. J receptors

55. Which of the following statements about obstructive sleep apnea (OSA) is true?
    a. OSA is most commonly caused by obesity
    b. OSA is associated with a decrease in ventilatory drive to the respiratory motor neurons
    c. OSA is associated with an absence of ventilatory effort
    d. OSA is associated with lower respiratory tract obstruction
    e. OSA is never associated with hypoxia.

56. Which of the following statements about mucus in chronic bronchitis is *not* true?
    a. Submucosal glands increase in number and size with chronic bronchitis
    b. Surface secretory cells increase in number and size with chronic bronchitis

c. The chemical composition of surface secretory cells changes with chronic bronchitis

d. The chemical composition of submucosal glands changes with chronic bronchitis

e. Particulate smoke deposition occurs in respiratory bronchioles in chronic bronchitis

57. Particle retention in the lung most often occurs:
   a. At the transition between the conducting airways and the terminal respiratory units
   b. At bifurcations in large airways
   c. At bifurcations in small airways
   d. In the nose
   e. In the trachea

58. Important defense systems in the respiratory system include:
   a. Mucociliary transport
   b. Innate immunity
   c. Adaptive immunity
   d. Migratory phagocytic and inflammatory cells
   e. All of the above

59. Alveolar macrophages:
   a. Are derived from blood monocytes
   b. Live 1 to 5 weeks in the respiratory tract
   c. Both dissolve and engulf foreign materials
   d. Are characterized by all of the above
   e. Are characterized by none of the above

60. Surfactants:
   a. Decrease surface tension at all lung volumes
   b. Increase surface tension at low lung volumes and decrease surface tension at high lung volumes
   c. Are resistant to hypoxia and sheer stress
   d. Are produced by type I epithelial cells
   e. Are characterized by all of the above

ANSWERS TO MULTIPLE–CHOICE EXAMINATION

1. a	13. b	25. a	37. e	49. e
2. e	14. e	26. b	38. a	50. c
3. e	15. b	27. c	39. b	51. d
4. b	16. d	28. b	40. e	52. b
5. f	17. b	29. b	41. a	53. d
6. b	18. b	30. c	42. a	54. c
7. g	19. d	31. e	43. b	55. a
8. a	20. c	32. b	44. d	56. d
9. d	21. c	33. a	45. d	57. a
10. e	22. b	34. a	46. a	58. e
11. a	23. b	35. c	47. c	59. d
12. e	24. b	36. d	48. a	60. a

INDEX

From STOREBOUGHT *to* HOMEMADE

From
Storebought
to Homemade

Secrets for cooking easy,
fabulous food in minutes

Emyl Jenkins
FOREWORD BY Jan Karon

QVC Publishing, Inc.

QVC Publishing, Inc.

Jill Cohen, *Vice President and Publisher*
Ellen Bruzelius, *General Manager*
Karen Murgolo, *Director of Acquisitions and Rights*
Cassandra Reynolds, *Publishing Assistant*

Design by Vertigo Design, NYC

Q Publishing and colophon are trademarks of QVC Publishing, Inc.

Published by QVC Publishing, Inc., 50 Main Street, Mt. Kisco, New York 10549

Manufactured in the United States of America

ISBN: 1-928998-43-7

First Edition

10 9 8 7 6 5 4 3 2 1

To all who, down through the years, have shared their families'
treasured recipes for the enjoyment of others.

If a man be gracious to strangers, it shows that he is a citizen
of the world, and his heart is no island, cut off from
other islands, but a continent that joins them.

—SIR FRANCIS BACON, 1561 1620

And to Charlotte Sizer. Thank you for your diligence,
good nature, and winning smile.
And to Benjamin and Matthew Hultzapple, the newest
generation at our family's dinner table.

Contents

Acknowledgments

Untold numbers of people contributed ideas, suggestions, and recommendations for this book—especially those who sent me recipes from their personal archives, and the patient grocery store managers and workers who listened to my questions and helped me track down products. Thank you, each and every one.

Thank you to those who helped to uncover much needed information, especially Joan Jacobsen and Dick Pretty, Jan Harris, Bill Satterfield, and Laura Wiletsky, and the very cooperative folks at Ragú, including Jim Stringfield and Helena Tregubov.

Thank you, Jackie Legg, food writer, hostess extraordinaire, and a very capable vice-president of Ukrops, that great food chain in Richmond, Virginia.

Thank you Larry Aaron, Cyndee Moore, Danny Vaden, Kim Demont, Nina Klinkenberg, and of course, my dear husband, Bob Sexton, for your patience and help in making it possible for me to have the time to pursue this project.

And thank you, especially, Jeanne Fredericks, my agent; photographer Monica Buck; Sarah Butterworth, who actually came up with the title, *From Store-bought to Homemade*; the book's designers at Vertigo Design, NYC; and my helpful and good friends at QVC, Jill Cohen, whose brainchild this was, Cassandra Reynolds, Rebecca Helmeczi, and most of all, Karen Murgolo.

Foreword

Thoughts on Cooking
—and Not Cooking

WHEN you've put one of Emyl's sensational dishes on the table, and after you've asked the blessing (you'll be amazed how this improves everyone's disposition), try doing what the Europeans have always done far better than we: Talk! Tell jokes! Ask questions! (If you were going to be shot for treason in the morning, what would you request for your last meal?) Recite a poem! Tell your favorite experience of the day! Tell the one seated to your right what you love most about them. Then tell the one on your left, and ask the others to do the same. Focus on the food too—is it good? What do you like about it? Compliment the cook!

The next thing you know, dinner will be more than the same old blue-plate special. You may even find it well seasoned with laughter.

"Laughter doeth good like a medicine," Scripture tells us. In truth, I've found laughter to be the loveliest of all the aids to good digestion!

I haven't really "cooked" cooked in years. That's because I can make so many wonderful things by hardly cooking at all.

A great favorite with my family is Simple Roast Chicken:

Rinse a whole fryer and pat it dry.

Rub it with a good olive oil and season well with salt, cracked pepper, rosemary, and paprika.

Stuff the cavity with half a lemon and several cloves of garlic.

Put the chicken on its back in a well-seasoned black skillet, and set it on the middle rack of your oven, which you've turned to 450 degrees.

Roast at 450 degrees for 30 minutes and at 350 degrees for one hour.

This simple recipe has a great bonus:

It roasts while I write!

See? That's not cooking, that's just a little fooling around in the kitchen.

■ ■ ■ ■ ■ ■ ■ ■

So what would *you* request as your last meal if you were to be shot for treason in the morning?

Make mine fresh lobster with drawn butter and a glass of very dry, very fine Champagne from Champagne!

Failing that, how about fried chicken, mashed potatoes, gravy, and short, flaky biscuits?

Failing that, how about liver mush? Fried crisp and golden, thanks.

When in the world are you going on a picnic again? You talk about doing it, you occasionally daydream about doing it, but you don't do it! Right? This summer, take your kids and go on a picnic. *Please!*

Spread a quilt or a blanket.

Don't worry about ants.

Lie on your back. Look up at the branches of trees. Find faces in the clouds.

Tell your kids what kind of kid you were at their age. Find out what they really, really, really want to be or do someday—what are their dreams?

And don't just take peanut-butter-and-jelly sandwiches, take something special. Like cold roast chicken (see above recipe) and really good bread (how about some Incredibly Quick Cheese Biscuits on page 224) and butter and cookies (try cooking up a batch of young Allison's Vanilla Crisps on page 264) and sweet tea.

After you eat, get out a sketchbook and colored pencils and
draw your children. Then, let them draw you. This will make
everyone roll with laughter, and they will say,
"Let's go on a picnic again really soon."

—JAN KARON
AUTHOR OF *THE MITFORD YEARS*

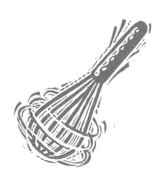

Introduction

The real art in food is flavor and not labor.

—GEORGES SPUNT,
*MEMOIRS & MENUS: THE CONFESSIONS
OF A CULINARY SNOB*, 1967

I LOVE TO COOK, but when I'm reading a recipe and I see the words "double boiler," my eyes glaze over. Mention a sieve, and I turn the page. Begin a recipe, "In a square of cheesecloth place a bouquet of herbs..." and I put the book down.

I love to cook, but I don't love the aggravation that comes with cooking. Never have. It's just not worth it, especially now that there are so many fabulous convenience foods to make the cook's job so much easier.

S till, who wants to lose the flavor and goodness of homemade cooking? Not I. Nor anybody else I know. Take my friendly UPS delivery man, for example. The other day, while he was putting an unusually large box inside for me, he said, "Don't know what you're cooking, but it sure smells good. Like when I was a little boy."

You see, I'm an old-fashioned cook, but with newfangled ways. With life so busy, I see no reason not to take advantage of the timesaving foods that are available to us. That's what our ancestors did.

Back in the nineteenth century, when women began clamoring for cookbooks, the cookbook writers took eighteenth-century recipes and modernized them to utilize new, nineteenth-century ingredients, equipment, and ways.

Same thing happened in the early twentieth century. Favorite family recipes that had once called for "a large legg of mutton," suddenly read, "take a 5-lb. leg of lamb."

Cookbooks no longer instructed the cook to "gather a peck of tomatoes," or my favorite, found scribbled in a late nineteenth-century cookbook, "buy 5 ct. worth of lemon extract." Instead, recipes now read, "Simmer 10 peeled and seeded tomatoes," or "use 1 teaspoon of lemon extract." And you better believe that once canned tomatoes were readily available from the local grocer, the recipes were changed to read, "Take a large can (16 oz.) of tomatoes...."

Trouble is, these days everyone is so anxious to cook everything *from scratch* that we've turned out a generation of frustrated cooks. It can take so long to prepare even the most basic meal that halfway through the process the weary cook asks, "Who wants pizza tonight?" or pulls out the remains of last night's Chinese takeout.

Somewhere along the way, we seem to have forgotten that it's okay to use storebought products to cook up delicious meals. That's what our mothers and grandmothers were doing in the 1950s and '60s when they made those mouthwatering dishes we still remember today.

Those mid-twentieth-century cooks had seen *their* mothers and grandmothers slaving in the kitchen, and they didn't want to follow suit. Anyway, by then, most of our mothers and grandmothers had jobs, just as we have today. Our mothers and grandmothers wanted maximum time with their families, and minimum time in the kitchen. It's time we learned what they knew.

Truth is, be it a family meal, a birthday party, a holiday gathering, or a special dinner party, family and friends and laughter are much more important than a homemade cake or a "from scratch" home-cooked meal, especially when you can turn so many ready-made storebought foods into delicious dishes with just a little doctoring.

That's what this book is all about—how to turn storebought food into delicious, easy to prepare, fun, and quick-to-make homemade dishes and meals.

Best of all, by using these recipes you'll end up having more time to spend as you wish, and fewer kitchen worries—a combination we can all use today. To top it all off, like the ice cream on pie à la mode, lots of these dishes bring back wonderful memories of bygone days. They tickle our nostalgic tastebuds.

"Cookbooks are not just for cooking...Cookbooks are for inspiration, for lifting the spirit and freeing the mind, for brightening your outlook as well as your parties and table conversation...for the understanding of people and places, for the revelation of the past and for the interpretation of the present...for culture, education, for inviting the soul, reviving memories, reliving experiences."

—"HOW, WHERE AND WHY TO READ A COOKBOOK"
HOUSE BEAUTIFUL, FEBRUARY 1957

"The culinary science is a progressive one, and many important discoveries are made every day, and new processes devised that add a new spice to life's enjoyments. This book is up with the times, and the experienced housewife will find in it many new ideas which will greatly add to her already charming methods of cooking."

—MRS. GRACE TOWNSEND, *THE STAR COOK BOOK*,
REVISED EDITION, 1895

Unfortunately, though, preparing the food isn't the hostess's only aggravation.

There are menus to be worked out—a task that can be more complicated than putting together a thousand-piece jigsaw puzzle. Then there's trying to figure out what to serve the food in—a task that is sometimes reason enough to call the whole thing off. And when you add thinking up and then arranging a centerpiece to the mix—well, no wonder you don't entertain more often.

That's why, in addition to these great, easy-to-prepare dishes, I've included menu suggestions, *The Finishing Touch* hints, *Sage Advice*, and even a guide to tell you *before you start*, the type of pots and pans you'll need to cook each dish. (How many times have you had the cake batter ready to go when suddenly you read, "pour the mixture into a bundt pan," and you haven't a clue where your bundt pan is, or if you even have one?)

So toss your kitchen aggravation to one side. Grind it up in the garbage disposal. Throw it out with the moldy cheese you never got around to grating. It's time to put frustrations away and to take the easy way out.

Your family will thank you.

Your friends will rave about your delicious fare.

And you'll look and feel better while enjoying your own meal or party—all with the absolute minimum of aggravation.

"Flower decorations on the table are to be in flat designs, so as not to obscure the view of the guests."

—*THE WHITE HOUSE COOK BOOK* BY HUGO ZIEMANN AND MRS. F. L. GILLETTE, 1926

This cook's words of comfort or You don't need a designer kitchen

I thoroughly enjoy watching the food programs on TV. Those shows are my soap operas—entertaining and fanciful. When I turn on the Food Network, I become a peeping Tom in someone else's kitchen. But my kitchen and cuisine bear no resemblance to what I'm watching.

I can assure you that my kitchen looks much more like your kitchen than it does any kitchen you'll see on TV, unless it's on a rerun of the 1960's *The Donna Reed Show*. For starters, our house was built in 1941, and the last (and probably only) time the kitchen was remodeled was in the early 1970s by a former owner. When I'm feeling defensive, I smugly say I have a "retro" kitchen. In truth, the poor thing's in desperate need of a face-lift *and* a makeover.

Like most kitchens of that era, my kitchen has practically no counter space. Or at least not enough for the type of cook that I am—the spread and clutter type.

It doesn't bother me one bit that I have to balance the cookie sheet (with the cookies still on it) on the edge of the old porcelain sink that is filled to overflowing with the measuring cups and mixing bowls I used to make the casserole that came out of the oven two hours ago.

You see, I come by my habits honestly. My mother was a messy cook too. But my fastidious father put everything into perspective for me.

"Your mother's mother kept the neatest kitchen I'd ever seen," he once told me, while surveying my own disaster of a kitchen. "She'd dirty a bowl and wash it before she went on to doing anything else. Your mother, on the other hand, started tearing the kitchen apart the moment she crossed the threshold to fix breakfast. But at the end of the day your grandmother's meals were as bland as her kitchen was clean. Your mother—well, she never cooked a bad meal in her life."

I assure you, I've cooked more than my share of bad meals, but Daddy's left-handed compliment is very comforting when I'm trying to keep a well-intended guest from taking the dirty dishes into my less-than-picture-perfect kitchen.

But, back to the kitchen itself.

I cook on a normal, kitchen-size, grill-less, electric stove. (I admit that it does have a convection oven, but I haven't figured out how to use it yet.) My only "gadgets" are the essential ones—microwave, toaster (for toasting toast, not bagels), food processor, Crock-Pot, and handheld mixer. Though I keep vowing to replace my parents' 1938 countertop Sunbeam Automatic Mixmaster (it has had an electrical short since 1989 that no one seems to know how to repair), I really don't need it. I've learned how to turn storebought goodies into home-made delicacies with a minimum of equipment.

So take comfort. You, too, can turn out great-tasting dishes in your own kitchen, no matter how old or new it, and your equipment, is. Today's fabulous food folks have made it possible. How big a mess you make in the process is up to you.

Restaurant Quality...
Restaurant Recipes...

In today's "let's eat out" mind-set, even grocery store products and cookbooks are cashing in on our love for restaurant fare. Have you noticed how many frozen foods are labeled "restaurant quality"? Even magazines and cookbooks are beginning to feature "restaurant" recipes.

I'll admit that I often say, "Bob, let's eat out tonight," even when I have the makings of a perfectly fine meal in my own kitchen. But that's more for a change of scenery than for a change of food.

Think about it. Do you know what you are getting when you're eating out?

Of course, if you live in L.A. and have reservations for Wolfgang Puck's famous restaurant, Spago, you can expect the sky to be the limit. Or, if you live in a large metropolitan area where neighborhood restaurants have innovative chefs who take great pride in their creations, you're probably in for a dining treat.

On the other hand, if you're going to one of the many chain restaurants that are the staples of American family life, chances are you will be eating preprepared food you could have served up at home—and made even tastier by adding your own "homemade" touch.

I found this out one night when I ordered a bowl of Tomato Florentine soup at one of the chain restaurants. In my mind's eye I saw a chef in the kitchen stirring up a steaming, aromatic pot of hearty stock, succulent onions, fresh tomatoes, secret herbs, and baby spinach leaves.

My dream came to an abrupt end when our young waiter said, "You're really going to like that. We just got in a new brand of soup and this one's a lot better than the Tomato Florentine soup we were serving last week." He was right. It was good. And it was right out of the can.

Want more evidence? Jackie Legg, the author of many cookbooks, once told me that one of the greatest marketing coups she'd ever seen pulled off was in one of America's famous restaurants where the customers lined up for bowls of hot corn. Hot *canned* corn, drained, to which butter had been added.

So, the next time you're thinking "restaurant," remember, you already have restaurant food in your own pantry, fridge, and freezer. And with the help of these recipes, you can come up with *improved* restaurant dishes—without the hassle of waiting in line, sending the wrong order back, and having to leave a tip.

"People sometimes praise a restaurant by saying it makes them feel at home…. I don't want to feel at home in a restaurant. I want to feel that I'm having a night out."

—ALVIN KERR, *GOURMET*, OCTOBER, 1960

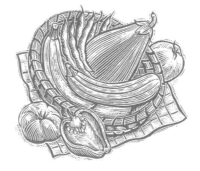

From STOREBOUGHT *to* HOMEMADE

How and When to Use This Book

The Well-Stocked Kitchen

MOTHER always said, "If you're going to be a good cook, first you have to have a good cookbook."

Really good cookbooks begin where every meal or party begins—in the kitchen, by which I mean the pantry, the fridge, even the cupboard shelves where you keep your china and glassware. That's why these next few pages are filled with suggestions for items you should keep on hand to help speed along the preparation of fast, fabulous food at home.

L et's begin with the pots and pans.
The day I tried to cook my first live lobster I learned that any meal can turn into a disaster if you don't have the right equipment.

There I was, a twenty-two-year-old bride, with a beady-eyed crustacean crawling around our Pullman-size apartment kitchen while I went running from door to door begging for a big pot. (I'd stupidly unleashed his claws before I began looking for the pot.) These days I'd know that just a large stock or pasta pot would do, but back then, we were eating spaghetti out of a can.

To avoid such culinary mishaps, here's a list of the basic cooking and baking equipment you'll need to prepare the recipes in this book:

BASIC COOKWARE

baking or casserole dishes—square and rectangular (Pyrex)

set of graduated glass mixing bowls that are also microwave/oven safe

cake, pie, and loaf pans

cookie sheet (the air-insulated variety goes a long way toward preventing burnt foods)

Crock-Pot

knives: a good set of kitchen knives, including a sharp paring knife and a serrated knife for slicing breads

one good set of measuring cups and spoons

molds: ring, individual

platter: at least one big enough to hold the holiday turkey or cut meats for a buffet

deep stock or pasta pot (8-quart)

pizza stone

saucepans: small (1-quart), medium (2-quart), and large (4 ½-quart), with lids

sauté pans: small and large

skillet, with lid

stovetop or oven roaster

The Well-Stocked Shelf

As important as the pots and pans are the staples you have in the pantry, refrigerator, freezer, and on your spice shelves.

Every well-stocked pantry should have an extra can or two of those foods that can dress up ordinary fare. These ready-made products are invaluable in two ways. Either they are used in the recipes as essential ingredients, or they help you make a great presentation.

In the essential ingredients category are the old standbys—cream of mushroom soup, chicken and beef broth, tomato paste, canned tomatoes.... Seasoned cooks find that their grocery carts go on automatic pilot when approaching the shelves where these staples are located.

But I also find some of the fancier, if not truly "gourmet" prepared foods are absolutely indispensable. When my children are coming home, I wouldn't dream of leaving the grocery store without picking up a couple of cans of artichoke hearts and at least one spare can of cilantro and lime juice–flavored chopped tomatoes—both ingredients in their favorite dishes.

Equally important to fast, fabulous food at home are wonderful pickles, jellies, and relishes. These not only add a sparkling flavor to ordinary foods, they also dress up a plate or platter, because you don't expect them to be there. And they add a bright splash of color to dishes that might otherwise look dull even though they are very tasty. Remember, we eat with our eyes as well as our taste buds.

You probably won't keep all these fancier ingredients on hand all the time. Yet, having a well-stocked larder really does make it possible to turn the mundane into something special on a moment's notice.

Now, if you never have more than four to six people (including yourself) at the table, one can or jar should suffice. But for larger groups, you should have a couple of cans or jars on hand.

(Though the following items are found on the grocery shelves, many need to be refrigerated after they are opened. Check the labels for instructions.)

IN YOUR PANTRY

bread crumbs—one canister

ketchup, mustard, and mayonnaise

crackers

> basic crackers such as Saltines or Triscuits
> more delicate crackers such as Carr's Table Water crackers

Melba toast (offered in many flavors)

cheese straws (the traditional Cheddar is now offered in an extra-spicy version, or try the blue cheese variety, if you're partial to that flavor)

salad dressings

a bottle each of Italian, Caesar, and Russian salad dressing

a few vinaigrettes (try these varieties: sun-dried tomato and red wine, balsamic, orange, garlic and herb)

fish (canned)

black caviar

minced clams

lump crab

shrimp

lump tuna

salmon

flour (self-rising) and/or Bisquick

fruits

a variety of canned fruits such as pears, peaches, mandarin oranges, and a mixed tropical fruit blend (Note: many fruits are now coming already flavored in the can, such as raspberry-flavored pears and cinnamon-flavored peaches)

Jell-O

What can I say? Jell-O, Jell-O, Jell-O in all sorts of flavors, for salads and desserts; and a box of instant vanilla and chocolate pudding mix too

meats

jar of dried beef

tin of deviled ham

nuts

sliced or slivered almonds

cashews

macadamia nuts

pecans

peanuts

pine nuts

sauces (see more on the varieties offered under convenience foods, but keep the following on hand)

a good barbeque sauce, sweet or vinegary, to your taste

Alfredo (which can be used when a basic white sauce is called for)

Cheddar cheese sauce

roasted garlic Parmesan cheese sauce

basic spaghetti sauce (tomato-based)

soups/stews

chicken broth and beef consommé

bouillon cubes (or Wyler's Shakers) in vegetable, chicken, beef, and ham flavors

cream of celery soup

cream of chicken soup

cream of mushroom soup

cream of shrimp soup

onion soup, both dried and canned

tomato soup

vegetable soup or stew

herbs and spices

dried basil

dried bay leaves

cinnamon

curry powder

Italian seasoning

If You're Just Beginning to Stock Your Spice Cabinet

THERE is seemingly no end to the number of herb and spice blends that are available today. But how often do you really use these specialty blends—Mediterranean, Eastern European, Cajun, Seafood Seasoning, Poultry Seasoning, Soul Seasoning, Garlic and Herb, All-Purpose Herb and Garlic, etc.? And do you have enough space to store several jars?

If you answered, "not often" and "not really" to those questions, here's my suggestion for a basic blend. Buy individual jars of dried thyme, basil, and bay leaf (crumbled). You'll use these herbs individually.

Then, buy an empty container and combine equal amounts of these three herbs to have on hand when you want a quick mixture.

About Pepper

I BELIEVE in cooking shortcuts and take them every chance I get. Still, there's a "closet" wanna-be chef lurking somewhere in me, and, I bet, in you. In truth, I haven't the time or the inclination, to make my own pie crust or learn how to handle phyllo dough, but there has to be a compromise.

The answer? The peppermill. I get great satisfaction from giving the fancy pepper mill a few bold turns, just the way all the great chefs do on TV!

Add to that the flavor freshly ground pepper gives to even the most mundane food and I wonder how we used to get through a meal shaking a few pitiful pepper grains from a paltry shaker.

So, when the recipes herein say, "Pepper to taste," and does not designate how much pepper to measure out, use this opportunity to become the chef you want to be and crank away to your heart's content. But, for your information, 1/4 teaspoon of

pepper equals approximately 12 to 15 robust grinds of the peppermill (the results will vary according to each pepper mill and your individual enthusiasm while turning).

My *Sage Advice* is to add pepper to stews and meats and vegetables early in the cooking process so the flavors will have time to blend. But, if your taste buds dictate, don't hesitate to add an extra twist of freshly ground pepper just before serving, or eating, as well.

squeeze bottle of lemon juice

at least one of the lemon-pepper blends mentioned under
   convenience foods

nutmeg

oregano

peppercorns

teriyaki and soy sauces

Tabasco or other hot sauce

thyme

vanilla and almond extract (real—not imitation—please)

Worcestershire sauce

spirits

bourbon

brandy

Madeira

sherry, dry

wine—a bottle of red and white for cooking (of as good a quality
   as if you were drinking it)

"What are the two drinks that can be served at any time of day and with any food?"

SHERRY AND
CHAMPAGNE

sugar

> brown
> confectioners'
> granulated

sweets

> a box of yellow cake mix
> chocolate, shortbread, and graham-cracker pie crusts
> a box or two of fancy cookies (Pirouettes are good)
> ice-cream toppings/sauces, such as chocolate or butterscotch
>> maple and/or a flavored syrup for pancakes

V-8 juice (canned), regular and spicy

vegetables

> French's Taste Toppers in the French Fried Onions flavor
> artichoke hearts, both marinated (jar) and in water (canned)
> prepared garlic
> can or jar of mushrooms
> can or jar of olives, ripe and Spanish (whole and sliced)

About Garlic

WHO says our taste buds can't change?

Garlic, once scorned, is now adored. It was so shied away from when I was growing up that *The Joy of Cooking*, the Bible for my generation of cooks, instructed us to "Learn to rest slivers of garlic clove on meat before cooking it."

These days we can't get enough of it—on our food or on our natural-remedy medicine shelves! We shamelessly order baked garlic in fancy restaurants (remember when you wouldn't go out in public if you'd had one slice of mild garlic bread?) and we are drawn by its delicious aroma into Asian restaurants, where we order garlic shrimp and broccoli.

Even the busiest cook can easily take the moment to tear away a couple of cloves from a plump garlic bulb, peel off the outer skin, and chop or press that now highly esteemed and oh-so-good-for-you herb into whatever dish she is preparing.

But there are times when prepared garlic will come in perfectly handy—especially if you don't cook very often, or if you've used up all your fresh garlic and haven't the time to dash to the store.

That's why you should always keep a jar of ready-to-use garlic in your pantry or, if opened, in the fridge. The basic exchange rule is: 1 garlic clove equals ¼ teaspoon garlic powder, 1 teaspoon garlic salt, or ½ teaspoon prepared garlic.

pesto, prepared (jar) and mix (envelope)

pimiento (small jar)

sun-dried tomatoes

canned whole and stewed tomatoes, plain and flavored or spicy
varieties

sliced water chestnuts

to add color and spice...

apple rings (red, in jar)

pickled beets

capers

chutney

pickled okra

olives (the "party" varieties, stuffed with almonds or cocktail onions)

spiced, pickled peaches (jar)

baby whole pickles in various flavors (sweet and/or dill)

relish

watermelon rind pickles

FROM THE FRIDGE

refrigerator biscuits and crescent rolls

cheeses

appetizer and/or party cheese such as Gouda, goat's milk, brie,
or a bag of Old Wisconsin Party Bites

bag of shredded Cheddar or blended cheeses

feta or blue cheese to sprinkle on salads

meat

long-life products such as Hormel already-cooked beef and pork,
Louis Rich Chicken Time Trimmers

FROM THE FREEZER

frozen meats you plan to use frequently, especially chicken, both
fresh and the ready-to-serve varieties like grilled breasts and breaded
and flavored strips

bag of frozen, cleaned, and cooked shrimp

diced or chopped onions

peppers: green, yellow, orange, and red strips, plus the diced
green variety

pizza crust, or a single-topping pizza

spinach soufflé

baked apples (for a side or dessert)

bruschetta (for instant hor d'oeuvres or appetizers)

vanilla ice cream

a couple of bags of the mixed vegetables listed under
    convenience foods

(Note: peep ahead to pages 14–18 under the Convenience Foods:

A Boon or a Boondoggle heading for other

ideas and suggestions.)

GARNISHES

Knowing that we eat with our eyes as well as our mouths, remember to include garnishes for both beauty and flavor. This final touch can turn "a bite to eat" into a "dining experience."

Herbs. The packaged herbs available today are a real boon to the cook who doesn't have an herb garden. But most don't keep very long, so buy them as near to using as possible. Dried herbs are usually called for in food preparation. If you are going to use fresh herbs, remember that they are not as strong or concentrated as dried. A general rule of thumb is to use 3 times as much fresh as dried.

The following are some ideas for garnishes that add flavor for the palate, as well as a touch of color for the eye:

slivered almonds

fresh basil leaves

fresh cilantro

eggs

lemons, limes, and oranges for decorative slices

fresh mint

sliced or diced onion or pepper, especially the colorful varieties

fresh parsley

fresh rosemary sprigs

To get ideas for unusual garnishes, study the photographs in the gourmet and lifestyle magazines. Often, you will see a single nasturtium blossom or marigold petals sprinkled on a dinner plate, or a soufflé topped with a spray of violets or violas. These are all edible flowers, so when thinking garnishes, remember to pluck a few fresh, edible flowers from your own garden and rinse them, or buy them as needed (read more about using garnishes in The Finishing Touch boxes).

Measurements

Did you know that the first cookbook to give exact measurements for recipes was the *Fannie Farmer Cookbook* published in 1895? Even back then, I'd wager that once the novice cook had tried a recipe a couple of times, she (most cooks were women in those days) would add a little here, take away a little there, and even toss some ingredients out while adding others—to please her family's tastes.

That's the wonderful thing about recipes. They aren't written in stone, only on paper. So take my *Sage Advice* based on years and years of cooking and entertaining. Use the measurements provided when first preparing a recipe. But once you've tried it, be ready to add your own very special touch.

A Tough Shell to Crack

NOPE. I'm not talking about walnuts or pecans, but hard-boiled eggs. I have never been very successful at removing that outer shell and coming up with a beautiful, unblemished white egg.

Rather, I manage to pull parts of the white away with the shell until the poor thing looks as if it has had a bad case of chicken pox and is permanently scarred.

However, thanks to that new kitchen gadget, the Egg Wave, I, and apparently millions of others, now break the egg directly into the microwave-safe container and turn out a boiled egg suitable for using as a garnish.

Even experienced cookbook writers have a difficult time with the many different products on the shelves these days. No longer can you instruct the reader to "open a can of tomato soup." Not only are there many different brands and varieties of tomato soup, but to complicate matters further, cans come in various sizes. Why, just the other day, when I was checking the ounces in a bag of tortilla chips, I had to decide whether to buy a 9-ounce, 12-ounce, 14-ounce, or 20-ounce bag.

Keeping this in mind, I have decided to round off most sizes in the recipes. Can sizes are meant to be guides—approximations. This means that when you read: "1 (14-ounce can)," it's okay to use a 13-ounce can, a 14.5-ounce can, or even a 16-ounce can. What you do not want to use is a 20-ounce can, or a 6-ounce can.

Along these same lines, generally I find it more convenient to purchase resealable *bags*, rather than boxes of frozen vegetables. Oftentimes I want to add a handful of lima beans to a soup or casserole. No reason to open a full box for that small quantity when I can reach into a bag, grab a few, reseal the bag, and save the rest for next time.

For that reason, many of these recipes will call for ½ cup frozen spinach, or ¾ cup yellow squash or zucchini, rather than ½ a 10-ounce box of frozen spinach, or 6 ounces of yellow squash or zucchini.

Equivalents and Conversions

No matter how carefully you plan, there isn't a cook—or even a chef—alive who hasn't scratched his head and wondered, "Now how many tablespoons are in a quarter of a cup," or "How many pounds of potatoes will it take to make two cups?"

Because *From Storebought to Homemade* is intended to provide a starting point for you to learn how to put together a meal at home easily and quickly, so that once you've seen how easy it is, you can venture out on your own, here are some charts you can refer to throughout your cooking adventures when you need to convert a measurement or determine an equivalent.

EQUIVALENTS

dash	less than ⅛ teaspoon
3 teaspoons	1 tablespoon
4 tablespoons	¼ cup
5 tablespoons plus 1 teaspoon	⅓ cup
8 tablespoons	½ cup
10 tablespoons plus 2 teaspoons	⅔ cup
12 tablespoons	¾ cup
16 tablespoons	1 cup
2 tablespoons	1 fluid ounce
1 cup	½ pint or 8 fluid ounces
2 cups	pint or 16 fluid ounces
4 cups	2 pints or 1 quart or 32 fluid ounces
4 quarts	1 gallon or 128 fluid ounces

THOSE PESKY POUND EQUIVALENTS

1 pound	equals approximately
brown sugar	3 cups
cheese	4 cups, shredded
confectioners' sugar	2 ½ cups
flour	4 cups
macaroni	4 cups
meat	2 cups, chopped
potatoes	2 cups, diced, or 2 large whole
rice, uncooked	8 cups, cooked
sugar	2 cups

HANDY SUBSTITUTIONS

1 slice bread	¼ cup dry bread crumbs
	½ cup soft bread crumbs
14 graham cracker squares	1 cup fine graham cracker crumbs
1 tablespoon fresh herbs	1 teaspoon dried herbs
1 cup honey	1 ¼ cups sugar
1 garlic clove	¼ teaspoon garlic powder
	1 teaspoon garlic salt
	½ teaspoon prepared garlic
1 medium lemon	2–3 tablespoons juice
	2 teaspoons grated rind
1 tablespoon prepared mustard	1 teaspoon dried mustard
1 medium orange	⅓ cup juice
	2 tablespoons grated rind
1 pound peanuts	2–3 cups nutmeats
22 vanilla wafers	1 cup fine vanilla wafer crumbs
⅓ onion	1 teaspoon onion powder
1 cup sour cream	3 tablespoons butter plus
	⅞ cup buttermilk
	or yogurt
¼ cup soy sauce	3 tablespoons Worcestershire plus 1 tablespoon water
1 quart whole strawberries	4 cups sliced strawberries
1 ⅓ cups chopped fresh tomatoes	1 cup canned tomatoes

Convenience Foods:
A Boon or a Boondoggle?

Another problem we face these days is the *names* products are given.

For example, almost every store brand and major frozen food company puts out a "mixed vegetable" product. But what a mixture! There's a broccoli, cauliflower, and red pepper mixture. There's a corn, onion, okra, celery, and tomato mixture. There's a 3-pepper mixture. The list goes on and on and on.

In fact, I long ago concluded that one reason more people aren't using today's fabulous convenience foods is because they simply have *too many choices.* Faced with too many choices, you turn away.

That's one way *From Storebought to Homemade* can be a real help to you. By guiding you to some of the best ready-made or convenience foods for these home-tested recipes, I hope to encourage you to try a few and become more adventuresome yourself.

But this book is in no way intended to be an endorsement of just one brand or series of products. For example, you may read in one recipe, "Bird's Eye Gourmet Potato Blend" (white potatoes, broccoli florets, petite carrots, baby cob corn, red pepper). Or you may read a more generic description in another recipe, "frozen, diced combo of onion and green pepper." The point is, if you can't find the exact product, don't give up. Simply make your own mix from individual packages of frozen, or even fresh, veggies you already have on hand.

Coping with GSVO (Grocery Store Visual Overload)

This brings up the question of how to deal with the overload, even panic, you experience when you're faced with so many choices.

I know that a trip to the grocery store these days can be absolutely daunting. New products are appearing not just monthly, it seems, but weekly. The food folks are learning that fast, fabulous food at home is the way to go.

How many times have you noticed, as I have, a package of beautifully trimmed, nice pink fresh pork chops lying in the grocery store cooler where the smoked pork chops are displayed, dropped by someone who didn't want to walk over and put the fresh ones back where they belonged.

Once the shopper spied the smoked ones, she no longer wanted the fresh chops. Not only do smoked chops have a stronger, more distinctive flavor, they have a longer shelf life, and can be turned into a meal more quickly than the fresh ones.

And what happens when you get to the chicken section? The choices are seemingly limitless. Just one quick run down the frozen chicken aisle will turn up Southwestern Glazed Chicken Breasts, Breaded Strips—crispy or regular—Barbecued Wings, Grilled Breast Fillets, Country Fried Chicken Nuggets, Chicken Tenderloins, even Diced Chicken Breast, which could be the harried cook's shortcut to distinctive, almost homemade chicken salad! And those are just a few of the selections!

These days, many of those fabulous specialties we love to order when we're eating out are now as close as our home freezer. What a boon! We can combine these familiar "name brand" convenience foods with home-cooked dishes when we're craving the taste of fast food, or when we want a quick meal but don't have time to stand in line waiting for a table at a restaurant.

These foods have become a real staple in my kitchen. Today's selections of already prepared foods have made it possible to bring back dishes I stopped preparing long ago because they were just too much trouble and too time-consuming.

For example, I used to spend hours slaving over a particular favorite of mine, stuffed pasta. When the kids were young we had it on weekends because that was when I could steal enough time to boil the pasta, prepare the stuffing, and tackle the tedious task of trying to fill the shells without splitting or tearing them. Once the kids left home, I no longer bothered.

These days I buy cheese-stuffed manicotti or meat-stuffed shells, smother them with my favorite already prepared sauce—to which I've added a few extra ingredients—and I've saved hours while enjoying the process.

Although some of you know that these twenty-first-century time-savers exist, many of you may shy away from such newfangled foods simply because there are just too many of them to decide which ones to buy.

Or, maybe you haven't tried them because you're spending hours at a time trying to prepare gourmet dishes from scratch. Or, you may be stuck in the old rut of roast beef on Monday, pork chops on Tuesday, leftover roast on Wednesday, chicken pot pies on Thursday, and fish sticks on Friday. Whatever the reason, don't feel bad. I've been in your shoes, but then I saw the light. That's why I've written this book—to help you.

For starters, here's a quick guide to a *few* (just the tip of the iceberg) of the untold numbers of shortcut products to look for and use in your cooking. These products are ones that can be found in small towns and large metropolitan areas alike, and in no way does the list begin to cover all the brand names or varieties available.

generic brands offered in the following combinations:

Italian veggies	zucchini, broccoli, carrots, green beans, limas
California	broccoli, carrots, cauliflower
winter	broccoli, cauliflower
stir-fry	sugar snap peas, broccoli, green beans, carrots, celery, onion, peppers, water chestnuts
Oriental style	green beans, broccoli, onion, mushrooms
fiesta blend	broccoli, carrots, Italian green beans, white beans, kidney beans, garbanzo beans, red pepper
stew veggies	potato, carrots, onions, celery
veggie soup mix	carrots, potato, green peas, green beans, corn, limas, okra, celery, onion
gumbo soup mix	okra, corn, onions, celery, red pepper

Bird's Eye

gourmet potato blend	white potatoes, broccoli florets, petite carrots, baby cob corn, red pepper
corn blend	white corn, broccoli, baby cob corn, Parisian carrots
mixed	corn, carrots, green beans, green peas
broccoli stir-fry	broccoli, carrots, onions, red pepper, celery, water chestnuts, mushrooms

broccoli, carrots, cauliflower

broccoli, corn, red pepper

broccoli, carrots, water chestnuts

cauliflower, carrots, pea pods

three-pepper combination

Green Giant "Create A Meal" (Green Giant also offers a "Complete Skillet Meal" with meat added)

Parmesan herb chicken

Szechwan

teriyaki

sweet and sour

garlic herb chicken

cheesy pasta and herbs

lo mein

lemon pepper

Stouffer's "Skillet Sensations" (Stouffer's also offers "Oven Sensations" with meat added, but I always seem to add more meat to these)

teriyaki chicken

grilled chicken and vegetables

beef fajita

frozen meats

meatballs

Armour and Tyson offer 18-ounce bags of chicken pieces in
the following varieties:

    southwestern glazed chicken breasts

    breaded strips

    barbecued wings

    grilled breast fillets

    country fried chicken nuggets

    chicken tenderloins

    diced chicken breast

ready-to-serve sauces

Ragú® "Cheese Creations!"™

    Roasted Garlic Parmesan

    Parmesan and Mozzarella

    Double Cheddar

    Classic Alfredo

    Light Parmesan Alfredo

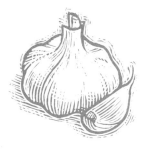

Ragú® "Robusto!"™

    Classic Italian Meat

    Chopped Tomato, Olive Oil, and Garlic

    Six Cheese

    Parmesan and Romano

    Sautéed Onion and Garlic

    Sweet Italian Sausage and Cheese

    Sautéed Onion and Mushroom

seasonings

Lawry's Seasoning Salt

flavor packs such as Knorr's Peppercorn Gravy or fajita
    and meat loaf varieties

dried lemon seasonings made by Knorr, Sun Bird, and McCormick

flavored cheeses

Philadelphia Cream Cheese blends, offered in regular, whipped, fat-free, light, and soft—and in flavors such as strawberry, honey nut (with pecans), chive, onion, and cheesecake

preblended juices

Welch's

    grape (both white and red varieties)

    strawberry breeze (5-juice blend)

    wild raspberry (3-juice blend)

    tropical carrot (carrot plus 5 juices)

Dole

    pineapple-orange

    orange-strawberry-banana

    pineapple-orange-banana

Minute Maid

    fruit punch (grape, pear)

    tropical punch (pineapple, grape, passion fruit)

Tropicana

    orange-tangerine

    orange-strawberry

    orange-pineapple

    white grape-peach

Excuse Me!

I'LL ALWAYS remember the conversation I had with a very well-known cookbook author and food critic. She didn't like my use of convenience foods one bit and told me so in no uncertain terms.

But, later in the day, when in the company of several other fine cooks, chefs, and writers, she said this: "I always chop my onions first, and then freeze them so I'll have them on hand."

I was dying to ask her what she did when chopping her onions that made them so much better than the already frozen chopped onions I use! But, having been raised always to be respectful of my elders, I demurred.

When you are considering frozen and convenience foods, think about it this way: We've been using frozen vegetables for years. But it's a new cooking day out there. So for those meals when time's at a premium, the choices listed earlier are there to help you out.

And here, to get you in the right mind-set, are just a few shortcuts to keep in mind as you begin to prepare fast, fabulous food at home.

TIME-CONSUMING	TIME-SAVING
peeling and chopping onions	frozen, chopped onions
peeling and chopping green peppers	frozen, chopped peppers
washing and slicing mushrooms	frozen, or canned, sliced mushrooms; or sliced mushrooms from the produce section or salad bar
washing and preparing lettuce	ready-to-eat, bagged lettuce
washing and shredding cabbage	shredded, bagged cabbage for slaw
washing and cleaning celery for chopping	already washed, bagged celery, or salad-bar celery
mincing and pressing garlic	prepared garlic in jars
washing, peeling, and preparing fruit	salad-bar fruits or jarred fresh fruits
washing, peeling, and preparing carrots, cauliflower, and broccoli	bagged or salad-bar veggies
preparing and baking a whole chicken	ready-to-eat rotisserie chicken
preparing and cooking chicken strips and pieces	frozen, or ready-to-eat chicken strips and cubes
cooking bacon	ready-to-serve bacon
preparing, slicing, or cubing ham	fully cooked ham slices and cubes
cubing or grating cheese	ready-to-use or -serve grated or cubed cheeses
cooking, shelling, deveining shrimp	ready-to-use shrimp
preparing custards	ready-to-eat individual servings
cooking and stuffing pastas	prestuffed manicotti and shells
mixing, shaping, and browning meatballs	cooked and frozen meatballs
removing, then dicing leftover turkey	ready-to-prepare turkey breast steaks or small turkey roasts
peeling, dicing, slicing, shredding, even mashing potatoes	ready-to-prepare potatoes, frozen or from the deli or refrigerator section

Ingredients

When Fresh Is Best—and When It Isn't

"Use only the freshest ingredients." How often do you hear these words of advice from today's leading chefs? I would agree, except for a few basic problems. Fresh vegetables do not grow everywhere yearround.

In my part of the world—Virginia—local tomatoes do not come in until the very end of June or the first of July. This means that in December most of the tomatoes in the grocery store have been shipped in from Mexico—a trip that takes days of hard, bruising travel. Tomatoes that have been picked at their prime (when they're the most flavorful) have only a two or three-day shelf-life. By the time tomatoes picked in their prime are shipped halfway across the country, they're already mushy and overripe.

Of course, climate and weather conditions make every growing season slightly different as you move from South to North and from East to West. I remember how amazed a Yankee friend of mine was when she ate freshly picked, plump, succulent strawberries in Florida in February. She thought you had to wait until June for such a rich culinary treat. So you don't miss the best of what nature has to offer, here's a quick guide to the best fruits and vegetables of each season.

winter

    the citrus fruits: grapefruit, oranges, tangerines

    greens: the kale, collards, mustard, and turnip greens that
        Southerners love and the rest of the world passes by

spring

    fruit: strawberries and blueberries

    vegetables: early peas, asparagus, fresh lettuces

    root vegetables: beets, carrots, potatoes, turnips

summer

    beans: every variety of beans, from pole and green beans to lima
        beans...even October beans come in the summer!

    fruit: blackberries, melons, peaches, apricots

    vegetables: eggplant, peppers, zucchini, and tomatoes, of course—
        you might try growing them yourself, even if just one or two
        patio-variety plants

autumn

    fruit: apples, grapes, pears, apricots

    vegetables: pumpkins, winter squash

Presentation: The Magic Ingredient

If you think the two main ingredients that go into a successful meal, be it a special Wednesday night family meal or a Saturday night company dinner, are color and flavor, you're right. *But*, a stressed-out cook can ruin even the prettiest, most flavorful event.

It takes more than a trip to the grocery store to turn storebought food into a homemade meal. The shopping list helps take care of the first "p" in cooking—"preparation,"—but there's the second "p" in cooking, and I've already hinted at it—"presentation."

Think about it. Your eyes linger over beautifully set tables. You watch in amazement as the chefs on the Food Network flick confetti-like slivers of pimiento and green peppers around an entrée, or top a dessert with a thin layer of lacy chocolate.

"I could never do that," you're already protesting.

Oh yes you can...*if* the rest of the meal is made in just minutes with already prepared food products, or even purchased at a local restaurant, café, or deli.

You see, a great meal can be remarkably simple. Often it takes only two steps:

1. Add a surprise ingredient to an already, or very easily, prepared food.

2. Add your own finishing touch to its presentation.

Throughout this book, you'll find side notes labeled *The Finishing Touch*. These contain short, quick suggestions for giving a special flair to your food's presentation. I've said it before, I'll say it again: Always remember, we also eat with our eyes.

A Word on Tomatoes

ONE of the saddest food days at our house comes some time in October when the first frost nips at the still-green tomatoes hanging on for dear life on the spindly tomato vine.

Of course, it's time for the plants to be yanked up and for the soil to rest. But what is a sandwich without a tomato?

These days, new and improved storebought cherry, grape, and Roma varieties add flavor and color to sandwiches and salads the rest of the year...until the homegrown summertime tomatoes come in.

When to Use This Book

"You don't eat like this every day do you?" I was asked when explaining the concept of *From Storebought to Homemade*.

Of course I don't. I like to eat out just as much as the next person. Further, there are those days when I roll up my sleeves to make some exotic concoction from scratch. And I don't expect you to cook this way every day either.

A Word about *The Finishing Touch*

WHEN IT COMES to creating your own finishing touches, let your imagination run away with you—especially when you're standing in front of a beautiful display of colorful fruits and vegetables in the grocery store or farmer's market.

Literally any fruit or vegetable that can be hollowed out can be used to enhance the presentation of your meal, and, in many instances, be eaten as well. A perfect example of this are the recipes, Peas in a Boat (page 168) and Peas in Tomatoes (page 169), and Shrimp-Filled Avocado Salad (page138).

To help get you started thinking creatively, here are some suggestions, many already familiar to you, but others that I hope you'll find a little more imaginative and different.

Fill the cavity of a pear or peach with cottage cheese or a flavored cream cheese and top it with a cherry, fresh berries, or mint sprig.

Pineapple halves, or even canned pineapple rings, are perfect "containers" for any variety of fruits or cheese.

Lemons, limes, and oranges make great "cups," either cut crosswise or lengthwise. What could be more colorful and spirit-lifting than seeing a scooped-out lemon shell filled with mint jelly or a scooped-out lime shell filled to the brim with salsa? Try putting apple sauce in an orange or tangerine shell to delight the children in your family.

Bake acorn squash in the microwave (5 to 6 minutes) or oven (350 degrees for 25 to 30 minutes) by cutting it in half, scooping out the seeds, and placing it in a baking dish with enough water to cover the bottom third of the vegetable. When done,

fill it with ready-to-serve mashed potatoes, stovetop dressing, or flavored rice.

Here's another idea. Scoop out a thick-skinned small, uncooked pumpkin and use it as an individual soup bowl. Or use a much larger one as a tureen.

Tomatoes, either the cherry or grape varieties, or the traditional, beefsteak variety, can be topped with any number of fillings, from a single small shrimp placed fancifully in a large cherry tomato, to crabmeat salad in a large, round one.

Boats made from yellow or green squash can be filled with anything from rice to cooked sausage. A head of cabbage filled with slaw...a small cantaloupe filled with ice cream...the possibilities are almost limitless.

The one drawback is that these presentations do take a little time. But I think of it

But when you want to bring the family or friends together at home, over a kitchen or dining-room table, but you haven't the time (or the energy) to make a true, homecooked meal from scratch, these recipes and suggestions can turn a laborious chore into a pleasant task.

this way. These are unexpected touches, gifts, so to speak, that tell volumes about you as a hostess. They say that you're witty, caring, and imaginative.

Presentation isn't just the decorative touches added to plates and serving dishes. The plates, platters, and bowls themselves can also enhance the total dining experience. Never fear. You don't have to dash out and buy a new set of china or serving dishes, but you can add, one by one, the pieces that will complement what you already have.

So let's peek inside the china and crystal cabinet for some versatile pieces you can use at an individual place setting or on a buffet table to add charm and distinction to any meal or party.

You may not have all these pieces right now, but I assure you that, as you accumulate them over time, they will pay for themselves in conven-

ience and appearance.

Individual ramekin dishes can be used for everything from rich desserts to spoon bread to minisoufflés to fruit garnish to nuts. *Individual seafood shells* are an alternative to ramekins, but they aren't quite as versatile. Both are inexpensive and make a nice showing.

A pretty crystal bowl can be used for the basic tossed salad, the incomparable holiday trifle, or any range of dishes in between, from potato salad to jelled salads.

Platters are indispensable for serving meats surrounded by garnish or accompanying fruits and vegetables. But small servings get lost on an oversized platter, so try to have various sizes to fit various needs.

Attractive casserole dishes that can go from the oven or microwave to the table are a staple in these days of casual entertaining. Though the highly decorated ones are ex-

tremely attractive, if you change your china pattern or even the wallpaper in your dining room, you may find that your favorite casserole dishes suddenly clash with the surroundings. I recommend basic white dishes that will go with everything. That way you can spiff up your presentation with an imaginative centerpiece of flowers or fruit, or with the food itself.

Young cooks who are just beginning to collect their "party essentials," and even more experienced folk, can come up lacking the perfect serving utensil at the last minute. So, before settling on the menu for a party or company dinner, think what you will need to serve each dish—fork, spoon, slotted spoon, etc. If you love antiques, you'll have fun searching for the proper cold meat fork or pastry server as you rummage through yard sales, flea markets, antique shops, even your grandmother's silver chest!

I say this more than once...if you will just take the time to do a little menu planning, the way you do when you're planning your shopping list, and figure out *where* you want to put your emphasis—on the entrée, the dessert, an interesting salad—you can turn out a meal with a minimum of effort that will bring in the maximum of compliments. By making just one special, or signature, dish you can tilt the tables. If you make a simple ice cream pie (page 257), that fantastic finale can turn your storebought rotisserie chicken garnished

For the Love of Food

BEFORE serving any meal, for company, or to your family, ask yourself three simple questions:

Does it look good?

Does it smell good?

Does it taste good?

Does it look good? If it doesn't, no one will want to eat it. Think about it. Why does mush look so uninviting? Because it looks like mush!

To make the food you are serving look good, arrange it prettily on the plate or platter. Don't just plop the food on the plate at random. Arrange it to show off the colors and textures of the food to their best advantage.

If the food is colorless—and even delicious items like chicken, pork, rice, and potatoes can be colorless and boring to look at—brighten it up with an eye-catching garnish.

How? Well, even if you aren't serving carrots, if you have a handheld grater and a fresh carrot (remember, you can buy just one carrot or a handful of presliced carrots from the salad bar), you can create a colorful garnish that will bring the whole plate or platter to life.

Or how about keeping a jar of sliced olives with pimientos in the fridge? Use them as garnish, or take thirty seconds and dice a couple of them into smaller pieces to create red and green "confetti." Use it alone or in combination with the carrots.

And what brings the chicken to life in the Cranberry-Sauce Chicken recipe? The red cranberry sauce, of course.

You'll find other items that can be used as garnish listed on page 9. Let your eyes, taste buds, and imagination be your guide.

Does it smell good? What makes you begin to salivate when your neighbor is grilling outside? The aroma, of course. What makes pumpkin pie, pumpkin pie? It isn't just the pumpkin. It's the aroma of the fabulous spices mixed with the pumpkin custard.

You can't bottle the delicious smells that come from the kitchen. The lesson here is that heating up or baking just one dish for your meal can fill your whole home with that "homemade" feeling (even if you've just doctored up a storebought product with one added ingredient).

But a word of warning! Don't overwhelm those rich kitchen smells by lighting scented candles. Nothing is worse than the rich beef-and-tomato aroma of a stew with pickled peach slices, deli potato wedges, and salad-bar salad into a special meal indeed.

And for those of you who are watching sodium and sugar and cholesterol, using storebought items at home actually can give you *greater* control over your choices and diet than eating at a restaurant or fast-food chain.

When to use this book? When you're looking for a quick and easy way to gather everyone together, enjoy your kitchen, and share your best.

combined with a light, sweet, gardenia-scented candle. Conversely, a heavily scented Christmas bay candle will completely smother the smell of delicate lemon zest.

The rule is simple. Use unscented candles on your dining table to create ambiance, not fragrance. Unscented votives are best because they don't cut off the across-the-table view of the diners, and they send out a low, romantic glow that relaxes everyone.

Does it taste good? Taste, after all, is what food is all about. But our tastes and taste buds vary. That's surely how the old saying "too many cooks spoil the broth" came into being. Mix together too many individual likes and dislikes, and you end up with a hodgepodge instead of a well-flavored delicacy.

Just as individual taste buds are different, so are the tastes of different brand-name foods. Simply put, not all canned tomatoes taste alike. And not everyone likes the same brand.

Throughout these pages I've suggested some specific products because they provide a quick and easy way to get around those time-consuming steps that might keep you from trying a recipe in the first place. Though I've tried to use products that are easily found, not all brands are available in every store.

If you can't find a product, speak to your grocery store manager. He or she should be able to help you locate it if it is available in that store, or even in the region, or to help you find an acceptable substitute.

I live in a small town, an hour's drive from the closest "big city." If you're in my situation, you've probably learned to keep a shopping list of specialty items to pick up when you're somewhere that has more choices than you can find at home. I anticipate those grocery store trips with as much enthusiasm as I do shopping trips for a special dress, a pair of shoes, or even toys for the grandkids.

Whether or not you have the perfect ingredient, or a good substitute, to make every dish taste its best, you still must do some tasting yourself. As you taste, make adjustments if necessary. If you think a dish needs more pepper, start grinding. If thyme is your favorite herb, toss in an extra ¼ teaspoon. If a dish calling for cream of mushroom soup seems a little dry to you, add ¼ or ⅓ cup of milk.

And all the time you're tasting, remember these words of wisdom: "Cooking is like love. It should be entered into with abandon, or not at all."

Menus That Work

In America, even your menus have the gift of language...
"The Chef's own Vienna Roast. A hearty, rich meatloaf,
gently seasoned to perfection and served in a creamy nest of
mashed farm potatoes and strictly fresh garden vegetables."
Of course, what you get is cole slaw and a slab of meat, but
that doesn't matter because the menu has already started your
juices going. Oh, those menus. In America, they are poetry.

—LAURIE LEE, BRITISH AUTHOR, *NEWSWEEK*, OCTOBER 24, 1960

THINK ABOUT IT. Take any shelf of cookbooks. Pick a book. Turn to the index. Look under "M." What do you find? "Meat...Meatballs...Meatloaf...Melon... Meringue...Minestrone...Mocha...Mousse...Muffins... Mushrooms...Mustard...." There's everything from Mamaliga (a Romanian cornmeal dish similar to Mexico's polenta) to Mixed Grill. All the "M" food words, but seldom *Menu*.

But what do you have to have before you can begin cooking a meal, be it supper for two or a buffet for twenty? A plan. A menu.

Without a menu that provides complementary tastes, colors, and food groups, even the fanciest meal will fall short. No matter how delicious each individual dish may be, a menu consisting of two cream of mushroom soup vegetable casseroles, a chicken dish, white rice, and a vanilla ice cream dessert will be...*boring*...from taste to color.

Of course, today's great "salad in a bag" selections make it much easier to add color and nutrition to any meal. But who wants to eat a mixed green salad twice a day, every day?

All in all, putting together easy, time efficient, and delicious complementary dishes can be difficult. Yet, I really can't overemphasize how important it is to match up foods properly. It's so important that food stylists are paid huge salaries to put together eye-appealing displays for magazines, books, and television shows.

As a quick rule of thumb, a mixture of colors will provide variety in taste and nutrition while pleasing the eye. You see this rule put into practice on your favorite television cooking show when a white fish and rice entree is brought to life by arranging strips of yellow and red peppers on top and green baby Brussels sprouts all around, or when a few blueberries are sprinkled around a vanilla pudding or ice cream dish.

Once you have chosen the food fare, there's yet another consideration—the pots and pans you'll need to prepare each course, and where each item needs to be cooked. A menu that calls for three casseroles to be cooked at different oven temperatures is useless to the young New York bride who owns only two baking dishes and cooks on an apartment-size ministove. That's why I've included a list of cookware needed at the end of the ingredients list for each recipe. In this menu section, if there's more than one item that requires an oven, I've made sure they can be cooked together.

Here, now, are menu suggestions to lighten up your kitchen duties while turning storebought items into homemade meals. As you read through these menus, note that there are two symbols to help you with your planning. A white box (□) denotes ready-to-serve selections that involve no more than opening a can or cello bag or microwaving a frozen item. A green box (■) denotes a *From Storebought to Homemade* recipe that can be easily and quickly prepared.

Here's another tip to keep in mind. The addition of a simple relish, a favorite pickle, or even a raw vegetable dish such as chow-chow, pickled peaches, watermelon rind pickles, or marinated carrots, can be a real pick-me-up at any table. They add unexpected flavor, they're filled with vitamins, and they add the splash of color that cooks are always looking for. What more could you ask?

Sage Advice

When planning a menu, write it out. Next, visualize it in your mind, making sure you have a pleasing blend of colors, tastes, and textures. Finally, think about what equipment you'll need to cook each item in and how you will serve it. These steps only take a few seconds and can keep you from last minute panic attacks.

Family Dinner Menus

I'm a great proponent of the old-fashioned family meal. These days, when the kids have soccer practice and music lessons and the parents find themselves getting home later and later from work or civic meetings or volunteer activities, we're losing more than just the family dinner, or supper (depending on what your family calls it), time. Families are losing the art of conversation, lessons in manners, and the chance to get to know one another—yes, even your own family—better. They are missing out on the wonderful joie de vivre that comes from sitting around the family dinner table and having fun.

I've never seen any studies done on the subject, but I'd wager that children whose families converse during the evening meal do better in school. When I was a little girl, the evening meal was when we talked about what I had learned in school that day. It's a tradition that was continued when my children were young too. We discussed their history, literature, science, and current events topics, and suddenly school lessons became fun and were reinforced as part of a relaxed dinnertime conversation.

But, back to the food. It's always easy to settle for pasta. Everyone likes it and it's so quick and effortless to prepare that you can have it every night. But it doesn't have to be that way, as these family dinner menus testify. The suggestions I make don't involve hours of preparation, and the menus combine ready-to-serve selections with quickly pulled together courses eveyone will enjoy.

And then there's yet another bonus. I promise that the delicious aroma of just one *From Storebought to Homemade* dish will whet everyone's appetite and make the entire meal special.

The
Finishing Touch

You'll save so much time using the menus, recipes, and ideas in this book, that you'll have time to add a distinctive finishing touch to special dinners and parties. Why not write out the menu on a heavy stock card that fits the occasion's mood, or that matches your décor. To save even more time, do it on your computer, using a whimsical font. You might even take a hint from Laurie Lee's quote at the beginning of the chapter and give your dishes a fancy name and elaborate description.

Family Menus

□ Denotes ready-to-serve selections that involve no more than opening a can or cello bag or microwaving a frozen item.

■ Denotes a *From Storebought to Homemade* recipe that can be easily and quickly prepared.

- ■ Orange-Pineapple Mold (page 147)
- □ Simple buttered broccoli
- □ Rotisserie roasted chicken
- ■ Bouillon Rice (page 179)
- □ Parker House dinner rolls
- ■ Brown Sugar Pie (page 255)

- □ Tossed salad (your favorite packaged, ready-to-serve salad and salad dressing.)
- ■ Chicken Marsala (page 90)
- □ Mashed potatoes
- □ Peas
- ■ Fruit Pizza (page 247)

- ■ Quick Chicken Pie (page 204)
- ■ Cheerful Green Beans (page 165)
- □ Sliced tomatoes
- ■ Marmalade Muffins (page 222)
- □ Chocolate chip or butter pecan ice cream

- ■ Quickly Assembled Chicken Meal-in-One (page 203)
- □ Garlic bread
- ■ Cake Mix Cookies (pages 276–277) and fruit

Sage Advice

Smart cooks perfect 3 or 4 dishes in every category—appetizers, soups, salads, entrees, accompaniments, desserts—and mix and match these when they need to serve up a spectacular meal at a moment's notice.

■ Everybody's Mother's Pork Chop Casserole (page 114)

□ Rice

□ Le Seur peas

□ Applesauce (one of the flavored varieties)

□ Carrot cake

□ Tossed salad

■ Mexican Chicken Casserole (page 199)

■ Mango Soufflé (page 146)

■ Old-Fashioned Pot Roast (page 103)

■ Bouillon Rice (page 179)

■ Green Bean Casserole (page 164)

□ Apple turnovers

■ Sweet and Sour Pork, American-Style (page 112)

□ Rice

□ Vegetable sauté

□ Caramel frosted cake

■ Tangy Tomato Aspic (page 148)

■ The Picky Eater's Beef Stew (page 209)

□ Noodles

□ French bread

□ Raspberry sherbet and cookies

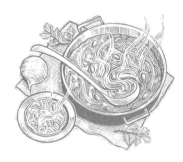

- Lime Yogurt Salad (page 145)

- Quick-Quick Brunswick Stew (pages 210–211)

- ☐ Biscuits

- Serendipity Pumpkin Cake (pages 268–269)

- Pickled Cole Slaw (page 131)
- ☐ Your favorite storebought fried chicken

- Jalapeño Corn Bread (page 230)

- A Side of Beans (page 281)

- You'll-Never-Guess-It's-Made-with-Cookies Ice Box Dessert
  (page 275)

When it comes to having a family dinner, and there are children in the house, don't forget the leftovers from an adult dinner party—casual or formal. This is a great way to begin to introduce children to fancier dishes without going to the trouble to specially prepare them.

- ☐ Tossed salad

- Pork and Cherry Supreme (page 113)

- Vidalia Onion Casserole (pages 166–167)

- Peas in Tomatoes (page 169)

- ☐ Chocolate cake (as a reward for trying the fancy dishes)

- Pepper and Mushroom Chicken Delight (page 96)

- ☐ Mashed potatoes

- ☐ Peas and carrots

- Bread Pudding (pages 270–271)

- ■ Corned Beef (page 102)
- ■ No-Fail Potatoes (page 184)
- □ Applesauce (perhaps one of the flavored ones)
- □ Green beans
- ■ Allison's Vanilla Crisps (page 264)

- □ Tossed salad
- ■ Old-Fashioned Pot Roast (page 103)
- ■ Dressed-Up Noodles (page 189)
- ■ Green Bean Casserole (page 164)
- ■ Chinese Chews (page 265)

Company Dinner Parties, Served Formally or Informally

"I hadn't realized that throwing a party was quite so much hard work. Perhaps that's why Mummy and Gran never throw parties in London."

—LUCY, IN *WINTER SOLSTICE* BY ROSAMUNDE PILCHER

Hard work aside, I decided a long time ago that one of the reasons people may be hesitant to entertain at home these days is that we've all been spoiled by cafeterias and buffet lines. They provide such abundance and variety that the poor hostess feels she just can't prepare enough food for her guests. (If, perchance, you are a Southerner, as I am, and are used to the three-meat, five-vegetable spread associated with Southern hospitality, the problem is compounded.)

In truth, however, your guests don't *care* how many items you're serving! They're coming to your home for the friendship and fellowship (and the chance to get out of their own kitchens). So rather than burden yourself with four appetizers, two entrées, and three vegetables, keep it simple. In these calorie-conscious days, many of your guests will secretly thank you!

Try any of the following easy-to-prepare, timesaving menus for a memorable dinner party. You can serve the meal yourself, but that might make you a disgruntled host or hostess—heaven forbid! So relax. Have a buffet. Or prepare a simple meal you can serve up on a plate and keep warm in the oven, or on a warming tray, while you fix the other plates. Or even serve the food in pretty bowls and on nice platters...family style.

With a little planning, and the use of prepared foods as a starting point, you'll find that throwing a party really doesn't have to be such hard work after all.

Just one more word of *sage advice* that my mother gave me. She'd say, "You know all your friends who lead such exciting lives? They're always busy going here and there and doing such interesting things in faraway places? Well, dear, invite them to dinner—and I bet they can all come!"

A SAMPLE MENU AND HOW TO THINK IT THROUGH.

Pretend it's a nice late-spring or early-summer Saturday and you decide you'd like to have some friends over for an early night, light Sunday supper. You don't have much time to plan, but you can still prepare an impressive and delicious, but almost effortless get-together. This is how.

Menu:
- Anything Goes Fruit Soup (page 83)
- Shrimp-Filled Avocado (page 135)
- □ Petite peas on a small leaf lettuce
- □ Sliced Roma tomatoes garnished with fresh basil leaves
- □ Dainty buttered biscuits from the frozen section served with butter and crab-apple jelly
- English Trifle (page 266)

The shrimp filling takes all of 5 minutes to stir together and should be prepared the night before. It's best if you mix the pudding and sherry together so the tastes have time to blend. But do not assemble the trifle yet.

The morning of the supper, whip the cream, cut the pound cake, and assemble the trifle. Place it in the refrigerator. The peas can be cooked in the microwave in 3 to 4 minutes while you're dishing the shrimp into the avocados or putting the lettuce to hold the peas on the plates.

The delicious combination of hot buttery biscuits served with storebought crab-apple jelly on individual bread and butter plates is always a hit, so plan to have plenty of biscuits on hand.

Company Menus

☐ Assorted nuts (from a can)

■ Cream Cheese and Olive Spread with crackers and celery stalks (page 43)

■ Lamb Chops in Sherry Marinade (page 124)

☐ Instant long grain and wild rice

■ Celery Casserole (page 159)

☐ Tomato with Mozarella and Basil Salad

☐ Peach sherbet and cookies

☐ Cocktail olives stuffed with almonds or jalapeño, kalamata olives, and caper berries

■ Pimiento Surprise with crackers and celery sticks (page 51)

■ Lettuce, Orange, and Almond Salad (page 129)

■ Timeless Chicken (page 97)

☐ Herb-flavored rice

☐ Green beans and almonds

■ Incredibly Quick Cheese Biscuits (page 224)

☐ Vanilla ice cream with Grand Marnier drizzled on top

■ Zesty Tomato Starter with Incredibly Quick Cheese Biscuits (pages 76)

■ Cranberry Sauce Chicken (page 92)

■ No-Fail Potatoes (page 184)

☐ Broccoli

■ Sinful Butter Brickle Ice Cream Pie (page 257)

- Avocado and Tomato Salad (page 137)
- Chicken à la Simon and Garfunkle, served over rice (page 89)
- □ Petite whole green beans
- Glazed Carrots with Onions (page 158)
- □ Apple pie à la mode

- Antipasto American Style (page 61)
- Garlic Roasted Pork Tenderloin (page 118)
- Pecan Rice (page 180)
- Peas in Tomatoes (page 169)
- Baked Tipsy Apples with ice cream (page 242)

- Chilled Strawberry Soup Number 1 (page 81)
- Champagne Chicken (page 88)
- □ Rice
- □ Broccoli topped with buttered bread crumbs
- Old-Fashioned Lemon Chess Pie (page 250)

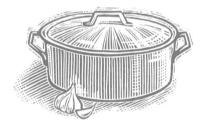

- □ Spinach salad
- Easy Beef Stroganoff (page 105)
- Dressed-Up Noodles (page 189)
- Tomato Puddin' (page 173)
- Sour Cream Biscuits (page 227)
- □ Fresh melon and fruit cup with Cointreau drizzled on top

- Virginia Cream of Peanut Soup (page 80)
- Beef Tenderloin (pages 106–107)
- Pureed Artichokes (page 151)
- Carrot Surprise (page 156)
- ☐ Whole string beans, buttered and garnished with pimiento
- Frozen Oranges and assorted chocolates (page 243)

From Storebought to Fabulous Retro-Modern Party

CAROL CARLISH was in a pickle of a mess. It was December 26th—enough to put anyone in a tizzy. A combination of Christmas traffic, long family good-byes, and nasty weather had delayed Carol and her husband, Robert, from getting back to their home in Danville until 3 P.M. Company was coming for supper at 7 P.M. What to do?

In her usual ingenious way, Carol headed for the grocery store while Robert helped on the home front.

While Carol was buying Knorr's Vegetable Soup Mix and Russian dressing, Cheese Whiz, and Moon Pies, Robert was gathering together recycled Christmas bows, half-burned candles, and a long-out-of-style Christmas tablecloth and napkins stored up in the attic.

By the time the company arrived, everything was cooked, and the decorations were in place.

Now, this was not your usual fancy party, but it was a night to remember, and it just goes to show what a little imagination can do. As Carol laughingly admits, her friends not only are still talking about the night, they are also copying her idea—now that they've gotten over their initial shock.

Here it is for you, too, to copy exactly what she did.

But first you have to know that behind her idea is a seldom-admitted, but very true food fact: *Foods have fads, and if you haven't eaten something in a while, you'll be amazed how good it is.* Or, in Carol's own words, "It's not that the foods taste bad, it's that they've gone out of fashion. Try them again, and they actually taste pretty good."

It's a fact I adhere to and often put to work myself. It's also why my kids are always asking me for their grand-

- Artichoke and Oyster Soup with cheese crackers (page 69)
- Pork and Cherry Supreme (page 113)
- ☐ Roasted potato wedges
- Green Bean Casserole (page 164)
- Flan, with whipped cream and raspberries (page 240)

mothers' recipes. And it's why I've updated so many "old-timey" recipes in these pages.

Now, this is what Carol's friends saw when they walked into her house.

In the living room the hors d'oeuvres were set out on the table for everyone to help themselves: Cheese Whiz in the jar, Saltines in the box, Vienna sausages and deviled ham in the tins, and a big bowl of veggie dip made by combining sour cream and Knorr's Vegetable Soup Mix surrounded by crudités— carrots, celery, broccoli, cauliflower...straight from the cello bags.

When they moved into the dining space, there on the once-stunning, but now-tacky Christmas tablecloth was quite a spread.

There was Spam—scored, glazed, and decorated with cloves; meatloaf; iceberg lettuce cut in quarters and "dressed" with bottled Russian dressing; green beans straight out of the can (which, Carol remembers, "Somebody actually said were good"); a broccoli casserole she had whipped up in no time with mushroom soup; a pretty, ready-to-serve jelled red fruit salad; mashed potatoes made straight from the box; as well as a casserole of Kraft's boxed macaroni and cheese (Carol's favorite "closet food"); and a loaf of white bread, still in its wrapper.

And for dessert...that Southern favorite—Moon Pies served with RC Cola and peanuts. (For those of you who don't know, you put the peanuts in the RC bottle and the salt makes the soda fizz up.)

Needless to say, everyone is now wondering what Carol will do next. She's confided that she's thinking about offering everyone a choice of different microwaveable meals.

The moral of this story is that imagination can make any meal a joyful, memorable time—for who can live without friends and food!

■ Gazpacho Plus (page 84)

■ Easy Chicken Tetrazzini (page 91)

■ Peas in a Boat (page 168)

■ Cornmeal Biscuits (page 228)

□ Butter pecan ice cream over angel food cake

□ Biscotti

■ Spanish Pork Chops (page 115)

□ Wild Rice

□ Broccoli

□ Bread and preserves

■ English Trifle (page 266)

■ Love Apple Fromage Soup (page 77)

■ Baked Rainbow or Brook Trout (page 98)

■ Portobello Deluxe (page 170)

□ Asparagus

□ Dinner rolls

■ The Basic Poached Pear (pages 244–245)

■ Avocado and Tomato Salad (page 137)

■ Garlic Roasted Pork Tenderloin (page 118)

□ Peas and almonds

■ Very Good Winter Squash (page 172)

□ Cheese straws

□ Raspberry ice cream and hazelnut pirouettes

"Civilized man cannot live without cooks."

—BULWER-LYTTON,
19TH-CENTURY ENGLISH
POET AND NOVELIST

Appetizers and Hors d'oeuvres

WHICH IS IT? An appetizer or an hors d'oeuvre? Check any dozen cookbooks and you'll find that half of them call cocktail meatballs an "appetizer," while the other half call them an "hors d'oeuvre." Does it really matter? The recipes are the same.

Further, the particular recipe (whether it's for cocktail meatballs or hot crab dip) is intended to whet your appetite, to make you want more.

So the difference between an appetizer and an hors d'oeuvre really comes down to this: *When* are you going to serve it?

An appetizer is traditionally served before a full meal. It's supposed to provide a nibble or two—something to stave off your hunger, but not so much that it fills you up while you are anticipating the main event.

On the other hand, an hors d'oeuvre is traditionally served at a cocktail party or before sitting down at the dinner table.

In reality, any of the selections given here can be served either as an appetizer before a real meal, or as part of a larger "cocktail spread."

Here's an interesting sidenote, though. The term "hors d'oeuvre" literally translates to "out of (the) work," meaning that these goodies are outside of the "work" required to prepare the rest of the meal. But wait. That means that hors d'oeuvres add more work to the cook's duties.

With that in mind, I've tried to assemble recipes for appetizers or hors d'oeuvres that are practically no work at all.

"At the moment of dining, the assembled group stands for a little while as a safe unit, under a safe roof, against the perils and enmities of the world. The group will break up and scatter, later. For this short time, let them eat, drink and be merry."

—MARJORIE KINNAN RAWLINGS, *CROSS CREEK COOKERY*, 1942

Hors d'oeuvres Aren't Just for Cocktail Parties

Setting the tone for a meal can be just as important as the food you serve. That's why there's no better way to begin a special family or company meal than with a fabulous (but easy) first course, leisurely presented. All the appetizer (and most hors d'oeuvre) recipes included in this chapter can be easily adapted to serving as a first course at a dinner party.

These days, a casual first course, served in the living room, den, or even the kitchen, is a great way to keep everyone occupied until all the guests or family members have arrived.

Further, the first course can be the cook's best friend. A tray of nibbles can be an instant icebreaker when all your guests don't know one another well. (Everyone loves to talk about food these days!)

Sage Advice

The thing about cocktail party food is that it's made up of all those foods you never fix for yourself at home, so everything tastes delicious. Here's another comforting thought. The cocktail hour conveniently arrives just as your guests' stomachs begin to grumble. And when you're hungry, everything tastes delicious. Remember that and your next cocktail party will be much easier. The way I see it, the preparations for a cocktail party—getting glasses and napkins together, putting flowers or seasonal decorations all around, seeing about ice—can be sufficiently time-consuming, so my rule for cocktail food is, keep it as simple as possible.

Or, a soup course served at the table can give the cook time to assemble the entrée plates, or even to make last-minute dessert preparations. (Suggestions for a variety of delicious and unusual soups suitable for serving as a light first course follow in the *Soups* chapter.)

To my way of thinking, a first course is very important.

A fabulous first course is the host or hostess's way of extending warm hospitality. It's something extra. Something special. Something unnecessary. Something that you took the time to do.

Whichever direction you choose—a finger-food appetizer or a soup served at the table—remember that the first course sets the tone of the meal to come.

An appetizer should be like a pretty bow on a nicely wrapped package that is yet to be opened.

Only you will know that the preparation took almost no time at all!

Sage Advice

A note on servings. There's really no way to figure out how many servings a dip or spread will yield. Dieters in the crowd will put a tiny morsel on the corner of a cracker, while those who are craving cream cheese and olives will dig deep into the bowl and heap the cracker high. So when preparing appetizers, ask yourself, how much would I eat and then remember, it is better to have too much than too little.

A Word about Time

TO HELP YOU conserve your valuable time, approximate preparation and total time guides are given for each recipe, except in the case where a "variation" creates no appreciable time difference.

Needless to say, the exact time it will take you to make any of the recipes will vary according to how many times your phone (or doorbell) rings (or you remember a call you forgot to make); how many times your kids, pets, friends, or other family members interrupt you; how

long it takes you to put your hands on the ingredient you're looking for; and whatever other of life's little distractions come along.

But when you're reading through a recipe and checking the time it requires, remember this: The PREPARATION TIME given in *From Storebought to Homemade* is based on using convenience foods. If you decide to peel potatoes, dice onions, and grate a pound of cheese, my estimated times will be far off. Further, the preparation times are the minutes

required to prepare the food *prior* to its cooking (or serving, if no cooking is required.) Cooking or chilling (in the case of several jelled salads and desserts) time is added to the preparation time to arrive at the approximate TOTAL TIME.

I've included these time gauges because I'm the type who likes to know what to expect. The fewer surprises, the better! I hope they will be helpful to you.

In short, I like my kitchen time to be pleasurable, and I'd like for yours to be too.

Cream Cheese: Better Than Sliced Bread

As any seasoned host or hostess will tell you, the 8-ounce package of cream cheese is a cocktail party lifesaver.

It doesn't matter whether you decide to use traditional cream cheese, one of the lighter varieties, or, my personal favorite, Neufchâtel (it has few calories but rich flavor). Tubs of whipped or soft cream cheese make these tasty treats easier than ever to stir up. Whichever variety you choose, this staple makes it possible to turn out any number of flavorful appetizers quickly and easily.

The secret to preparing any of the following recipes in no time is simple. Keep some cream cheese in the fridge and several toppings and items to combine with it in the pantry.

So, the next time you need a quick appetizer, just flip through these recipes, match the ingredients in the recipes with those you have on hand, and you're set to go. But don't stop there. While gathering those ingredients, use your imagination.

Roquefort Cheese Spread

BLEND the cheeses together. For a creamier consistency, you can add a tablespoon of heavy cream or a teaspoon or so of milk. Or, for variety, add 2 tablespoons of good cognac or brandy in place of the cream or milk.

YIELDS APPROXIMATELY 1¾ CUPS

1 (8-ounce) package soft cream cheese

4 ounces Roquefort cheese

1 tablespoon heavy cream or a teaspoon milk (optional)

2 tablespoons cognac or brandy (optional)

Cookware needed: mixing bowl

PREPARATION TIME: *3 to 5 minutes*
TOTAL TIME: *3 to 5 minutes*

Cream Cheese and Olive Spread

READY-TO-ADD and highly flavorful diced olive spreads make this delicious treat a cinch. But if you're using a jar of olives rather than a prepared olive spread, add just enough of the liquid from the olives to give the spread the consistency you desire. Also remember it will take longer to prepare, since you have to dice the olives.

YIELDS APPROXIMATELY 1 CUP

1 (8-ounce) package soft cream cheese

½ cup diced olive product such as Vine Country Food's garlic and herb olive spread, or a tapenade (or, use a 4-ounce jar of sliced olives with pimiento)

Cookware needed: mixing bowl

Blend the cheese and olives together.

PREPARATION TIME: *5 minutes*
TOTAL TIME: *5 minutes*

"The great thing about entertaining is being with the people you have invited. It is a bit discomfiting for your guests if you are slaving over the stove, and emerge, hot and rather martyred, just in time to sit down at the table with your guests!"

—CLAIRE MACDONALD,
THE HARRODS BOOK OF ENTERTAINING, 1986

Sage Advice

The Cream Cheese and Olive, and Pimiento Surprise (pages 48 and 51) spreads aren't for cocktail parties only. They also make delicious lunchtime or picnic sandwiches.

Date Cheese Ball

WHEN I BEGAN writing this book, I had no idea what a sentimental journey it would be. But I've learned that just the mention of a particular food can bring on a flood of memories of a meal, a trip, and very often of friends, family, and loved ones. This, of course, speaks volumes about what is really important in life.

Imagine going on like this just because the moment I began to type out "1 (8-ounce) box chopped dates" I remembered how much my father liked dates, especially around Christmas time.

Years ago, Christmas was the only time you could find dates in the stores. Today, they are available year-round, which makes this easy appetizer a perennial favorite at my house—and it always brings back precious memories.

YIELDS 1 LARGE, OR 2 SMALL BALLS

2 (8-ounce) packages soft cream cheese

1 (8-ounce) box chopped dates

1 cup chopped pecans

Cookware needed: mixing bowl

The Finishing Touch

Serve this with ginger snaps and Ritz crackers.

Combine the cream cheese and chopped dates.

Shape the mixture into one or two balls and roll each one in the chopped pecans.

Chill at least 24 hours before serving. The longer this spread has to "mellow," the better it tastes.

PREPARATION TIME: *15 minutes*
TOTAL TIME: *15 minutes, plus the chilling time*

Russian Delight

TO SERVE this for a cocktail party, you simply put the cream cheese on a plate, gently spread it with the caviar taken straight from the jar (being careful not to break the bubbly eggs), and sprinkle the onions on top. But to make individual appetizers, follow the directions below. For a variation on Russian Delight, try the next recipe.

SERVES 8

1 or 2 tablespoons frozen, diced onions

1 (8-ounce package) soft cream cheese

1 (2-ounce) jar red caviar

Spread a handful of frozen, diced onions on a paper towel to defrost.

Put a dollop of the soft cream cheese on each of 8 plates.

Cover the cheese with a liberal helping of caviar and top each serving with a sprinkling of the now-defrosted diced onions.

PREPARATION TIME: *10 minutes*
TOTAL TIME: *10 minutes*

The
Finishing Touch

Add yet another color and texture by garnishing with a curly parsley leaf. Put a few small crackers on each plate, or pass them.

Caviar Pâté

YIELDS APPROXIMATELY 1¾ CUPS

1 (8-ounce) package soft cream cheese

½ cup sour cream

1 teaspoon onion flakes or finely diced, frozen onions

⅛ teaspoon prepared garlic, or one small clove minced

1 (2-ounce) jar red caviar

Cookware needed: mixing bowl

Combine all the ingredients in a small bowl and chill well before serving with your favorite crackers or cocktail bread.

PREPARATION TIME: *10 minutes*
TOTAL TIME: *10 minutes plus chilling time*

Instant, No-Mixing-Required Cheese Spreads

Sage Advice

Be brave. In addition to the usual hot-pepper jelly or caviar toppings, which everyone seems to serve, try peach chutney or apricot or black cherry preserves.

WHAT COULD BE simpler than unwrapping a block of cream cheese, or turning it out of the tub, and topping it with a flavorful addition? I've already suggested you do that in the Russian Delight recipe given earlier, but not everyone is going to serve caviar. If you're one of those who won't, consider using one of these alternatives.

YIELDS VARY ACCORDING TO GUESTS

1 (8-ounce) package soft cream cheese

1 jar of your favorite chutney, preserves, or marmalade

or

1 medium-size bar creamy goat cheese (chèvre)

1 jar sun-dried tomato tapenade, with olive oil added for taste and consistency

or

1 medium wedge brie

1 jar fruit salsa (raspberry is good)

The Finishing Touch

Garnish any of these plates with a sprig of parsley or a twist of lemon peel.

To serve any of these instant, no-mixing-required cheese spreads, just take the wrapping off the cheese, place it on a pretty plate or in a bowl, and spoon the topping gently over the top.

PREPARATION TIME: *4 to 5 minutes*
TOTAL TIME: *4 to 5 minutes*

"You should never think of a recipe as more than the basic foundation upon which you can build a dish which is exactly right for yourself and your family. Imagination, originality, experimentation, all these play a part in the kitchen."

—PAMELA FRY, *THE GOOD COOK'S ENCYCLOPEDIA*, 1962

Cheddar Cheese
Comes to the Rescue

Though cream cheese may be the staple of the cocktail party buffet, Cheddar cheese runs a close second. There may be times when you have either a block of trusty "rat" cheese on hand, or even a resealable, already grated cheese mixture on hand, but no cream cheese.

For such emergencies, or to include in your menu if you're planning ahead, try these hors d'oeuvres.

Sage Advice

Too many cheese-based hors d'oeuvres or appetizers are boring and similar in taste. Unless you are preparing a true cocktail buffet to be spread through several rooms— your living room, dining room, and kitchen, for example—do not put out more than one cream cheese and one other cheese selection.

Crackers

SERVE WITH CRACKERS. But what kind of crackers? Here's a guide.

For spicy, salty, or meat or seafood spreads, try Carr's Table Water Crackers with Cracked Pepper, Rye (Wasa) crackers, and flavored Melba toast.

When serving highly flavored dips or strong cheeses (slices or cubes), serve a variety of the blander (but absolutely delicious) crackers—Saltines, Triscuits, Wheatsworth, or Pepperidge Farm Butterfly Crackers.

And don't overlook those sweet crackers. Not only can they add variety to your cocktail buffet, but they can actually take the place of a dessert. How? Try this.

Create your own instant, no-mixing-required cheese spread by topping a fruit-flavored spread (like the Philadelphia Cream Cheese varieties or Brummel and Brown Spreads) with a complementary fruit (for example, fresh strawberries or strawberry preserves atop a strawberry cream cheese), and serve it with wheat crackers (Carr's or Breton are examples) or thin ginger snaps.

Cheese and Olive Ball

YIELDS 1 LARGE BALL
■ ■ ■ ■ ■ ■ ■ ■

¼ cup tapenade, or sliced ripe olives, or Spanish olive pieces, drained

1 (8-ounce) package sharp Cheddar cheese, grated

¼ stick soft butter

⅛ to ¼ teaspoon minced garlic

Few drops Tabasco sauce

Dash cayenne

Cookware needed: mixing bowl, food processor

The
Finishing Touch

If you wish, once the mixture is thoroughly chilled, you can make small, individual cheese balls and put out party picks for serving.

If using olives (not tapenade), chop in a food processor so they will be finer in consistency.

Combine them with the other ingredients and chill the mixture in the refrigerator until it is firm enough to be formed into a ball.

Serve with a spreader and crackers.

■ ■ ■ ■ ■ ■ ■ ■
PREPARATION TIME: *5 minutes*
TOTAL TIME: *10 minutes,*
unless you make the bite-sized balls

Say Cheese!

THE MANY, and ever increasing, varieties of already grated cheese found in the refrigerator section of grocery stores today should make you smile.

Pick up a bag of mozzarella, Parmesan, or a Colby-Jack blend to top a casserole. Buy some Cheddar—from mild to sharp according to your taste—to toss with a salad or to make a fondue. Select from a variety of seasoned cheeses when preparing Mexican or Italian dishes. In addition, there are low-fat options and both finely and coarsely grated cheeses.

When figuring out how much of an already grated cheese to buy, remember that 4 ounces of grated cheese equals 1 cup. Most recipes found in these pages call for either 8- or 16-ounce packages of cheese. Sometimes the packages give cup measurements. In that case, a 2-cup bag will yield 8 ounces of grated cheese, and a 4-cup bag 16 ounces. So just pick up a 2- or 4-cup resealable bag and you're done. Another storebought convenience to take home.

Cheese Dip in the Round

IF YOU LIKE my suggestions about using fruits and vegetables as "containers" in *A Word about The Finishing Touch* on page 22, you'll enjoy fixing and serving this imaginative and very tasty Cheddar cheese dip.

YIELDS APPROXIMATELY 3 CUPS

1 loaf round bread—white, dark, or rye, from the bakery

1 (16-ounce) package sharp Cheddar cheese, grated

4 ounces blue cheese (or Roquefort)

½ teaspoon dry mustard

1 teaspoon butter, softened or whipped

2 teaspoons frozen, diced onion

½ to ¾ teaspoon Worcestershire sauce

1 (8-ounce) bottle beer

Cookware needed: mixing bowl

Cut the top off the round loaf of bread the way you would cut the top off a pumpkin. Hollow out the interior, saving as much of the bread as possible to use for dipping (as in a fondue).

Blend the cheeses, mustard, butter, onion, and Worcestershire sauce in a mixing bowl, and allow the mixture to stand for at least 30 minutes. (If you plan ahead, you can use this time to prepare the bread loaf.)

When you are ready to fill the bread loaf with the mixture and put it out for your guests, slowly beat the beer into the mixture, until the dip is smooth and airy.

Fill the hollowed-out bread round, and serve with the reserved bread bits, along with additional cubes of rye, wheat, or grain breads for dipping.

The
Finishing Touch

Garnish this fanciful spread with chopped chives, paprika, or parsley.

PREPARATION TIME: *15 minutes*
TOTAL TIME: *approximately 45 minutes*

Cheddar Cheese with Strawberry Preserves

SURPRISE. That's what gives zing to a recipe. Like serving a dip in a round of bread. Or serving strawberry preserves with a cheese appetizer. That unexpected combination seems to have originated around Augusta, Georgia, the home of the famed Master's Tournament. That's where I had it the first time.

The tasty combination was probably thought up by some desperate hostess who found out she was having last-minute guests drop by after a day on the golf course. Don't wait for that to happen to you to prepare it. It's a great appetizer to serve while you're getting dinner on the table, or as part of a cocktail party spread.

YIELDS APPROXIMATELY 3 CUPS

1 (16-ounce) package sharp, grated Cheddar cheese

1 cup chopped pecans

½ cup mayonnaise

¼ cup frozen, minced onion

1 clove garlic, or 1 teaspoon prepared garlic

½ teaspoon Tabasco sauce

1 cup strawberry preserves (your favorite brand)

Cookware needed: mixing bowl

Combine all the ingredients except the strawberry preserves. Mix well and chill for 2 to 3 hours.

Shape the mixture into a ball, or put it in an attractive serving dish. Or, if you have time, press it into a lightly greased ring mold.

If served as a cheese ball or spread, surround it with the strawberry preserves or put the preserves on the side. If served as a mold, fill the center with the preserves.

Serve with crackers. Melba toast rounds or Triscuits are good choices.

PREPARATION TIME: *15 minutes*
TOTAL TIME: *2 to 3 hours*

Pimiento Surprise

BOBBYE INGRAM used her imagination one day when she was putting out a tray of pimiento cheese and crackers. "What would happen if I added a little horseradish to dress up my storebought pimiento cheese," she wondered. She tried it and had an instant success on her hands.

Keeping this story in mind, read on.

YIELDS APPROXIMATELY 1 CUP

8 ounces pimiento cheese, from the deli

4 tablespoons prepared horseradish

Cookware needed: a mixing bowl

Stir together, adjusting the amount of horseradish to your taste. Serve with your favorite crackers or bread.

PREPARATION TIME: *2 to 3 minutes*
TOTAL TIME: *2 to 3 minutes*

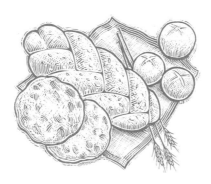

"'What about using that great recipe of yours for a parsley dip as a sandwich filing?' she asked. ...And what about that stuff you do with chopped ripe olives and garlic?'"

—VIRGINIA RICH,
THE NANTUCKET DIET MURDERS, 1985

Hot Cheese Pie

LOOKING for a simple Cheddar cheese appetizer that's hot? This will fill the bill. It is hot both temperature- and taste-wise. Though this recipe will serve a crowd, you can easily halve or quarter it to meet your needs.

SERVES 8 TO 12

3 (4-ounce) cans diced or sliced jalapeño peppers, mild or hot to your taste

1 (16-ounce) package sharp Cheddar cheese, grated

8 eggs

Cookware needed: pizza pan, mixing bowl

Sage Advice

To make this a heartier appetizer, add a layer of cooked ground beef (1/2 to 1 pound) after the cheese and before the eggs.

Preheat the oven to 350 degrees.

Drain the jalapeño peppers and spread them out on paper towels. Be sure to pick out any remaining seeds.

Spread the peppers in a shallow, throwaway aluminum pizza pan.

Top the peppers with a layer of cheese.

Beat the eggs until foamy and pour them over the cheese and peppers.

Bake in the preheated oven for 35 minutes.

PREPARATION TIME: *10 minutes, if you don't add the meat (see Sage Advice)*
TOTAL TIME: *45 minutes*

Dressed-up English Muffin Appetizers

Sage Advice

Use plain, wheat, or sourdough muffins, but not any of the sweeter varieties.

HERE'S another Cheddar cheese appetizer you can easily prepare in the twinkling of an eye. In fact, it takes more time to grab up the necessary ingredients at the grocery store than it does to assemble the mixture.

True, the spreading and cutting may take a little while, but once that's done, these appetizers are easily frozen. Then you'll have a "homemade" appetizer that can be served as quickly as a minipizza or any other snack you could have bought at the store and stashed in your freezer.

These are guaranteed to come in handy for a spur-of-the-moment casual evening with friends, if someone drops by unexpectedly, or if you happen to crave a salty snack while watching late-night TV.

MAKES 72 APPETIZERS

2 cups olive spread or tapenade

1 (8-ounce) package sharp Cheddar cheese, grated

¼ cup diced onion, fresh or frozen

½ cup mayonnaise

1 teaspoon curry powder

6 English muffins, halved

Cookware needed: mixing bowl, cookie sheet

Preheat the oven to 375 degrees.

Combine the olive spread, cheese, onion, mayonnaise, and curry powder.

Spoon an ample amount onto each muffin half and cut each half into 6 pie-shaped wedges.

Put these on a cookie sheet, cover, and freeze. Once frozen, transfer them to freezer baggies until needed.

When ready to serve, bake them, still frozen, at 375 degrees for 10 to 12 minutes, or until bubbly.

PREPARATION TIME: *30 minutes*
TOTAL TIME: *45 minutes*

Sausage-Cheese Balls

IF YOU HAVE the time to make them, it is nice to serve bite-sized appetizers (in addition to nuts—which guests actually seem to eat by the fistful, rather than one by one).

I like these three-ingredient, quick-cooking sausage-cheese balls because the ingredients can be sort of "mixed or matched" according to what you have on hand—hot or mild sausage, mild or highly seasoned cheese. I'll give you the basic recipe first, and then show how you can alter it.

MAKES 10 TO 12 DOZEN

16 ounces hot sausage, uncooked
1 (16-ounce) package mild Cheddar cheese, shredded

3 cups biscuit mix

Cookware needed: mixing bowl, cookie sheet

Sage Advice

Even though these take some time to prepare, after baking, they can be frozen in moisture-proof containers. To serve, remove them from the freezer and heat at 350 degrees until warm.

Preheat the oven to 350 degrees.

Crumble the sausage into a large bowl.

Add the cheese and mix well.

Blend the biscuit mix into the sausage and cheese.

Shape the mixture into walnut-sized balls and place them on an ungreased, air-insulated cookie sheet.

Bake for 10 to 12 minutes.

Options: If you have mild sausage on hand, use a jalapeño cheese in place of the mild Cheddar; or if you have only mild sausage and mild cheese on hand, add paprika or even chili powder to taste.

PREPARATION TIME: *approximately 30 minutes*
TOTAL TIME: *approximately 1 hour*

Parsley, Sage, Rosemary, and Wine

SEASONED butters are a treat often associated with fine restaurant dining, but they can also add a special touch to your own dining or buffet table, especially for a first course or appetizer.

Try serving honey-flavored butter (Land O Lakes makes a good one) with wedges of good dark pumpernickle or marble rye bread for a sweet savory.

YIELDS 1 CUP

If you are unable to find a ready-to-serve honey-flavored butter, simply stir 3 to 5 tablespoons of honey into 8 ounces of softened butter and mix well.

To make your own herbed butter, soak 2 tablespoons of mixed herbs (McCormick makes many blends) in 2 tablespoons of dry white wine for 2 hours. The herbs will absorb the wine flavor. Then mix the herb mixture with an 8-ounce tub of whipped butter or spread.

Served with crackers or bread, just as you would offer cream cheese with bagels, these flavored butters make a nice addition to an individual appetizer plate. Or, used in place of mayonnaise or mustard, they can dress up any sandwich.

PREPARATION TIME: *5 minutes*
TOTAL TIME: *5 minutes to 2 hours, depending on the blend*

"There is so much wine made all over Italy that I wouldn't have been surprised if I had turned on a faucet in a particularly luxurious hotel, and found a luscious red wine coming out!"

—MORRISON WOOD.
THROUGH EUROPE WITH A JUG OF WINE, 1964

Cheddar-Crab Spread

RANKING right up there with cheese as a favorite appetizer is crabmeat. Add the cheese to the crabmeat and you have a spread that's sure to please.

Many crab appetizers are intended to be served hot—which can be a drawback. But this one can be served at room temperature immediately after you've stirred it together, or it can be made earlier in the day and served chilled.

Sage Advice

Don't forget the horseradish. That's what gives this its zip!

YIELDS APPROXIMATELY 2 CUPS

1 ¼ cups mayonnaise

1 (6 ½-ounce) can crabmeat

4 ounces sharp Cheddar cheese, grated

1 teaspoon prepared horseradish

4 tablespoons French dressing

¼ cup frozen diced onion, or to taste

1 tablespoon dried parsley

1 teaspoon dried dill

1 teaspoon Durkee's seasoned salt

Cookware needed: mixing bowl

Combine all the ingredients and stir until well blended. Serve at once, or refrigerate.

PREPARATION TIME: *5 to 10 minutes*
TOTAL TIME: *5 to 10 minutes*

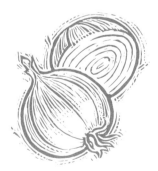

Crabmeat Spread

WHAT *is* it about seafood that makes it so appealing as an appetizer?

Well, in the days before it was possible to ship fresh fish, or freshly frozen fish, to inland locations, canned fish—shrimp, crab, minced clams, even sardines—was often the only fish available. These selections were much better suited for preparing a delicious appetizer than they were for making a full entrée.

Times and food availability may have changed, but crab and shrimp and clam appetizers are just as good as ever. The trick is to serve them in a snazzy way. You've read some ideas in *Hints and Tips* and *A Word about The Finishing Touch* in Chapter 1, but check *The Finishing Touch* to this recipe for yet another.

YIELDS APPROXIMATELY 2 CUPS

1 (8-ounce) package cream cheese

½ (10-ounce) can cream of chicken soup

2 teaspoons Wyler's Shakers, chicken flavored

1 (6-ounce) can crabmeat, drained

Cookware needed: mixing bowl

The
Finishing Touch

This is a perfect time to put into practice my suggestion for using a vegetable in place of a ceramic or glass serving bowl. How about using a pepper—yellow, orange, red, green, or purple—whatever complements your party's décor—to hold the Crabmeat Spread.

Stir all the ingredients together to blend well.

Serve with cracker rounds or crinkled potato chips.

PREPARATION TIME: *5 minutes*
TOTAL TIME: *5 minutes*

Yummy Shrimp Spread

YIELDS APPROXIMATELY 1 CUP

1 (8-ounce) package cream cheese

½ cup frozen salad-size shrimp, defrosted or 1 (6-ounce) can shrimp, drained

2 tablespoons cocktail sauce

or

1 (8-ounce) package cream cheese

½ cup frozen salad-size shrimp, defrosted or 1 (6-ounce) can shrimp, drained

2 tablespoons ketchup plus ¼ teaspoon Worcestershire sauce, 1 teaspoon lemon juice, and ⅛ teaspoon prepared garlic

or

1 (8-ounce) package cream cheese

1 individual jar ready-to-eat shrimp cocktail

Cookware needed: food processor or blender

Toss all the ingredients into your food processor or blender and mix to a pastelike consistency.

Chill and serve with crackers.

PREPARATION TIME: *about 5 minutes*
TOTAL TIME: *5 minutes, plus time to chill*

Never Underestimate the Power of Celery

VIRTUALLY any of the spreads or balls in this chapter can be spread in celery stalks and passed as an extra treat before or even during dinner. Remember this when you have leftovers after a cocktail party.

Smoky Salmon Ball

THE EVIDENCE is in and the verdict is salmon is *really* good for you. So why not serve it as an appetizer when you're having beef for an entrée?

Actually, it isn't the salmon, but rather the liquid smoke that turns this inexpensive and otherwise pretty bland food combination into a recipe that will have everyone clamoring for more.

YIELDS 2 CUPS

1 (8-ounce) can red salmon, drained and "cleaned up"

1 (8-ounce) package cream cheese

2 tablespoons lemon juice

2 teaspoons well diced or even grated onion

¼ teaspoon salt

1 teaspoon liquid smoke, or to taste

Cookware needed: mixing bowl

Prepare the salmon by removing any bones or discolored flesh. (FYI, the bones are very good for you and the discolored flesh is natural, but you don't want to include these in the ball. Personally, I always gobble these up on the spot.)

Combine all the ingredients until totally blended. Let the mixture sit for a while at room temperature and then taste to check the flavoring. The liquid smoke taste should be present but not overpowering.

Shape it into a ball for serving. (Cover and refrigerate if not serving at once.)

PREPARATION TIME: *10 minutes*
TOTAL TIME: *10 minutes, or longer if you elect to use one of the suggestions in The Finishing Touch.*

Sage Advice

This is one of my favorite spreads so I do lots of tasting while preparing it. Fresh lemon juice is best, but the bottled type will do. And I don't like the onions to dominate or compete with the salmon, lemon, and liquid smoke flavor, so I go easy on those, depending on how potent the onion is.

The Finishing Touch

If you wish, chill the ball before serving and roll it either in finely chopped fresh parsley or in finely chopped pecans for a dressier appearance.

Pineapple-Cheese Ball

MY FORMER sister-in-law, Janet Kimsey, introduced me to this pineapple and cream cheese appetizer back in the early '70s. I don't remember anything else about her party that particular night. Probably because I never moved from my spot in front of this truly delicious and rather "different" cocktail food. From that night on, it's been standard fare in my home.

Over the years, thanks to the introduction of frozen onions and green peppers, I can make it more quickly than ever. And if I tossed the cream cheese and pineapple in the food processor or blender, it would go even more quickly. Actually, I'm sure you could make this recipe using pineapple-flavored cream cheese and that would cut the prep time down even more. But I like to use my handheld electric mixer to blend the pineapple and cream cheese, just the way I did the first time I made it...as sort of a tribute to the old days.

YIELDS APPROXIMATELY 3 CUPS

The Finishing Touch

Like the Smoky Salmon Ball, after chilling, when it is easier to handle, this Pineapple-Cheese Ball can be rolled in a topping— in this case either finely chopped fresh parsley or finely chopped pecans. But, it's much zippier if you serve it in a pineapple boat. To do this, slice the pineapple lengthwise (leaving the leaves attached) and scoop out the fruit. Then fill the shell to overflowing with the Pineapple-Cheese mixture. Sprinkle additional pecans and green pepper on top as a garnish, if you wish. Serve with wheat thin crackers.

2 (8-ounce) packages cream cheese

1 (8-ounce) can crushed pineapple, drained

or

2 (8-ounce) containers pineapple-flavored cream cheese

⅓ cup diced green pepper

2 tablespoons frozen, diced onion

2 heaping tablespoons Durkee's seasoned salt

½ cup pecans, chopped

Finely chopped parsley or pecans (see *The Finishing Touch*)

Cookware needed: mixing bowl

Either thoroughly mix the cream cheese and drained, crushed pineapple together, or begin with the pineapple-flavored cream cheese.

To this, add the green pepper, onion, seasoned salt, and pecans.

Roll into a ball, cover, and chill.

PREPARATION TIME: *5 to 10 minutes*
TOTAL TIME: *5 to 10 minutes, plus time to chill*

Antipasto Appetizers

Years ago, many fine restaurants—and they weren't necessarily Italian—served an "antipasto" appetizer. (Though it appeared to be free, the cost was hidden in the price of the entrée.)

Sometimes one large antipasto plate was presented for the table. Other times each person was treated to an individual plate of goodies. Either way, it was a delightful way to begin a meal, and much healthier and prettier than today's usual bread, a couple of crackers still in their packaging, and aluminum foil-wrapped butter or margarine pats served in a brown plastic basket.

I think it's time to bring the antipasto plate back, but this time to your dining table—whether for a Wednesday night family meal, a Saturday night company dinner, or a cocktail party.

If you'd like a traditional antipasto plate, see The Traditional Antipasto Plate on page 62. The one below is lighter and simpler.

Antipasto American Style

FOR A QUICK, light antipasto-type appetizer course, all you need are some pickles and olives (either from jars or selected from the deli section of the grocery store), a few crudités (a French word for healthy veggies—carrot, celery, cherry or grape tomatoes, broccoli florets, even crisp, blanched green beans) from ready-to-serve packages or the salad bar, plus a few crackers (taken out of the cellophane, please) or rounds of good bread.

Arrange these items on a "commonly-shared" platter, or on individual plates.

The
Finishing Touch

A good-sized dab of an easily spreadable flavored cheese or butter gives the antipasto platter or plates an air of elegance and your taste buds a real treat. Or, if you wish, you can fill the cavities of ready-to-serve celery stalks with some of the spreads found in this chapter. Remember, any of the spreads can be made ahead of time and kept in the refrigerator.

The Traditional Antipasto Plate

THERE isn't a drop of Italian blood on either side of my family, even by marriage—a fact that I greatly regret. So to learn the ingredients for a traditional antipasto plate, I had to ask around.

In the process, I found that everyone I asked had a slightly different version of what constitutes a truly authentic antipasto. For example, both Karen Murgolo, at QVC Publishing, and my Danville friend, Pete Castiglione, have Southern Italian roots. In that warm area of Italy, the traditional antipasto plate always includes some wonderful native-grown citrus fruit, such as grapefruit or orange.

Here, as best I can determine, are the most popular ingredients used for a traditional antipasto. Make your selections from this list when preparing yours.

YIELD VARIES ACCORDING TO QUANTITY
AND NUMBER OF ITEMS INCLUDED

artichoke hearts—use the marinated ones out of a jar

olives—both Spanish and black, pitted or not

hard-boiled eggs—this is the only potentially time-consuming ingredient

slices of pepperoni or salami

sardines or anchovies

tomatoes—either whole cherry or grape tomatoes or sliced large tomatoes

green peppers

cold vegetables—green beans, celery, asparagus, even beets

a few beans—preferably chickpeas or garbanzo beans, but lentils work, too

cheese cubes

and, of course, some colorful and delicious citrus sections or slices

Cookware needed: individual plates or large platter

The Finishing Touch

After you've made your antipasto selections according to your (and your guests') tastes, you get to the fun part—arranging the plate attractively. Try beginning with either the beans or sliced hard-boiled eggs in the center. Top these with a strip or two of green peppers, or a couple of anchovies or sardines. Surround the beans or eggs with pepperoni, olives, artichoke hearts, tomatoes, cheese cubes, or whatever. Sprinkle the entire plate lightly with an oil-based (not creamy) Italian dressing and a few turns (to taste) of freshly ground pepper. I often use the marinade from the jar of artichokes as the dressing.

Curried Chicken Bits

LOOKING for a different finger food to serve as an appetizer? Try these Curried Chicken Bits accompanied by a bowl of duck sauce taken right out of the bottle.

SERVES 12 PLUS

1 cup white wine

1 teaspoon curry powder

1 teaspoon celery salt

1 to 2 tablespoons duck, or egg roll sauce, plus additional for serving

2 pounds fresh or frozen chicken cubes, strips, or tenders, unflavored and unbreaded, uncooked

Cookware needed: skillet

Combine the wine, curry powder, celery salt, and 1 or 2 tablespoons of the duck or egg roll sauce in a deep skillet, and bring the mixture to a gentle bubble.

Add the chicken to the pan and, if necessary, just enough water so that the chicken is completely covered.

Cover the pan and cook for 2 to 3 minutes. Turn the pieces over and cook another few minutes, until done.

Remove from the heat and refrigerate the chicken in the liquid for 2 to 3 hours or longer. When ready to serve, drain the chicken and cube it into bite-size pieces.

Serve it with toothpicks and duck sauce on the side.

The
Finishing Touch

Wondering what to put the toothpicks in? Think fancifully. A silver cordial glass, a miniature vase, even an empty spice jar disguised with a few strands of colored raffia tied at the throat.

PREPARATION TIME: *30 minutes*
TOTAL TIME: *about 3 hours, or until well chilled*

1, 2, 3 Appetizer

WHO says that deli meats have to be paper-thin slivers and used only for sandwiches? Not I. Especially when I need a quick and easy appetizer.

Now, if you're thinking of one of those chunky cheese-and-mystery-meat-cube platters served with toothpicks, think again.

You can present a nice appetizer by taking a hint from the way fancy restaurants do it. It's as easy as 1, 2, 3 and the key word is "presentation."

1. Ask for ⅛-inch-thick slices of specialty deli meats.

2. Select a vinaigrette that complements the flavor of the meat to give it an elegant and distinctive touch.

3. Arrange everything prettily on a salad plate for individual servings.

SERVES 4

1 pound sun-dried turkey breast, peppered beef, or other specialty deli meat, sliced ⅛ inch thick; or smoked salmon

4 ounces organic greens (mesclun) or several small lettuce leaves

1 jar tomato basil, balsamic, Dijon mustard, lime-cilantro,

orange, or another bottled vinaigrette or dressing that will complement the taste of the meat

Coarsely grated Parmesan cheese, to taste

Freshly ground black pepper, to taste

Slice the deli meat into quarter pieces.

To serve, cluster some of the greens at one side of the plate. Beginning where the leaves end, layer 3 or 4 pieces of the meat so they slightly overlap. Add a few more greens at the outside edge of the meat.

Drizzle a tablespoon or so of the vinaigrette over each serving. Sprinkle with a little coarsely grated Parmesan cheese and finish off with a turn or two of fresh pepper.

PREPARATION TIME: *10 minutes*
TOTAL TIME: *10 minutes*

Everyone's Favorite...Meatballs

MY MOTHER-IN-LAW Margaret Rich eats her dessert first. "Why save the best for last?" she asks.

Maybe it was the New England influence in my childhood, but I was brought up to believe you *must* save the best for last. That's why I've saved the quickest, easiest, and absolutely no-fail best appetizer for last.

And, if you aren't at the feeding trough first when these are on the menu, I can guarantee there won't be any left for the latecomers. What are they?

Meatballs.

Already you're conjuring up visions of chopping, dicing, stirring, mixing, and oh no...sautéing.

Forget it. Hop in the car and drive to the nearest store where you can buy already cooked, ready-to-serve plain old meatballs...the type you can toss into spaghetti or, as you'll see, turn into an instant appetizer.

SERVES APPROXIMATELY 20

1 (18-ounce) package fully
    cooked meatballs, frozen

1 (10-ounce) jar grape jelly

1 (16-ounce) bottle ketchup

Combine the grape jelly and ketchup in a large, heavy saucepan.

Stir over medium heat to blend the jelly and ketchup.

Add the meatballs and simmer for 20 to 30 minutes, so the wonderful flavors will be absorbed.

PREPARATION TIME: *5 minutes*
TOTAL TIME: *approximately 30 minutes*

Sage Advice

The same jelly and ketchup formula can also be used with ready-to-eat ham cubes and cocktail franks. Also, usually plan on 3 to 5 "pieces" per person. This recipe is easily doubled.

Soups

"**SOUPS,**" said my friend, Jan Harris. Most everyone in town knows Jan. When she was in kindergarten her mother used to prop her up on a milk crate so she could reach the cash register and check customers out at her family's Midtown Market in Danville, Virginia. "I love soups, but I don't have time to spend hours watching over them. Please put some easy soups in your book," she begged. I promised I would, because when I'm eating out and am given the choice of soup *or* a salad, I'll take the soup, thank you very much.

A nd when planning a seated dinner at home, I almost always include a soup course. To my way of thinking, a flavorful soup starts the meal off on the right note and can add zest to an otherwise simple menu. It even sends a special, caring signal to your guests. (They think you've been slaving over the stove, mixing, stirring, and flavoring your magical concoction for hours— though none of mine require so much work.) Served as a first course, soup can be elegant.

Some like it hot;
Some like it cold;
Some like it
in the pot,
Nine days old.

—MOTHER GOOSE

Yet a hearty soup can be a meal in itself. Anytime there's a chill in the air, give me a bowl of soup, some bread, and sweet butter or cheese, and I'm set.

For that reason, you'll find soups in this chapter that work well as appetizers *and* heartier, full-meal soups that are perfect for serving with a salad or a sandwich.

Either way, when it comes to soup, count me in.

Dollops Don't Have to be Fattening

TIME and again in this chapter you'll read "sprinkle with Parmesan cheese," or "garnish with a teaspoon of sour cream," or " top with a small dollop of whipped cream."

If fat calories begin dancing in front of your eyes, don't dismay. You're only adding a little bit of those luscious ingredients, and that primarily for color. But if you're still concerned, use one of the reduced-fat substitutes that are available on the market.

Or, try this. Buy some sliced low-fat cheese and a couple of attractive, very small pastry or cookie cutters. A star or crescent moon, for example. Cut out a cheese shape and float it in your soup.

And remember that a thin slice of lemon or cucumber, a sprig of parsley or chives, a thin slice of pimiento-stuffed Spanish olive, even a few plain or flavored croutons, can always be used as a garnish.

2-Step Steak Soup

TRADITIONALLY, soups were made from leftovers, especially the remains of a pot roast, turkey, or ham. But unless you're cooking for a sizable group, chances are you won't have a roast around to begin with. Still, that shouldn't deter you from enjoying the hearty goodness of a meat-based soup, such as this quick and easy 2-Step Steak Soup.

SERVES 6

2 (14 ½-ounce) cans Progresso Vegetarian Vegetable soup

1 (17-ounce) package Hormel Always Tender beef tips with gravy

Dash of Tabasco or other hot sauce, to taste

Cookware needed: saucepan

Heat the soup on medium high until piping hot. Add the beef tips with their juices and hot sauce, to taste. Stir, and simmer for 10 to 15 minutes

PREPARATION TIME: *5 minutes*
TOTAL TIME: *20 to 25 minutes*

Sage Advice

If you prefer a less thick soup, toss in as much V-8 or tomato juice as you like.

"In these days, when a request on a postal card, will bring to a housekeeper the grocery catalogue of any of the great city stores, there is little excuse for the home caterer being ignorant in the matter of what is new and desirable in the line of canned goods…. An entire meal may be easily and quickly prepared, either using canned goods in connection with other materials at hand, or having the entire meal composed of food put up in glass or tin."

—*THE BUTTERICK COOK BOOK,* EDITED BY HELENA JUDSON, 1911

Artichoke and Oyster Soup

TRUST ME, my guests do. I never tell them the name of this soup until they've tasted it. By then they're hooked. Further, they don't believe me when I smile and say, oysters and artichokes. In truth, it's the garlic and the anise and the red pepper that bring the soup to life.

I first tasted this delicacy in Delaware. When I asked for the recipe, it was eagerly shared by my hostess. Though the soup is simple to make, it really does need a resting period, so don't plan to make it and dish it up immediately. Plan to let it sit in the refrigerator for at least 6 to 8 hours, or even a full day before serving. Then be ready for a real treat.

SERVES 8 TO 10

2 sticks butter

⅓ cup frozen, diced onions

3 (14-ounce) cans artichoke hearts, drained and quartered

3 tablespoons flour

4 (14-ounce) cans roasted garlic flavored chicken stock

1 teaspoon red pepper flakes

1 teaspoon anise seed, or to taste

1 teaspoon salt

1 tablespoon Worcestershire sauce

1 quart oysters

Fresh or prepared additional garlic, to taste

Cookware needed: large pot with lid, food processor

Melt the butter in a pot large enough to hold all the ingredients and sauté the onions until soft.

Add the artichokes and sprinkle the vegetables with the flour. Stir to coat everything well but do not allow the flour to brown.

Add the garlic flavored chicken stock, the red pepper flakes, anise seed, salt, and Worcestershire sauce.

Cover and simmer for about 15 minutes.

While the mixture cooks, drain the oysters, reserving their liquor, and check them for shells.

Mince the oysters in a blender or food processor. This can be done in just a whirl or two. Be sure not to overchop and turn them into puree. Add the oysters and oyster liquor to the pot and simmer for about 10 minutes longer. Do not allow the soup to boil.

Refrigerate for a minimum of 6 to 8 hours, or for a full day. (It keeps well for up to 3 days.) Reheat over medium-low to medium heat; do not allow the soup to boil. At this point, taste it and decide if you want to add a little garlic flavoring.

The Finishing Touch

To add a little color to this bland-appearing, though extremely flavorful, soup, sprinkle it with a little paprika or garnish it with some chopped parsley or chives. Or, in the center of each bowl, place a single parsley leaf or 2 chive leaves crossed to form an x.

PREPARATION TIME: *15 minutes*
TOTAL TIME: *25 minutes*

Chicken Chowder

THANKS to the availability of skinless, boneless, frozen chicken breasts and trusty cream of chicken soup, it's possible to put a filling bowl of chicken soup on the table in nothing flat.

The trick is to keep a resealable package of chicken in your freezer and, when you reach for the cream of mushroom soup at the grocery store, grab up a couple of extra cans of cream of chicken soup for your pantry, as well.

With these ingredients on hand, you only have to add a can of creamed corn and some evaporated milk and suddenly you've turned chicken soup into a delicious chowder.

SERVES 6 TO 8

The
Finishing Touch

Though you will have added pepper while the soup is cooking, add a couple of grinds to each bowl and pass peppered crackers with a mild cheese, such as Swiss or Camembert, as an accompaniment. The sharp pepper taste really sets off the creamy chicken chowder.

2 frozen (or fresh) boneless chicken breasts

1 ¼ cups water

½ cup frozen PickSweet Seasoning Blend (onion, celery, green and red pepper, and parsley mix)

2 tablespoons butter

2 (10-ounce) cans cream of chicken soup

1 (15-ounce) can creamed corn

1 (5-ounce) can evaporated milk

Freshly ground pepper, to taste

Cookware needed: large saucepan

Cook the chicken breasts in the microwave by placing them in a microwave-safe bowl and covering them with the water. Microwave on high for 4 to 5 minutes, or until they are no longer pink.

While they are cooking, sauté the Seasoning Blend in the butter in a heavy saucepan over medium heat.

Stir in the soup, corn, milk, and pepper.

While the soup is heating and the flavors are blending, remove the chicken from the microwave. Pour the cooking water into the soup mixture and stir well.

Dice the chicken breasts and add them to the pan.

Bring the soup to a gentle bubble, stir, and then reduce the heat.

Simmer for 10 to 15 minutes.

PREPARATION TIME: *20 minutes*
TOTAL TIME: *30 to 40 minutes*

Cioppino

MANHATTAN clam chowder is good, but the presence of the shrimp and the absence of the potatoes and vegetables in this tomato-based clam soup make it a delicious, light alternative. The availability of shelled, cooked frozen shrimp and the convenience of canned minced clams make it possible to mix it up in nothing flat.

SERVES 6

2 tablespoons olive oil

⅔ cup frozen, diced combo of onion and green pepper

1 clove garlic, minced, or 1 teaspoon prepared garlic

3 (7 ½ ounce) cans minced clams with their juice

1 (14-ounce) can Italian-flavored diced tomatoes

½ cup dry white wine

1 (8-ounce) package raw shrimp

Salt, pepper, dried basil, and dried oregano, to taste

Cookware needed: large pot with lid

Heat the olive oil in a large, heavy pot.

Add the onion and pepper combination and sauté until transparent, then add the garlic.

While the vegetables are cooking, drain and reserve the clams, keeping the juice.

Add the clam juice, the tomatoes, and the wine to the pot.

Bring the mixture to a gentle boil and then reduce the heat to a simmer. Cook the soup, covered, for 10 minutes.

At this point add the shrimp and reserved clams. Simmer, uncovered, for 4 to 5 minutes.

Taste and adjust the seasonings. You can use a blended Italian seasoning instead of the basil and oregano.

PREPARATION TIME: *10 minutes*
TOTAL TIME: *20 to 25 minutes*

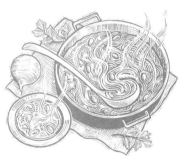

Improved Minestrone Soup

A **GOOD** bowl of minestrone served with a crusty French or a dark rye bread and a salad is my idea of the perfect cold-weather lunch. Problem is, the canned minestrone soups don't have the hearty flavor I like so much. How do you add that heartiness with a minimum of effort? Look to the freezer and the spice rack, gather a few ingredients, start these on the stove top, and *then* add the canned soup.

You'll need a little extra time to make the base to which you'll add the canned soup, but only a *little* extra time. In fact, once, when I learned that out-of-town guests were arriving (unexpectedly, naturally) at lunch-time, I pulled this soup off in 20 minutes flat. Everyone thought it was homemade and had taken hours.

The soup can be made the day before it is served, but don't over-cook it. Unlike many soups and stews, whose flavors blend through hours of cooking, this is one that blends perfectly well during the "resting" process.

SERVES 6 TO 8

1 (14-ounce) can onion-flavored beef broth

1 teaspoon olive oil

4 or 5 dried bay leaves

¼ teaspoon dried oregano

½ cup frozen Fordhook lima beans (they're the large variety)

½ cup small elbow or shell macaroni

1 (14-ounce) can cannellini (white kidney) beans

1 (14-ounce) can Italian-style diced tomatoes

½ cup frozen zucchini or yellow squash slices

1 (16-ounce) can ready-to-serve minestrone soup

Salt and freshly ground pepper, to taste

Grated Parmesan cheese, for serving

Cookware needed: large pot

In a large pot, combine the beef broth with the olive oil, bay leaves, and oregano and bring to a boil.

Add the lima beans and macaroni. Return the liquid to a boil while you open and rinse the beans.

Add the beans, tomatoes, and frozen squash slices and stir.

As soon as the soup begins to bubble, add the minestrone soup and reduce the heat to medium.

Cook for approximately 10 minutes to blend the flavors. Remove the bay leaves and add salt and pepper to taste.

Serve with grated Parmesan cheese passed in a bowl.

PREPARATION TIME: *10 minutes*

TOTAL TIME: *20 minutes*

Sage Advice

The wonderful thing about this recipe is that it is so flexible. If you don't have onion flavored beef broth, but you do have a can of French onion soup on hand, use that. You can use whatever small pasta you have in the pantry—little shells, elbow macaroni, small bow ties, even a few strands of angel hair pasta broken into small pieces if that's all you have. If you have Italian stewed tomatoes instead of the diced variety, use those. Or, if you're out of flavored Italian tomatoes, use a can of unflavored ones, but add a hefty amount of oregano, or an Italian spice blend, and even a little garlic. If you can't find cannellini, use white or red kidney beans.

Lentil Soup

MY GREEK FRIENDS tell me that lentil soup is from Greece. My German friends tell me their grandmothers made it in Germany. Actually, lentils have been found in Egyptian tombs that date from 2000 B.C., and they are as much a staple in Eastern European countries as they are in South America and the western reaches of the United States. It matters not where the lentils or the recipe originated. What matters is that this recipe is full of vitamins and fiber, is delicious, and can be made in less than half an hour.

SERVES 6 TO 8

1 cup diced potatoes from a 20-ounce package or 3 medium potatoes, diced

1 (8-ounce) package already diced ham bits, or frankfurters, finely chopped

2 (19-ounce) cans ready-to-serve lentil soup

¼ cup frozen, diced onion

8 to 10 grinds black pepper

½ teaspoon dried oregano

½ teaspoon dried thyme

2 or 3 dried bay leaves

Salt, to taste

Croutons

Cookware needed: small pot, large pot

In a small pot, cover the potatoes with water and boil the potatoes until tender, about 10 minutes. Meanwhile, chop the frankfurters, if using them, or open the package of ham, and empty the cans of lentil soup into a large pot. Drain the potatoes and add them to the soup along with the meat, onion, herbs, and spices. Simmer about 20 minutes.

Serve with a round of warm bread on the side or croutons as a garnish.

PREPARATION TIME: *15 to 25 minutes*
TOTAL TIME: *approximately 40 minutes*

The
Finishing Touch

A thin slice of lemon, with all the seeds removed, is a nice garnish if you're serving this soup for a special occasion.

Tell Me It's Homemade Clam Chowder

The Finishing Touch

Like so many delicious but cream-based soups, clam chowder needs a bright finishing touch. The usual choices are parsley and chives. But with colorful cherry and grape tomatoes now available year-round, try adding a very thin slice of one of these along with a small parsley leaf. Then surround the garnish with a couple of grind- ings of fresh pepper.

TALK ABOUT NERVE! That's what one notable food guru (who chooses to re- main anonymous) had when she served clam chowder to a family that's in the seafood restaurant business. In her defense, she didn't know that when she planned the menu. "I never would have been so brazen, or so foolish," she now laughingly admits.

Fortunately the story, or should I say the meal, had a happy ending—so happy that her guests begged for her homemade clam chowder recipe. When she hesi- tated, they backed off, knowing that special recipes are often well-guarded secrets.

Little did they know that she was serving them canned clam chowder...with an extra touch she had learned from another friend who worked for a clam chowder specialty house in Maine!

Proof once again that you can have the best restaurant food right in your own home—straight out of the can.

SERVES 4 TO 5

2 (15-ounce) cans Snow's Clam Chowder

1 (6-ounce) can minced clams with juice

½ cup cream

Fresh ground pepper, to taste

Cookware needed: large saucepan

Blend and heat all the ingredients.

PREPARATION TIME: *10 minutes*
TOTAL TIME: *15 minutes (until well heated)*

Tomato Soup Collage

Think soup and tomatoes come to mind. As well they should. Tomato soups are always crowd pleasers, in addition to which they are colorful and start the meal off on a cheerful note. Here are three varieties of tomato soup that can be formal or casual, depending on how you serve them.

Too Easy Spicy Tomato Soup

WHO'D EVER THINK of serving a favorite cocktail as soup? They did it in the 1970s, but Bloody Mary Soup seems to have been forgotten in recent years. Back then, the cook chopped and sautéed onions and celery, which were then added to tomatoes. The mixture was then pureed and strained. No wonder it passed out of fashion!

These days, try serving your favorite bottled or canned Bloody Mary mix as a soup—either chilled or heated. Whether or not you add the vodka is your choice.

The Finishing Touch

This cocktail/soup makes a great first course when served in mugs with a leafy stalk of celery for garnish. If you're serving it in traditional soup bowls, a couple of pretty green leaves, be they cilantro, parsley, or celery, add a dressy touch.

Zesty Tomato Starter

TOMATO SOUP has a real affinity for beef bouillon. Years ago, everyone served that simple combination as an appetizer, and it's as good today as ever, especially if you dress it up a little. Do this by adding a couple of large fistsfuls of frozen, diced onions and green peppers and an ample sprinkling of dried basil to the soup while it's heating. The flavors punch up the taste, and the diced onion and pepper give the soup that "homemade" look.

Garnish it with a teaspoon of sour cream, straight out of the squeezable bottle, and chives.

SERVES 6

1 (10-ounce) can tomato soup
2 (10-ounce) cans beef bouillon, or broth
½ cup frozen, diced combo of onion and green pepper

1 heaping teaspoon dried basil
¼ teaspoon sugar
Sour cream, for garnish
Cookware needed: large pot

Sage Advice

If you are not going to add the sour-cream garnish, stir in a tablespoon of butter while the soup is cooking for added richness of flavor.

Combine all the ingredients except the sour cream in a large pot. Stir, and bring the soup to a gentle bubble over medium-high heat. Immediately turn down the heat and allow the soup to simmer for 10 to 15 minutes.

PREPARATION TIME: *5 minutes*
TOTAL TIME: *15 to 20 minutes*

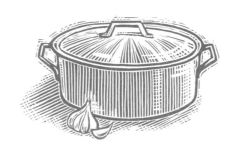

Love Apple Fromage Soup

WHEN my friend Jean Carol Vernon isn't entertaining audiences with her beautiful voice, presiding over a civic club meeting, or traveling with her grandchildren, she is preparing lunch for her church or theater or club friends. This delicious starter always helps to start things off on the right foot. It's simple to cube a block of Velveeta cheese, but you can use the already cubed variety to save even more time.

SERVES 4 TO 8,
DEPENDING ON SIZE OF CUP OR BOWL

1 (10 ¾-ounce) can tomato soup

1 soup can whole milk, not skim or low fat

4 (1-ounce) cubes Mild Mexican Kraft Velveeta or another mildly spicy cheese

Cookware needed: microwave-safe mixing bowl

Combine the soup and milk in a microwave-safe mixing bowl. Add the cheese pieces and set the microwave to 4 minutes on 50% power. After 30 seconds, stir, and continue to stir the mixture every 30 seconds, until thoroughly blended and heated. (The time may vary according to individual microwaves.)

PREPARATION TIME: *5 to 10 minutes*
TOTAL TIME: *10 to 15 minutes*

The Finishing Touch

Serve the soup in individual punch or demitasse cups, or in mugs (no spoon needed) or a bowl (spoon needed). Garnish each serving with a few seasoned croutons and serve the soup with cheese straws, or a slice of bruschetta (broiled bread with salsa and cheese) right on top.

When the tomato was introduced to France,
the Parisians called it "pomme d'amour,"
and imbued it with aphrodisiac qualities, which
is why, in Elizabethan times, it was
known as the "love apple."

Tomato and Chili Bean Soup

LIKE so many of the recipes in this book, this one grew out of "desperation." It started out with that panicked question, "What on earth can I *feed* them?" I'm sure you know the feeling well.

Even when I was writing this book and definitely had a well-stocked pantry, just such a panic set in. A business acquaintance, who lives some 30 miles away, ran by just a little after 12 o'clock noon one February day. At five minutes to two, I felt compelled to fix a bite of lunch. The day called for soup.

There was a problem with every idea I had in mind. Clam chowder—no clams. Brunswick stew—no more cans of Mrs. Fearnow's stew. Peanut butter? Two jars of extra crunchy, but no smooth.

I grabbed a can of Roasted Garlic Tomato soup, a new product I'd bought to try out, and some hot chili beans. It was that simple. In fact, deciding what to have took longer than mixing up the soup.

SERVES 4

1 (10-ounce) can Roasted Garlic Tomato soup

1 can water

1 (14-ounce) can hot chili beans (red kidney beans)

Cookware needed: pot

The Finishing Touch

Add some Parmesan cheese—a few hefty shakes, or a heaping tablespoon of the finely grated type is fine. Or, if you have it on hand, use some grated Cheddar cheese from the bag. And don't forget the tortilla chips, or, if you have time to make it, corn bread.

Combine the tomato soup and water and mix well.

Pour off and reserve the top juices from the can of chili beans.

Add the beans and the juices that naturally cling to them to the soup and stir.

Add half the reserved bean liquid. Cook for 3 to 4 minutes, until the flavors begin to blend.

Taste, and add additional reserved kidney bean liquid to your liking.

PREPARATION TIME: *5 minutes*
TOTAL TIME: *15 minutes*

Lady Wellington's Summertime Soup

MINA WOOD serves this soup in the summer, when she's having a lunchtime committee meeting as President of the Garden Club of Virginia. Try it, and everyone will think you slaved for hours. (It's the addition of the fresh tomatoes that does the trick.)

SERVES 8 TO 10

3 to 5 ripe, homegrown, medium-size tomatoes

1 (48-ounce) can V-8 juice

1 cup sour cream

Dried basil, salt, and pepper, to taste

Cookware needed: blender or food processor, large bowl

Coarsely chop the juicy, summertime tomatoes in a blender or food processor.

Combine the tomato pieces (removing the seeds that will have separated in the chopping process), the V-8 juice, and the sour cream in a large bowl.

Stir together and season to taste with the basil, salt, and pepper.

Chill for 2 to 3 hours before serving.

PREPARATION TIME: *10 minutes*
TOTAL TIME: *2 to 3 hours to chill*

The Finishing Touch

Garnish the soup with a sprinkling of chopped chives or a sprig of parsley.

Virginia Cream of Peanut Soup

CREAM of peanut soup is a legendary Virginia delicacy, served at many restaurants and inns, including those in Williamsburg. Recipes are found in countless Virginia cookbooks, but they all call for chopping and straining and all those steps that I'm trying to avoid these days.

Although you can buy canned peanut soup in some gourmet shops or departments, it's not on every grocery shelf. For those of you who can find it, skip the recipe below and go straight to *The Finishing Touch*.

For those less fortunate, here is a really simple recipe that requires only a little patient stirring and is guaranteed to delight your guests with its delicate flavor.

SERVES 6 TO 8

1 quart whole milk, not skim or low fat

2 tablespoons butter, softened (honey-flavored, if available)

1 tablespoon flour

1 cup creamy or smooth peanut butter, not crunchy

Salt, to taste

Cookware needed: large pot, small bowl

The Finishing Touch

Though optional, a little sherry enhances the soup's flavor. Whether you use dry or sweet sherry depends on your taste. Once the soup is ladled into soup bowls, top each serving with a small dollop of whipped cream.

Heat the milk over medium-low to medium heat. Do not allow it to boil.

Combine the butter and flour in a small bowl or measuring cup. Add a little of the hot milk and blend until smooth. Stir this paste, little by little, into the rest of the milk, blending it thoroughly.

Add the peanut butter by large spoonfuls, stirring each one into the milk until completely blended. Keep the soup hot, but do not allow it to boil. Add salt to taste.

PREPARATION TIME: *15 minutes*
TOTAL TIME: *25 minutes*

Chilled Soups

There are times, especially in the hot summer, when nothing is more refreshing than a chilled soup. Gazpacho has become a universal favorite, but for variety, why not try serving a fruit-based chilled soup?

I did, back in the 1980s, when I found a recipe for a fruit and Champagne soup in one of the women's magazines. It was incredibly easy to make and entailed little more than combining a bottle of Champagne with some fruity ingredients. Everyone wanted the recipe, and I shared it—obviously one time too many because, though I've searched high and low, I can't find it. (If you know it, please send it to me!)

Luckily, the following delicious chilled soups come close to that lost Champagne delight. They're light, delicious, and colorful.

Chilled Strawberry Soup Number 1

SERVES 6

2 cups Dole's orange-strawberry-banana juice

⅓ cup sifted powdered sugar

2 (10-ounce) packages frozen sliced strawberries, defrosted

½ cup Burgundy or other dry red wine (optional)

½ cup sour cream

Cookware needed: blender, pitcher

Combine the juice, powdered sugar, and strawberries in an electric blender and process until smooth. Add the Burgundy, if using it, and sour cream and process 2 more minutes.

Cover and chill for several hours.

PREPARATION TIME: *10 minutes*
TOTAL TIME: *only however much longer as it takes to defrost the strawberries*

Sage Advice

Experienced cooks will tell you, "If you won't drink it, don't cook with it." They're referring to "cooking wine," of course, and who would drink that! Remember these words when you add the Burgundy or another dry red wine to this soup.

The Finishing Touch

If you refrigerate the soup in a pretty glass, or even plastic, pitcher, you can pour it straight into cups, mugs, or small bowls at the table. Top off each cup or mug of this chilled fruit soup with a slice of a strawberry or mint leaves.

Chilled Strawberry Soup Number 2

JUST in case you're looking for a lighter, and even easier soup, try this.

SERVES 6

2 (10-ounce) packages sliced frozen strawberries, slightly defrosted

1 cup ginger ale, or, why not... Champagne

Cookware needed: blender, large mixing bowl or pitcher

In an electric blender, reduce the slightly defrosted strawberries to a crushed, not pureed, consistency.

Combine the strawberries with the liquid, either in a large bowl or in a pitcher, and refrigerate.

See *The Finishing Touch* for Chilled Strawberry Soup Number 1 (page 81).

PREPARATION TIME: *5 minutes*
TOTAL TIME: *5 minutes*

Summer Peach and Apricot Delight

SERVES 6

2 (11 ½-ounce) cans apricot nectar

2 (6-ounce) jars pureed baby-food peaches

¾ cup orange juice

½ cup whipping cream

½ cup sour cream

1 (10-ounce) package frozen sliced strawberries, defrosted

Pinch cinnamon

Cookware needed: mixing bowl

Stir all the ingredients together in a bowl, and refrigerate.

PREPARATION TIME: *5 minutes*
TOTAL TIME: *5 minutes*

Anything-Goes Fruit Soup

BY NOW you see how easy it is to make chilled soup, and you've realized, Hey! there's no cooking involved. So tuck this generic recipe away and prepare it according to your taste and the ingredients you have on hand.

SERVES 4

- 1 medium banana
- 1 (8-ounce) can crushed pineapple, drained
- 1 cup of any of the numerous varieties of fruit blends available today, such as Welch's wild raspberry, Minute Maid tropical fruit punch, or Tropicana orange-tangerine blend
- ½ cup half-and-half
- **Cookware needed:** large mixing bowl

In a large mixing bowl, mash the banana.

Add the drained crushed pineapple and stir.

Add the fruit blend and half-and-half, and mix well.

Refrigerate until thoroughly chilled.

PREPARATION TIME: *5 minutes*
TOTAL TIME: *as long as it takes to thoroughly chill, approximately 3 to 4 hours.*

The Finishing Touch

Garnish with Cool Whip or whipped cream topped with a small piece of fruit—strawberry, cherry, kiwi, peach, mango, banana, whatever.

Gazpacho Plus

SPEAKING of gazpacho, it's the perfect starter for a relaxed buffet when you're serving the Mexican-Chicken Casserole (page 199), or almost any other entrée. Unlike the summertime chilled fruit soups, gazpacho is a soup for all seasons. To give the canned variety a homemade touch, try the following.

SERVES 4 TO 6

¼ cup frozen, diced combo of onion and green pepper

1 (5.5-ounce) can spicy V-8 juice

2 tablespoons wine vinegar

1 tablespoon lemon (or lime) juice

2 (15-ounce) cans gazpacho

Worcestershire sauce, to taste

Cookware needed: large mixing bowl

The Finishing Touch

The usual dollop of sour cream is fine, of course, but a thin slice of lemon, lime, or cucumber is equally attractive.

While the frozen onion and green pepper mix is defrosting on a paper towel, open the cans and combine all the other ingredients in a large mixing bowl.

Pat the onions and green peppers dry and add them to the bowl.

Stir, and refrigerate for 3 to 4 hours minimum.

PREPARATION TIME: *5 minutes*
TOTAL TIME: *as long as it takes to chill thoroughly*

Mock Vichyssoise

VICHYSSOISE is another one of those once-popular soups that seems to have faded into the past. When you look at the old recipes that call for a sieve and a blender, well, you know why.

But our mothers were pretty cunning, and sometime during the vichyssoise era, someone came up with this "mock" vichyssoise recipe that I found scribbled on a card in my mother's recipe box. It doesn't have the leek flavor of a true vichyssoise, but when garnished with chopped chives, it's close. Still, this soup is awfully good and easy, doesn't need any cooking, and requires only a mixing bowl to prepare. That's my kind of "cooking."

SERVES 8 TO 10

2 (10-ounce) cans chicken broth
2 (10-ounce) cans cream of
  potato soup
2 (8-ounce) cartons sour cream

2 teaspoons frozen, diced onion
Chopped chives, for garnish
Cookware needed: large mixing
  bowl

Thoroughly combine all the ingredients, except the chives, and chill for several hours. Serve garnished with the chopped chives.

PREPARATION TIME: *6 to 7 minutes*
TOTAL TIME: *6 to 7 hours to chill*

"A circle of chairs is never provocative of good talk unless there is a table in the middle. In France when conversation was even more of an art than it is now they never rose at the end of a meal fearing to break the flow of thought with the flow of [the] bowl."

—LOUISE HALE,
*WE DISCOVER THE
OLD DOMINION,* 1916

Easy Entrées

HOW MANY TIMES have you complimented a delicious entrée only to have the cook tell you, "It's so easy. There's nothing to it."

"But there *is* something to it," you've thought, all the time knowing that deep down you would be *afraid* to try it.

Or maybe you're the one who orders salmon every time you eat out. Only a professional chef can prepare it, you've reasoned. Certainly you couldn't.

Well, it's time to shed those fears.

I myself, never fixed a pork tenderloin until one day when I dropped by to visit with my friend Charlotte Pennell, who was putting one in the oven. We talked so long that the roast was finished before we were! Charlotte carved a slice for me on the spot. It melted in my mouth. When I realized how sinfully simple pork tenderloin is to prepare—and how many ways it can be fixed, it became a regular at my house.

And as far as salmon goes—when I was young, all the cookbooks gave instructions for poaching a *whole* salmon, not just a couple of fillets. Why, it would have taken the two of us a month to finish off an 8-pound fish, and I didn't know enough just to ask for a smaller piece!

The message here is: Be brave. Remember, this chapter is named *Easy Entrées*.

Don't be afraid to try the entrée recipes that require only baking or poaching, such as pork tenderloin or salmon. They are like Jan Karon's favorite roasted chicken recipe in the Foreword. These entrées will cook by themselves while you tend to the other items on the menu.

"You see, we can't always do things the same way.
...If a favorite recipe calls for celery or other
seasoning, and it isn't on hand, we have our own
dried and crushed celery leaves in jars, or we grate
orange rinds, etc. as needed. We may not have the
same things on hand the next time we make
something, so we improvise."

—LILIAN BRITT HEINSOHN, *SOUTHERN PLANTATION*, 1962

Champagne Chicken

WHAT would we do without chicken? Actually, a better question is, how do you give chicken a distinctive flavor?

Dress up that everyday bird in an easy and succulent sauce made of cream and Champagne. It's a dish suitable for the gods.

This is one of the few recipes in this book that requires a little more time to prepare. But it's easy, and because you won't find these flavors in any already prepared sauce, everyone will think that you've been slaving in the kitchen for hours, instead of spending just a few minutes "assembling" the dish. Plan to serve it over wild rice or noodles.

SERVES 6 TO 12, DEPENDING ON APPETITES AND THE ACCOMPANIMENTS

Sage Advice

Don't scrimp on the cream. This is a rich, flavorful sauce and one that blends beautifully with broccoli or asparagus when those vegetables are served as an accompaniment on the plate.

4 tablespoons butter

6 whole chicken breasts, fresh or frozen, but uncooked

3 cups dry (brut) Champagne

1 quart heavy cream

1 (4- or 6-ounce) can or jar sliced mushrooms, drained

1 cup frozen, diced onion

4 to 5 dried whole bay leaves

½ teaspoon dried thyme

1 teaspoon nutmeg

Cookware needed: skillet with a lid

Place 3 tablespoons of the butter, the chicken breasts, and 2 cups of the Champagne in a covered skillet. Cook over medium-low heat for 15 to 20 minutes.

Turn the chicken, baste well, and continue to cook it for another 15 to 20 minutes, or until it is golden brown.

Remove the chicken and wrap it in a piece of heavy aluminum foil to keep warm while you prepare the sauce.

Blend the cream into the liquid in the skillet.

Add the mushrooms, onions, bay leaves, and thyme. When the mixture begins to bubble ever so slightly, turn the heat to low and simmer the sauce for about 15 minutes, stirring occasionally.

At the end of this time, remove the bay leaves and add the remaining tablespoon of butter, the remaining cup of Champagne, and the nutmeg. Stir, and return the chicken breasts to the skillet to warm in this succulent sauce while you prepare the plates.

PREPARATION TIME: *15 minutes*
TOTAL TIME: *approximately 1 hour*

Chicken à la Simon and Garfunkel

MINISTERS' WIVES must have an endless supply of delicious, quick, easy-to-prepare recipes. Considering all the entertaining that they are called on to do and the frequency with which they have to take a dish to church functions—well, it's a necessity.

But where do *they* get them? And what if you *are* the minister—*and* a woman?

This is the case for Becky Powell, Assistant Minister of The First Presbyterian Church in Danville, Virginia. When in need, Becky called on her aunt, Bea Garrett, a caterer in Richmond, Virginia. Aunt Bea gave her this handy recipe, but doesn't have a clue where it got its name.

Do you? Read the ingredients: parsley, sage, rosemary, and thyme. It's the name of the old Simon and Garfunkel hit.

SERVES 4

½ stick margarine or butter

2 tablespoons chopped parsley

¼ teaspoon dried sage

¼ teaspoon dried rosemary

¼ teaspoon dried thyme

4 ready-to-serve grilled chicken breasts

1 cup dry white wine

4 slices mozzarella cheese

2 cups cooked instant rice (½ cup per person)

Cookware needed: saucepan, skillet with a lid

Melt the butter in a small saucepan.

Add the herbs and stir. (This step can also be done in a measuring cup in the microwave.)

Lay the chicken breasts in a skillet and pour the herb mixture over them.

Cover the skillet and simmer on low heat for 10 to 15 minutes.

Add the wine and cook another 10 or so minutes, until the flavors have blended.

Lay the slices of mozzarella cheese on top of the chicken.

Cover the skillet just long enough to melt the cheese, approximately 4 minutes.

Serve over white rice, pouring the remaining pan sauce over the chicken and prepared rice.

PREPARATION TIME: *10 minutes*
TOTAL TIME: *30 minutes*

Chicken Marsala

SO MUCH FOR THE OLD RULE: white wine with white meat, red wine with red meat. It is well known that tastes truly do complement one another, and it can be vitally important to blend the grape with the meal. Perhaps it is because I am hardly a wine expert that I, personally, belong to the school that says, eat what you like, drink what you like—and red wines are usually my choice.

This recipe is one instance where the flavor of a little red wine greatly enhances the mild taste of the chicken. And by using ready-to-serve flavored chicken strips, this entrée can be prepared in just a few minutes.

SERVES 4 TO 6

2 tablespoons olive oil

½ cup frozen, diced onion

1 clove garlic, or ½ teaspoon prepared garlic

1 (4-ounce) can sliced mushrooms

2 tablespoons flour

½ cup Marsala wine

1 ½ cups red table wine

2 (10-ounce) packages ready-to-serve (fully cooked, breaded) Italian, or herbed chicken breast strips

Cookware needed: skillet

The Finishing Touch

Good served either on top of, or next to, pecan rice. Be sure to spoon up liberal amounts of the tasty Marsala sauce over the chicken for color and flavor.

In a skillet large enough to hold all the ingredients, heat the olive oil and sauté the onion and garlic for approximately 3 minutes. Add the mushrooms and sauté another 2 minutes, tossing lightly.

Sprinkle the onion and mushrooms with the flour, blending well.

Gradually add the 2 wines, stir well, and simmer on low heat for 15 minutes.

Add the chicken strips and heat thoroughly on medium-low for approximately 10 minutes.

PREPARATION TIME: *Approximately 10 minutes*
TOTAL TIME: *30 minutes*

Easy Chicken Tetrazzini

IN MY storehouse of memories of culinary delights is the wonderful turkey tetrazzini that Virginia Vincent, one of Mother's lifelong friends, made. Whether we ate it at the Vincents' house, or she brought it as a casserole to our house for a potluck supper—any time, any place, it was one of my favorites.

And with good reason. When made the old-fashioned way, it took hours to prepare—beginning with roasting a turkey (usually around the holidays) so there'd be leftovers for the tetrazzini. By using ready-to-serve chicken and other modern convenience foods, tetrazzini is now an easy-to-prepare treat any time of the year.

SERVES 6 TO 8

¾ cup frozen, diced combo of onion and green pepper

¼ cup chopped celery (optional)

1 tablespoon butter

2 tablespoons diced pimiento

1 (10-ounce) can cream of mushroom soup

1 (10-ounce) package ready-to-serve unflavored chicken pieces

1 box chicken and noodle dinner

1 cup herbed stuffing (crumbled), not croutons

4 ounces Cheddar cheese, grated

Cookware needed: large skillet, baking dish or casserole

Sage Advice

The celery adds a lot of crunch and flavor to this dish, even though it takes a little extra time and effort to chop. Rather than leave it out, remember to pick some up from the salad bar at the grocery store. Or, substitute a can of chopped water chestnuts (drained) from your well-stocked pantry.

Sauté the onion, green pepper, and celery in the butter over medium heat until tender and transparent.

Add the diced pimiento, soup, chicken, and chicken and noodle dinner and stir to combine.

Turn the mixture into a greased 3-quart baking dish or casserole.

Combine the stuffing and cheese and sprinkle the mixture on top of the chicken.

Bake at 350 degrees for 30 minutes.

PREPARATION TIME: *10 to 12 minutes*
TOTAL TIME: *approximately 45 minutes*

Cranberry-Sauce Chicken

Sage Advice

If desired, assemble the recipe in advance and refrigerate until ready to cook later in the day.

"**YOU** absolutely have to put in the pretty chicken dish!" Judie Bennett exclaimed as we piled my suitcases into the back of her SUV in the parking lot of the Civic Center in Beaumont, Texas, where I'd just given a talk.

"Yes, yes!" echoed her good friend Susan Kent, who was along for the ride and the fun. "It's just beautiful."

"You mean 'lovely,'" Judie Bennett corrected her. "That's what Lady Jan would say. 'Lovely. It's lovely.'"

"Who's Lady Jan? What chicken dish? What makes it so pretty...I mean, lovely?" I asked my two new friends.

Seems Lady Jan is Susan's sister, who married a real-life English Lord. The chicken dish is this easy chicken, and it's the cranberries that make it so lovely and, I quickly add, delicious.

Put it on your must-try list. It will become an instant hit, especially when you learn that you can assemble it hours, or even a day ahead.

SERVES 6 TO 8

The Finishing Touch

Surely you've come up with this one yourself by now. For a festive, trouble-free dinner, serve the chicken with rice and your favorite green vegetable accompaniment—perfect during the Thanksgiving or Christmas season.

8 boneless chicken breast halves, frozen or fresh

Garlic powder

1 (8-ounce) bottle Russian dressing

1 (2-ounce) envelope Lipton's dry onion soup mix

1 (16-ounce) can cranberry sauce, the whole berry variety

½ cup water

Cookware needed: baking dish or casserole, mixing bowl

Preheat the oven to 350 degrees.

Place the chicken breasts in a greased baking dish and sprinkle them lightly with garlic powder.

Combine the Russian dressing, dry onion soup mix, cranberry sauce, and water and pour the mixture over the chicken.

Bake for 1 hour, basting occasionally to ensure that the chicken absorbs the delicious cranberry flavor.

PREPARATION TIME: *10 minutes*
TOTAL TIME: *a little more than 1 hour*

Russian Apricot Chicken

THERE ARE LOTS of recipes that make you say to yourself when you read them, "Why didn't I think of that?"

This is not one of those. For who would ever dream of combining Russian dressing and apricot preserves? Well, someone did, and the result is mouth watering, and easy to make.

SERVES 6

6 to 8 fresh or frozen chicken breasts, thawed

1 (8-ounce) bottle Russian salad dressing

1 envelope dry onion soup mix

1 (10-ounce) jar apricot preserves

Cookware needed: covered baking dish or casserole

Preheat the oven to 350 degrees.

Place the chicken in a baking dish.

Combine the other ingredients, and pour the mixture over the chicken.

Cover and bake for 45 minutes. Uncover and cook for an additional 15 minutes, or until browned.

PREPARATION TIME: *5 to 10 minutes*
TOTAL TIME: *1 hour 10 minutes*

The
Finishing Touch

Of course, this is one of those chicken dishes that's just fine served over rice. But it is equally good with pecan rice (page 180) served on the side or a box of dressing "dressed up" with the addition of pecans or pine nuts to give it an extra crunch.

Suzy's Microwave BBQ Chicken

SUZY BARILE, a North Carolina writer friend of mine, cooks a mean barbeque chicken. The recipe is one that goes back a couple of generations in her family— well, sort of. When you read Suzy's story, you'll realize that every generation looks for shortcuts to help them pass treasured mealtime traditions down through the years.

Dear Emyl...One of my favorite meals when I was growing up was my mom's BBQ chicken served with white rice and corn on the cob. Looking back, it wasn't a difficult meal that she prepared, and her family history explains why: She grew up in Orlando, Florida, in the days when the city was considered a part of the "Old South." Her family had a full-time cook, Mamie.

Mamie prepared all the family's meals, even working Saturday morning to fix the roast or ham or whatever the family was having for Sunday dinner. I have no recollection as to whether my grandmother could cook. With someone else to prepare the family's meals, however, Mom didn't learn to cook until after she graduated from college and married.

By then it was the early 1950s, and "instant" rice and potato flakes, canned soups, and frozen vegetables were making their way onto supermarket shelves. As a novice cook, Mom must have been thrilled! It's for that reason that many of her recipes reflect the availability of those convenience foods. Perhaps those "instant" foods came in handiest after a long day spent meeting the needs of seven children.

I can certainly understand the allure. When my daughter, Jennifer, was in elementary school and I was a single mom working full time at a community newspaper, it was tough for me to get home in the evening, get her settled doing homework, and still have dinner prepared quickly enough to suit my seemingly starving child.

That's when I took my Mom's BBQ chicken recipe a step further, adapting it for cooking in a microwave oven. It doesn't quite have her special touch, but when served with the "juice" poured over white rice as she used to do, and corn or sweet peas added to the menu, my daughter is in heaven. To her, it's still Granny's BBQ chicken!

Mom used to brown a 2-pound cut-up, frying chicken in ¼ cup of shortening, add 1 can of tomato soup (canned tomatoes work, as well), ¼ cup of pickle relish, ¼ cup chopped onion, and 1 teaspoon Worcestershire sauce, then reduce heat to simmer, cover, and cook for 1 hour.

I do it this way:

SERVES 4 TO 6

1 cup ketchup
1 cup mustard
1 cup molasses

1 chicken, precut

Cookware needed: mixing bowl, microwave-safe baking dish or casserole

Combine the ketchup, mustard, and molasses in a bowl.

Place the precut chicken pieces (from a whole chicken) in a microwaveable dish.

Pour the sauce over the chicken.

Cover the dish with wax paper and cook in a microwave oven on high for 18 minutes, turning the dish every 6 minutes for even cooking.

PREPARATION TIME: *7 to 10 minutes*
TOTAL TIME: *approximately 30 minutes*

Sage Advice

To Suzy's instructions, I'll add that by using the precut whole chicken, you're carrying on the look and feel of the original, old-fashioned recipe. You'd lose that if you used all boneless breasts, something our moms and grannies didn't have at their disposal.

Pepper and Mushroom Chicken Delight

THIS CHICKEN entrée is one of those dishes that is sinfully easy to prepare. Further, you can serve it over rice or with a side of potatoes, pasta, or noodles as a starch. Add a simple green salad with a dressing of your choice, or, if you're tired of salad and your taste buds are craving peas, broccoli, or asparagus, fix those. With all these choices, there's no excuse to not have dinner taken care of.

SERVES 6 TO 8

½ to 1 teaspoon prepared garlic, or 2 or 3 garlic cloves, minced

1 cup frozen red pepper, onion, and mushroom combo (Bird's Eye makes this), or make the mixture from individual packages

¼ cup olive oil

2 (14-ounce) cans Italian-flavored tomatoes

8 already grilled chicken breasts

Salt, pepper, and dried oregano to taste

Cookware needed: skillet, with lid

Sauté the garlic, pepper, onion, and mushrooms in the olive oil until the vegetables are lightly browned.

Add the Italian-flavored tomatoes and simmer on medium-low heat to blend the flavors, approximately 5 minutes.

Add the already grilled chicken breasts and continue to simmer for 10 to 15 minutes. Adjust the seasoning with additional salt, pepper, and oregano, if desired.

PREPARATION TIME: *10 minutes*
TOTAL TIME: *25 minutes*

Timeless Chicken

THERE are times when even food writers need help, and this was one of them! I had agreed to introduce a speaker at a 4 PM event, and, without thinking, had invited several people to a sit-down dinner in his honor at 6 PM.

I wanted it to be a lovely occasion, but time was working against me. Why, I'd be lucky to get home and put on fresh lipstick before the guests arrived. This truly had to be a do-ahead event.

The more I looked through my supply of recently purchased cookbooks for a special entrée, the worse it got. All the recipes ended with "serve immediately." Then I remembered a company dish that once had been regular fare at my parties.

When I found the recipe, the page was splattered with food stains—proof of its success.

I made the recipe in 2000 the same way I had made it in 1962—down to the last ingredient. And my guests enjoyed it just as much as they had thirty-eight years earlier—down to the last morsel.

That's when I decided to name it Timeless Chicken.

SERVES 6 TO 8

1 (10-ounce) can cream of mushroom soup

1 (8-ounce) carton sour cream

8 to 10 chicken breast halves, frozen or fresh

8 to 10 thin slices of ham, prosciutto, or dried chipped beef

½ cup dry sherry

1 can mushrooms, drained

Paprika

Cookware needed: mixing bowl, rectangular baking dish or casserole

Preheat the oven to 350 degrees.

Combine the mushroom soup and sour cream. Spoon a small amount in the bottom of a baking dish and spread it out to cover.

Sprinkle the chicken breasts with a little paprika.

Wrap a piece of the ham, prosciutto, or chipped beef around each breast.

Place the wrapped breasts in the baking dish in a single layer.

Add the sherry and mushrooms to the remaining soup and sour cream mixture. Pour this over the chicken.

Bake 1 to 1 ½ hours until bubbly and crusty around the sides.

PREPARATION TIME: *10 minutes*
TOTAL TIME: *approximately 1 ½ hours*

Sage Advice

Use the saltiest ham you can for this dish. That's a Virginia, Smithfield, or Country ham, in my part of the world. What you don't want is a sweet, honey-baked ham. That's why the choices of prosciutto or chipped beef (right out of a jar) are offered as alternatives.

The Finishing Touch

Serve with a wild rice mix to dress the meal up a little more; otherwise, long-grain rice is just fine. But this is a "white" entrée, so be sure to serve it with a colorful accompaniment such as green beans garnished with red peppers, or well-seasoned zucchini, spinach, or asparagus garnished with pimiento or small tomatoes, sliced or quartered.

Baked Rainbow or Brook Trout

FRESH TROUT is the best reason I know of to go to the mountains. Years ago, that was the only time lots of people could get trout. Of course, these days we can pop into the local grocery store and pick up good trout, even if it's not fresh out of a brook.

Though I love simple, pan-cooked trout lightly seasoned with lemon, it can be hard to watch the skillet when you're chasing the kids, finishing up a phone call, or just tending to the rest of your dinner menu. Not having to stand by the stove makes this quick, oven-baked trout a handy, and good, fish entrée.

SERVES 6

Sage Advice

When I gave a friend this recipe, she asked why I didn't use the prepared Roasted Garlic Parmesan Cheese Sauce. It's because I think the garlic is a little heavy for the delicate flavor of trout.

¼ cup chopped parsley
¼ cup chopped chives
Salt and pepper, to taste
6 to 8 dressed trout
¼ cup Alfredo sauce of your liking

¼ cup grated Parmesan cheese, plus additional for cracker crumbs (optional)
½ cup fine cracker crumbs
Cookware needed: baking dish or casserole, mixing bowl

Preheat the oven to 375 degrees.

Sprinkle the parsley and chives over the bottom of a buttered shallow baking dish large enough to hold the fish in a single layer.

Salt and pepper the fish, and place them on the bed of parsley and chives.

Combine the sauce and ¼ cup of grated Parmesan cheese, and gently spread the mixture on the fish.

Sprinkle the cracker crumbs (to which you may add additional cheese, if desired) over the fish.

Bake the trout for 15 minutes, or until it is easily flaked with a fork.

PREPARATION TIME: *5 to 10 minutes*
TOTAL TIME: *25 minutes*

Crab Imperial

COOKS, especially those with sterling reputations, sometimes have to cross their fingers behind their backs when asked if a particularly delicious item is "homemade." Of course, polite guests really shouldn't ask.

Charlotte Pennell, whose culinary talents put most of us to shame, was caught in such a predicament when she served this adaptation of an old Charleston, South Carolina, recipe (or receipt, as they called recipes back in the eighteenth century). Seems that a particularly persistent guest kept raving about this Crab Imperial and insisting that Charlotte tell where she had bought the fresh crabmeat. Luckily, the store where she bought the canned crabmeat also had a fresh fish department.

This recipe is a sure winner for a special company dinner. Yes, crabmeat is expensive, but this is a special dish.

SERVES 6

4 (4-ounce) cans lump crabmeat (Orleans Lump)

½ teaspoon Worcestershire sauce

1 tablespoon horseradish

¼ teaspoon salt

¼ stick softened butter

1 beaten egg

½ cup mayonnaise

1 tablespoon sherry

4 ounces mild Cheddar cheese, grated

Cookware needed: mixing bowl, baking dish or casserole

Rinse the crabmeat under cold water and gently press it dry between paper towels or in a strainer.

In a mixing bowl, combine all the other ingredients except the cheese, then add the crabmeat.

Refrigerate the mixture for 30 to 60 minutes. During this time, preheat the oven to 300 degrees.

After it has chilled, divide the mixture among individual scallop shells or ramekins, or turn it into a baking dish or casserole.

Sprinkle the cheese on top and bake for 30 minutes.

Accept the compliments graciously.

The
Finishing Touch

The individual, inexpensive scallop shells available in kitchen stores add a special touch to Crab Imperial. And to dress up your dinner plates further, place the shell on a lettuce leaf just before serving. Boston or "living" lettuce is usually the right size and shape to curl up around the shell.

PREPARATION TIME: *15 minutes*
TOTAL TIME: *about 1 hour and 30 minutes*

Crabmeat in Shells

Sage Advice

Carolyn suggests that capers (2 to 3 heaping tablespoons) and frozen petite peas (½ to ⅔ cup) can be added, as well. If adding the peas, cook them in boiling water for only about 1 to 2 minutes before draining and combining with the crabmeat mixture.

YOU KNOW it's going to be a good recipe when a friend is so anxious to tell you about it that she calls you from her car phone! Grace Litzenberg did just that as she was leaving Greensboro, North Carolina, after having breakfast with her cousin, Carolyn Hill Hesselbach.

Carolyn has lived in the Grand Cayman Islands for some twenty-five-plus years, but as a constant reminder of her North Carolina roots, she prepares this delicious crabmeat entrée in serving shells from the North Carolina coast.

Put away your fears that the recipe will call for fresh crabmeat, because even though the Caymans are surrounded by water, fresh seafood, especially crab, can be as hard to come by there as it is here, so Carolyn uses canned crabmeat. But, she confessed, she does use fresh parsley, which she grows in her small garden. Luckily for us, fresh parsley is now available in the produce section of most grocery stores.

SERVES 6

The Finishing Touch

Don't forget to garnish with a pretty sprig of parsley and even a lemon curl or slice. This dish can be served in store-bought pastry puffs, if you don't have the shells or ramekins.

¼ cup diced celery
2 tablespoons butter
Several sprigs fresh parsley
2 (6-ounce) cans crabmeat drained
⅔ cup mayonnaise

Juice of half a lemon
Salt and pepper, to taste
½ to 1 cup Parmesan cheese, grated
Cookware needed: mixing bowl, individual serving shells

Preheat the oven to 350 degrees.

Sauté the celery in the butter, then add the parsley.

Remove from heat and combine with the crabmeat, the mayonnaise, the lemon juice, and salt and pepper, to taste.

Put into individual shells or ramekins and top with an ample amount of grated Parmesan cheese.

Bake for 15 minutes.

PREPARATION TIME: *15 minutes*
TOTAL TIME: *30 minutes*

Navy Wives Shrimp Curry

I'M TOLD that this shrimp dish got its name because Navy wives served it so frequently. The use of curry and fresh seafood certainly qualifies it as the sort of dish that these ladies would have concocted when living in a foreign port. Add to that the tradition of serving "toppings" along with the dish, and this is clearly a variation on the traditional East Indian curry.

It's a tasty dish and one that's easy to make, now that cream of shrimp soup is once again on the grocery store shelves. (For a few years, it was very hard to find.) If you can't find the shrimp, substitute canned lobster bisque. That seems to be in most stores.

To guarantee that you're getting the plumpest, most tender shrimp, consider purchasing ready-to-eat shrimp from the grocery store. Otherwise, rely on fully dressed, tails-off, frozen shrimp.

SERVES 6

¼ cup frozen, chopped onions

3 teaspoons (or more to taste) curry powder

1 tablespoon butter or olive oil

1 (10-ounce) can cream of shrimp soup

1 cup sour cream or half-and-half

8 ounces (or more) cooked shrimp

Cookware needed: skillet

If using frozen shrimp, allow them to defrost.

Sauté the onion and curry powder in the butter till the onion is tender.

Add the soup and stir, then the sour cream or half-and-half, and stir again.

Add the shrimp and cook just until they are heated thoroughly—3 to 5 minutes.

Serve the shrimp curry over hot rice (the instant variety, of course) with the following condiments, or others of your choice, set out in individual bowls, each with its own spoon:

- chopped tomato
- chopped green pepper
- chopped cucumbers
- chopped scallions
- raisins soaked in brandy
- chutney
- grated coconut
- chopped nuts

PREPARATION TIME: *15 minutes*
TOTAL TIME: *15 minutes plus, depending on your choice of condiments*

Sage Advice

Don't let the list of condiments frighten you off with visions of chopping and dicing. Much of this work has already been done for you. Think about it. Many of the items can be found in any well-stocked salad bar. You can open a can of chopped tomato and green pepper and drain off some of the extra liquid. Or you can quickly defrost frozen green peppers by spreading them out on a paper towel while you prepare the curried shrimp. Even coconut comes already grated these days, and there is a great variety of canned, chopped nuts.

The Finishing Touch

Tart, citrusy, fresh lime juice is the perfect finishing touch for this creamy curried seafood dish. Garnish individual plates with large lime wedges, or for a buffet, include a bowl of lime wedges with the condiments. And for the easiest centerpiece ever, fill a bowl with whole limes and lemons and stick in sprays of darker greenery gathered from shrubs.

Corned Beef

AT THE TOP of my list of easy-to-prepare, but usually-not-in-your-repertoire of quick entrées is corned beef.

I can't count how many times people have asked, "Hhmmmm, what are you cooking?" only to reply, "I've never tried that," when I've told them it was corned beef.

All it takes is water, beef, spices, and time. If you're a Crock-Pot cook, this is an ideal meat with which to vary your usual fare. And if you're one of those cooks who loves the smell of good food, but you don't like to spend a lot of time in the kitchen, corned beef is just the ticket.

Do try it. It is very good when served with an onion casserole (try the Vidalia Onion Casserole, page 166), a vegetable dish, and good bread—especially on a weekend, since there is usually some left over for another busy day.

SERVES 12 TO 16,
BUT YOU'LL WANT THE LEFTOVERS FOR SANDWICHES,
SO DON'T SKIMP WHEN YOU'RE COOKING.

2 onions, peeled and halved

2 to 3 celery stalks, or ½ cup diced celery from the salad bar

3 heaping tablespoons pickling spices (the spices from the package of corned beef, plus more from a jar of pickling spices)

4 quarts water

1 (4-pound) corned beef, with spices included in the packaging

Cookware needed: Crock-Pot or large (8-quart) covered pot

Put the onions, celery, and spices in the water; cover and bring to a boil.

Add the meat, cover and, when the water has returned to a boil, turn the heat down to low.

Simmer for approximately 4 hours, or until the center of the corned beef is eas-ily pierced with a long, sharp fork. Check occasionally to see if more water is needed in the pot.

PREPARATION TIME: *15 minutes*
TOTAL TIME: *approximately 4 hours, 15 minutes*

Old-Fashioned Pot Roast

MY STEPDAUGHTER, ERIKA, can be hard to please at mealtime, but it's really not her fault. She inherited her picky eating habits from her father, my husband.

Trying to be a good stepmother, I always ask her what she'd like to eat when she's coming in from graduate school. Knowing that I'm not going to settle for the usual "pizza" request, she answers, "How about one of your good pot roasts?"

That's the same answer I get when I ask other young folks who are coming to dinner what they'd like to eat.

It makes sense. Few young folks will take the time to cook a roast. And if they did, chances are the leftovers would grow mold in their refrigerators. One day, though, things will be different.

So, for Erika, and others like her, here's how to cook your own pot roast and make it flavorful by using prepared seasoning mixes right off the grocery store shelf. You won't cook it today, and maybe not even this year or next. But you'll have it on record for when you do need it, because you won't find this recipe in today's nouvelle cuisine or gourmet cookbooks.

YIELDS 3-4 SERVINGS PER POUND

2 tablespoons olive oil

1 (3-to-5 pound) chuck roast

1 cup water

1 medium onion, halved or quartered

2 stalks celery, or an ample handful-size serving of pieces from the salad bar

5 or 6 dried bay leaves

1 envelope seasoning mix (see *Sage Advice*)

⅔ cup red wine

Cookware needed: covered skillet or heavy 4-quart pot

Heat the oil in a heavy skillet over medium-high heat.

Sear the roast quickly on all four sides, if you wish. (Some cooks insist on searing roasts before cooking them to hold in the juices; others don't.)

Add the water, onion, celery, and bay leaves. Cover and bring to a boil.

Thoroughly mix the envelope of seasoning with the red wine. Add the mixture to the pot.

Turn the heat to low and allow the roast to simmer for 2 ½ to 3 hours or longer, depending on how tender you want the meat to be.

PREPARATION TIME: *10 minutes*
TOTAL TIME: *approximately 3 hours*

Chipped Beef Deluxe

THOUGH I find it hard to believe, I used to push the plate aside when Mother served chipped beef. It must have been the name, surely not the taste. These days, there are times when I absolutely crave a hearty serving of chipped beef with a fresh, juicy tomato on the side as the perfect complement.

Chipped beef is a cinch to fix, thanks to Stouffer's, and so good that I serve it to company—most of whom used to push their plates aside when their mothers served it, too. To dress up this old standby, try this recipe.

SERVES 6

2 boxes frozen, creamed chipped beef

¼ cup (or more) sliced Spanish olives with pimiento

½ teaspoon Angostura bitters

Pepper, to taste

Cookware needed: medium saucepan or microwave-safe bowl

The
Finishing Touch

Older cookbooks always say "serve over toast points." But English muffins, waffles, noodles, or even rice work equally well.

Follow the package directions for cooking the creamed chipped beef on the stovetop.

When done, open the packages and pour the contents into a microwave-safe serving bowl.

Stir in the olives, bitters, and pepper, to taste.

Cover with plastic wrap, being sure to leave one corner open to vent, and microwave for 30 to 60 seconds. Or, if you prepared the frozen creamed chipped beef in a microwave oven, stir in the olives, bitters, and pepper, to taste, and microwave for 20 seconds.

PREPARATION TIME: *3 to 5 minutes*
TOTAL TIME: *15 minutes*

Easy Beef Stroganoff

FOOD is like fashion. What goes around comes around.

For years, no one even mentioned Beef Stroganoff. The rage was all Beef Wellington or London Broil or Beef Medallions.

Suddenly, Beef Stroganoff is beginning to make a comeback at dinner parties and even in some restaurants. It's about time.

This long-ago favorite is as good as ever, and much, much less time-consuming to make than it used to be. And for the generation that missed it—it's a brand-new taste!

SERVES 6

1 tablespoon butter

½ cup frozen, diced onion

1 (4-ounce) can sliced mushrooms, drained

½ teaspoon prepared garlic, or 1 garlic clove, minced

2 (17-ounce) packages Hormel Always Tender Beef Tips

1 ½ cups sour cream

½ cup dry white wine

Cookware needed: skillet with lid

Melt the butter in a heavy skillet.

Add the onion, mushrooms, and garlic, and sauté gently over medium-high heat for 3 to 4 minutes.

Gradually add the beef tips, blending them with the vegetables.

When the mixture is beginning to bubble, lower the heat to a simmer, cover, and cook for about 6 to 7 minutes longer.

In a large measuring cup, combine the sour cream and white wine.

Add the wine mixture to the meat and simmer just until blended, about 5 to 6 minutes.

PREPARATION TIME: *5 minutes*
TOTAL TIME: *20 minutes*

The
Finishing Touch

The traditional way to serve Beef Stroganoff is over wide egg noodles, but rice does just as well. Be sure to add a colorful garnish. Sprinkle the serving platter with freshly snipped chives, dill or parsley, or, if you're preparing individual servings, arrange a few herb leaves and cherry tomatoes on the side of each plate before you dish up the Stroganoff.

Beef Tenderloin

Sage Advice

The best tenderloins really are those that have had a chance to marinate at room temperature for a few hours, or, if refrigerated, overnight. Allow ample marinating time, and don't skimp on the marinade either.

FORGET "a rose is a rose is a rose." A tenderloin is a tenderloin is a tenderloin. Whether it's beef or pork, this cut of meat can't be beat for tenderness or ease of cooking. No wonder it's becoming a popular meat during the holidays for families where the tradition of eating a homecooked meal is important, but the cook is pressed for time.

In fact, one of the beauties of a tenderloin is that it can be served at a cocktail party, dinner party, or holiday event. It's good any time.

But if the tenderloin falls short, it's in the flavor category. Without a little help from spices or seasoning, the meat can be bland. That's where marinades get to show off.

There are countless delicious ready-to-use marinades, but when you consider how simple it is to stir together a few ingredients for a more distinctive taste, you may want to go that route.

The number of servings will vary greatly,
depending on how thin the meat is sliced
and how large a tenderloin you cook.
A general rule of thumb is to allow
⅛ to ¼ pound per person. Thus, a 3-pound
tenderloin will yield from 9 to 12 servings.

1 (2-to-3 pound) beef tenderloin
For marinade:
1 cup bourbon
½ cup soy sauce

½ cup brown sugar
Cookware needed: rectangular baking dish or casserole, mixing bowl

Place the tenderloin in a baking dish.

Thoroughly combine the bourbon, soy sauce, and brown sugar and pour the mixture over the tenderloin.

Cover the dish with aluminum foil and marinate the meat at room temperature for 3 to 4 hours, or in the refrigerator overnight. Turn the meat occasionally, so the full tenderloin will be immersed in the marinade. (If the meat was refrigerated after marinating, allow it to sit, uncovered at room temperature to take the chill off, or for about 1 hour, before cooking it.)

Preheat the oven to 425 degrees.

Baste the meat well before cooking and bake it, uncovered, in the marinade for 35 to 45 minutes.

For a larger tenderloin, weighing 4 to 6 pounds, increase the cooking time to 50 to 60 minutes.

(These cooking times are for a rare tenderloin. Of course, the time can be extended for a more well-done meat, but almost everyone agrees that tenderloin tastes best when it is pink, not brown, in the middle.)

Remove the pan from the oven, baste the tenderloin with the marinade and juices one last time, and allow it to rest for at least 10 to 15 minutes before carving. Or, allow it to cool, then refrigerate it for 2 to 3 hours before carving, and serve it chilled. Chilled, sliced beef tenderloin is an elegant addition to any cocktail party.

■ ■ ■ ■ ■ ■ ■ ■

PREPARATION TIME: *10 minutes*
TOTAL TIME: *from 45 to 60 plus minutes,*
depending on cooking time

The
Finishing Touch

Garnish your serving platter with parsley, fresh herbs, cherry or grape tomatoes—even lemon slices—whatever you have on hand to add color and a little pizzazz to this delicacy.

City-Style, Country-Style Steak

IT'S THE OLD SAYING that necessity is the mother of invention.

When Gene Brown couldn't find a recipe for Country-Style Steak, that old, delicious and reliable standby in many a Southern household, he decided it was time to share his. But not before jazzing it up a little.

Now, thanks to Gene, we Southerners will no longer be forced to go to our favorite "down home" diner or restaurant to order this favorite. And, if you're from another region of the county, Gene's addition of red wine takes the "country" out of the name and makes it acceptable anywhere! That's why we've renamed it City-Style, Country-Style Steak.

SERVES 4

2 tablespoons vegetable oil

4 pieces cube steak

Flour for dredging

Salt and freshly ground pepper, to taste

¼ to ½ cup dry red wine, or Madeira (optional)

1 (14-ounce) can beef broth

Cookware needed: large skillet with lid

While the oil is heating over medium to medium-high heat, dredge the steaks in flour, salt, and pepper. (I put a liberal amount of these 3 ingredients in a large plastic bag for this process. It keeps the flour from getting all over the countertop and floor.)

Shake the excess flour off each steak while holding over the plastic bag, then brown them on both sides in the oil. Remove steaks to a plate.

Splash in the wine and, using a wooden spoon, scrape the brown bits off the bottom of the pan, blending them into the wine.

Add the can of beef broth and, when the liquid returns to a gentle boil, put the steaks back in the skillet, cover, turn the heat to low, and allow them to simmer for an hour, or until very tender.

When the meat is done, if the liquid is a little too "runny," remove the skillet cover, put the meat on a plate and cover with aluminum foil to keep warm. Turn up the heat to medium and let the liquid cook down to the desired consistency.

Return the meat to the pan for just a couple of minutes to reheat, and then serve.

PREPARATION TIME: *15 minutes*

TOTAL TIME: *1 hour and 15 minutes, or until the meat is tender, which may vary according to the meat itself*

Sage Advice

Chopped or sliced onions can be added to the mixture during the browning process, or, instead of beef broth, use a can of French Onion soup, undiluted.

The Finishing Touch

Serve with instant rice or deli potatoes and a vegetable or two taken right out of the freezer or can and you have a true old-fashioned homemade meal that your family will request over and over again.

That Other White Meat

There's not much you can do to mess up pork (or ham). It lends itself equally well to tomato or cream sauces, fruits or vegetables, potatoes or rice.

Many pork recipes can be cooked either in a skillet on the stove top, or in a baking dish in the oven. Further, once you've assembled any one of these dishes, you can leave it alone to do its own thing—short of letting it burn. I guess I think of pork chops the same way I think of cream cheese. Whatever you do to it, chances are it will turn out just fine.

On top of those advantages, ham has long been a ready-to-serve favorite. Canned deviled ham, ham products like Spam, and even fully cooked canned hams have been around since the first part of the twentieth century. The recent addition of fully cooked ribs, already diced ham cubes, and even roast pork make the cook's job even simpler. In many instances, you can pull one of these products out of the refrigerator or freezer, combine it with whatever else you have on hand, and put together a delicious entrée.

To get you started, here are some of my own and other cooks' favorites that use either ready-to-serve or fresh pork.

"Please, if you don't mind, pass the pork chops."

—MORRIS MARKEY, "THE TASTY PIG," 1949

Sage Advice

Pork or ham? Most people call any cured or smoked pork "ham." But the reference books inform us that only the pig's hind leg is technically a ham. That still leaves a lot of delicious pork—the roasts, ribs, chops, tenderloins, and even bacon—to enjoy.

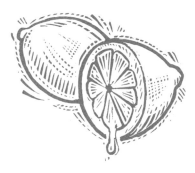

Pork Tenderloin with Sauerkraut

MY SON, Langdon, is a great cook. But his preference, as is true for lots of thirty-something guys, is for the grill. I, on the other hand, am more of a kitchen cook.

There's another difference in our culinary preferences. He loves sauerkraut, as does his sister. I'm not really sure where they cultivated that taste, since I never fixed sauerkraut for the family when they were growing up.

But when he fixes pork tenderloin with sauerkraut and easy dumplings, I know why they like it so much, and wish I had known about this recipe earlier.

SERVES 6 TO 8

The
Finishing Touch

Serve with baked apples or a spiced applesauce for a really easy **From Storebought to Homemade** *meal!*

1 (32-ounce) package sauerkraut, drained, with liquid reserved

1 (4-to-5-pound) pork tenderloin, sliced and tied

½ cup distilled white vinegar

For dumplings:

1 package frozen dumplings

2 quarts water

Cookware needed: skillet with lid, medium saucepan

Buy an already-sliced and tied pork tenderloin, or have the butcher slice and tie it for you (½-inch thick slices).

Spread ½ the drained sauerkraut in the bottom of a heavy skillet or a large saucepan.

Lay the tenderloin on this layer; then cover it with the remaining sauerkraut.

Add the sauerkraut liquid and the vinegar to the pan.

Cover, and bring to a boil; then simmer on medium-low heat for about 20 minutes or until done.

To prepare the dumplings, bring 2 quarts of water to a rolling boil. Drop the dumplings into the boiling water. They will rise to the top as they are done.

Remove the dumplings from the water with a slotted spoon and drop them into the pan with the tenderloin and sauerkraut. Cover the pan and simmer for 10 to 12 minutes.

PREPARATION TIME: *15 minutes*
TOTAL TIME: *40 to 45 minutes*

Apple-Kraut Pork Chops

FOR a slight variation on the basic Pork Tenderloin with Sauerkraut recipe, try this quick and easy dish.

SERVES 6 TO 8

1 (32-ounce) package sauerkraut, drained

1 (25-ounce) jar applesauce

6 to 8 pork medallions or chops

Cookware needed: baking dish or casserole

Line the bottom of a baking dish, large enough to hold the pork in a single layer, with all the sauerkraut.

Spoon the applesauce over the kraut and lay the pork on top.

Cover the pan and cook at 350 degrees for 1 hour, or until the chops are white in the center.

PREPARATION TIME: *5 minutes*
TOTAL TIME: *approximately 1 hour*

Sage Advice

For whatever reason, some people just don't like meat served on the bone. That pretty much eliminates pork chops and T-bone steaks. I, personally, love the bones and can be found sucking every last morsel of meat and juice off mine. But for those who do not share my enthusiasm, trimmed pork medallions are a perfectly good substitute to use in all these pork chop recipes.

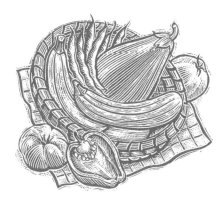

Sweet and Sour Pork, American Style

LOOKING for a way to jazz up pork chops? It's hard to imagine anything easier than this way of cooking the "other white meat." You can select whatever type of chop you prefer—center cut, thin, thick—or even pork medallions. Further, this quick dish can be prepared on the stovetop (or, if you wish, in the oven). Of course, the cooking time will vary according to the cut of meat and the method you use to cook it, but the taste will always be pleasing.

SERVES 6 TO 8

2 tablespoons canola or peanut oil

½ cup frozen, diced onion

6 to 8 pork chops of your choice

½ of an 11-ounce jar sweet and sour sauce

Cookware needed: skillet with lid, or baking dish or casserole

The
Finishing Touch

Take a hint from our Asian friends and serve these with egg rolls, fried rice, glazed carrots, green pepper strips, and pineapple.

Heat the oil in a skillet large enough to hold the chops in a single layer. Add the onion and sauté for 3 to 4 minutes.

Add the chops to the skillet and brown them on both sides.

Pour the sweet and sour sauce over the chops, cover the pan, and simmer for approximately 30 minutes, or until done (when the chops are white in the center). (If you wish to bake the chops in the oven, do so covered at 350 degrees for approximately 1 hour, or until done.)

PREPARATION TIME: *10 minutes*
TOTAL TIME: *40 to 45 minutes, or 70 minutes if baked*

Pork and Cherry Supreme

MY FATHER was partial to anything with cherries. Every Christmas he received a box of chocolate-covered cherries from anyone who couldn't think of anything else to give him. Cherry preserves were his favorite. (Blueberry preserves were a close second.)

This preference even extended to furniture. He much preferred "cherry wood" to walnut or even mahogany, and he always attributed this love for the tree and its fruit to his New England childhood.

In his later years, when Mother could no longer do the cooking, I'd ask him if there was something he'd particularly like me to prepare, and he'd often answer, "pork chops." After a moment's pause, he'd add, "You know, the ones with the cherries."

To prepare this dish you have to make the sauce, but that takes only a minute, and it cooks while you're browning the pork, so it's next to no effort.

SERVES 4 TO 6

2 tablespoons canola oil

6 to 8 pork chops or tenderloin medallions

½ cup orange juice

1 teaspoon lemon juice

¼ teaspoon allspice

½ teaspoon cinnamon

¼ cup brown sugar

1 teaspoon butter

⅔ cup cherry preserves

Cookware needed: skillet with lid, medium saucepan

Heat the oil in a skillet large enough to hold the pork chops in a single layer and brown the chops on both sides.

Combine the juices, spices, brown sugar, butter, and cherry preserves in a sauce pan and cook over medium-low heat until the ingredients have blended, or for about 5 to 7 minutes. (Do not boil.)

Pour the sauce over the browned pork chops, cover, and cook on low or medium-low heat for approximately 30 minutes, or until done.

PREPARATION TIME: *10 to 15 minutes*
TOTAL TIME: *approximately 45 minutes*

The
Finishing Touch

Just like the Cranberry-Sauce Chicken on page 92, this is a pretty (or lovely, if you prefer) entrée to serve at holiday time as a nice change from the usual turkey or baked ham.

Everybody's Mother's Pork Chop Casserole

WHEN I was growing up, this pork-chop-and-creamed soup–based casserole was such a standby that it actually became known as "everybody's mother's pork chop casserole." But like so many of our mother's recipes that were quick and easy, it seems to have been forgotten or lost in our attempts to serve fancier fare.

It is still just as good as it was 50 years ago, and, take it from this grandmother, it's a real favorite with the up-and-coming kiddie generation. They'll even eat their green beans if you smother them in some of the "sauce" from the casserole (though you might have to pick out some of the larger bits of mushrooms for the very pickiest eaters!).

SERVES 6 TO 8

The Finishing Touch

Serve this over rice, with something spicy, like a pickled peach or cinnamon-flavored apples, whose zingy flavor will really pick up the mellower pork and rice tastes.

1 (10-ounce) can cream of mushroom soup

Salt and pepper, to taste

6 to 8 pork chops or tenderloin medallions

Cookware needed: baking dish or casserole

Preheat the oven to 350 degrees.

Spoon enough of the mushroom soup into the bottom of a baking dish to cover it.

Salt and pepper the pork chops and place them on top of the soup.

Spoon the remaining soup over the pork and cover the pan with aluminum foil.

Bake for 45 minutes to 1 hour. Halfway through baking, either baste or turn over the pork.

PREPARATION TIME: *5 minutes*
TOTAL TIME: *approximately 1 hour*

Spanish Pork Chops

IF YOUR MOTHER, or your friend's mother, served the pork chops baked in mushroom soup, you can bet she also served "Spanish" pork chops. The green peppers, onions, and tomatoes gave the dish an "exotic" flavor back in those days when people didn't jet about the way they do today.

Mother, who loved peppercorns, always tossed a handful of them into her version of Spanish pork chops. I discovered my friends' mothers didn't do this when they whispered to me, "What are these black bullets?" or, heaven forbid, they unexpectedly bit down on one.

These days, rather than chopping and dicing the onions and adding the peppercorns, I smother the pork chops with Rotel Tomatoes and Green Chilies and add some diced celery for the extra crunch I've always liked. The dish would be equally tasty if you used Italian-flavored tomatoes, I'm sure.

In other words, once you have the pork chops, use whatever variety of canned tomatoes you find on your pantry shelf.

SERVES 6 TO 8

1 (14-ounce) can onion-flavored beef broth

6 to 8 pork chops of your choice

¼ cup chopped celery

1 (10-ounce) can Rotel Tomatoes and Green Chilies

Cookware needed: baking dish or casserole

Preheat the oven to 350 degrees.

Pour a little of the onion-flavored beef broth into the bottom of a baking dish.

Add the pork chops to the pan and sprinkle the celery over them.

Spread the tomatoes and chilies and the remaining beef broth on top of the chops.

Cover and bake for approximately 1 hour.

PREPARATION TIME: *10 minutes*
TOTAL TIME: *approximately 1 hour and 15 minutes*

Sage Advice

If you wish, you can cook this in a covered skillet on top of the stove. That usually cuts down on the cooking time by 15 to 20 minutes, or even more. Either way, serve the pork over rice to keep the broth from going to waste.

Quick as a Wink Roast Pork

Remember when pork was served with gravy and noodles? Or with dressing? I do, but I'm not sure my own children do. They always preferred roast beef to pork roast, so that's what we had.

But now the very convenient Hormel Pork Roast Au Jus makes it possible to return this old-fashioned favorite that skipped a generation to the family dinner table. Of course, you don't have to gussy it up at all, but I'm one of those cooks who can never leave anything alone—even a can of soup. So here are two ways to turn this storebought entrée into a homemade dinner.

Roast Pork with Noodles

SERVES 4 TO 6

■ ■ ■ ■ ■ ■ ■ ■ ■

The Finishing Touch

Serve the pork over hot buttered noodles and garnish it with fresh parsley.

2 (1-pound) packages Hormel Pork Roast Au Jus

¼ cup dry white wine

½ cup mushrooms, fresh or canned, drained

¼ cup sliced green olives

Cookware needed: skillet

Pour the au jus sauce from the roast pork pouches into a skillet.

Stir in the white wine, mushrooms, and green olives. Bring the liquid to a gentle simmer and add the pork. Continue to simmer for 5 to 7 minutes.

■ ■ ■ ■ ■ ■ ■ ■ ■

PREPARATION TIME: *10 minutes*
TOTAL TIME: *20 minutes (includes cooking noodles)*

Sunday Dinner Pork

SERVES 4 TO 6

2 (1-pound) packages Hormel
Pork Roast Au Jus

½ cup sour cream

1 teaspoon white vinegar or
white wine

3 to 4 dried bay leaves

Fresh ground pepper, to taste

Cookware needed: skillet with lid

Pour the au jus sauce from the roast pork pouches into a skillet.

Stir in the sour cream and vinegar or wine. Add the bay leaves and bring the liquid to a gentle simmer.

Cook for approximately 5 minutes, then add the pork and cover it well with the sauce.

Cover the skillet and continue to simmer the pork for 5 to 7 minutes.

Remove the bay leaves, add a few turns of freshly ground pepper, and serve.

PREPARATION TIME: *10 to 15 minutes*
TOTAL TIME: *15 minutes*

The
Finishing Touch

Serve this with stovetop dressing or pecan rice (page 180), mango soufflé (page 146), and string beans for a delicious, different, colorful, and satisfying meal.

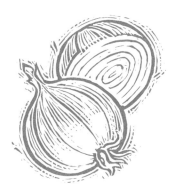

Garlic-Roasted Pork Tenderloin

THE ALREADY MARINATED pork tenderloins found in the meat section of the grocery store are real time savers. You don't have to take the time or trouble to marinate them, and they cook quickly, making it possible to serve a scrumptious appetizer or a company-quality meal on just a couple of hours' notice.

But if you have a couple of days' warning, buy a plain tenderloin and try this marinade. I think it's wonderful.

SERVES 8 TO 10

1 teaspoon salt

1 teaspoon pepper

1 teaspoon dried oregano

1 teaspoon dried thyme

4 to 5 cloves garlic, crushed, or 2 to 2 ½ teaspoons prepared garlic

1 (5- to-6-pound) pork tenderloin (not seasoned or marinated)

2 tablespoons distilled white vinegar

Cookware needed: rectangular baking dish or casserole

The Finishing Touch

Garnish the platter with orange, mango, lemon, and apple slices.

Two days before cooking, combine the salt, pepper, dried oregano, dried thyme, and garlic.

Put the meat in a baking dish and cut ½- to ¾-inch-deep slits every 2 to 3 inches down the length of the tenderloin.

With your hands, thoroughly rub the seasoning mixture over all sides of the tenderloin, pushing some of it down into the slits.

Pour the vinegar along the length of the tenderloin.

Cover the pan tightly with plastic wrap and refrigerate it for 2 days, turning the meat halfway through the time.

When you're ready to cook, preheat the oven to 350 degrees.

Remove the plastic wrap, turn the tenderloin, and cover it tightly with aluminum foil.

Puncture the foil in a few places to let the steam escape.

Bake for 2 hours.

Remove the pan from the oven and allow the tenderloin to sit, uncovered, for 10 to 15 minutes before slicing and serving.

PREPARATION TIME: *10 to 15 minutes*

TOTAL TIME: *2 days, plus 2 hours and 10 minutes*

Wild Rice and Sausage

VERSATILITY, that's what I like in a recipe. I've pointed out that experienced cooks have a repertoire of dishes they cook over and over again.

Wild rice and sausage fits the bill perfectly. It is equally at home on the breakfast table or a dinner buffet.

Though it calls for browning the sausage and cooking the rice instead of just "assembling" already prepared foods, the compliments you'll receive for this traditional Deep South dish will make it well worth the effort. It certainly isn't hard to make. It just takes a little time. Try using this as your "signature" piece on a menu with other, more quickly prepared, dishes.

SERVES 6 TO 8

1 (6-ounce) box wild rice, instant or regular

1 pound bulk pork sausage, not links or patties

¼ cup frozen, diced onions

1 (10-ounce) can cream of mushroom soup

1 teaspoon dried thyme

1 (4-ounce) jar pimientos

Cookware needed: saucepan, skillet, mixing bowl, baking dish or casserole

Sage Advice

Use either mild or hot bulk sausage, according to your preference. And, in case you're out of cream of mushroom soup, cream of chicken soup will work perfectly well.

Preheat the oven to 350 degrees.

Prepare the rice according to the package directions.

While the rice is cooking, brown the sausage in a skillet, stirring and breaking it up with a spoon. Add the diced onion at the end of the cooking so they are gently sautéed. Drain the sausage and onion and transfer the mixture to a bowl.

Add the rice, soup, dried thyme, and pimientos, and combine.

Pour the mixture into a greased baking dish.

Bake for approximately 25 to 30 minutes, or until bubbly.

PREPARATION TIME: *20 minutes*
TOTAL TIME: *50 to 60 minutes*

Veal Scaloppini Picatta

AT THE TOP of my top-ten favorite foods list (if David Letterman were ever to ask me) is Veal Picatta. But when I made it, though good, I just couldn't get it lemony and flavorful enough for my taste.

Then one day I thought, what if I were to add some dried lemon seasoning mix right out of the envelope? But how could I get this flavor into the veal itself, and not just make the sauce lemon flavored?

When I began cooking in the early 1960s, veal cutlets were so thick they had to be pounded between pieces of wax paper to thin them and make them tender. Although we now can buy veal scallops that are already paper thin, I decided to use the same technique to coat the veal with the seasoning.

I spread a layer of the lemon seasoning on a sheet of plastic wrap, placed the veal on this, and sprinkled more seasoning on top. After covering the veal with another sheet of plastic wrap, I gently pounded the meat just enough so some of the lemon seasoning was absorbed. It worked. Suddenly my veal picatta tasted like the dish I'd had in restaurants, especially when I used the rest of the dried lemon mix to make the sauce.

But there was yet another problem. Since the entrée was prepared in a skillet on top of the stove, sometimes the slices tended to dry out while I dished up the rest of the meal. Or, if I served up the veal first, the thin slices got cold.

This recipe both gives veal picatta the rich lemon flavor I love and also eliminates those last-minute worries. Though this is a two-step recipe, I find the results well worth the small amount of extra work.

SERVES 2 TO 3

The Veal:

1 envelope dried lemon seasoning mix (Knorr, Sun Bird, and McCormick make varieties)

6 veal scallops, thinly sliced

1 tablespoon butter

1 tablespoon olive oil

1 tablespoon (or more) lemon juice

Zest of one lemon (optional)

Salt and pepper, to taste (see *Sage Advice*)

The Sauce:

Remaining lemon seasoning mix

Water

1 cup chicken broth, easily made from instant bouillon crystals, or the canned variety

1 tablespoon (or more) lemon juice

White wine (optional)

Salt and pepper, to taste (see *Sage Advice*)

Cookware needed: skillet, rectangular baking dish or casserole, mixing bowl

Preheat the oven to 350 degrees.

Spread a couple of tablespoons of lemon seasoning on a piece of wax paper or plastic wrap.

Place two veal slices on top of the seasoning. Sprinkle the veal with a couple of more tablespoons of the lemon seasoning. Cover it with another sheet of wrap, and pound it gently. (The bowl of a serving spoon, the back of a spatula, or the handle of a chopping knife all work perfectly well.) Repeat this process until all the slices are coated.

Brown the veal in the butter and olive oil over medium to medium-high heat for just a minute or two on each side, or until lightly browned. You will probably have room in your skillet to cook only 3 or 4 slices at a time. When all the veal is cooked, turn the heat down to low.

As the slices are done, lay them in a baking or casserole dish lightly greased or sprayed with nonstick cooking oil.

To make the sauce: In a small mixing bowl combine the remaining lemon seasoning with just enough water to moisten it to a pastelike consistency.

Stir in the chicken broth and lemon juice. Add a little wine if you wish, and salt and pepper to taste.

Add this mixture to the skillet with the warm pan juices from cooking the veal and blend quickly, until the liquid begins to bubble gently.

Pour the sauce over the veal slices, scraping the bottom of the skillet well to get all the delicious brown bits.

Cover the pan with foil, and bake for 15 minutes, so the juices and veal blend well. If it is necessary to hold the veal longer, simply turn off the oven.

Sage Advice

If you prefer, use a lemon-pepper seasoning in place of the usual pepper to add even more lemon flavor.

■ ■ ■ ■ ■ ■ ■ ■ ■

PREPARATION TIME: *15 minutes*
TOTAL TIME: *30 minutes*

Elegant Veal Scalloppini Picatta

SERVES 2 TO 3

6 slices prosciutto, sliced thin

6 slices Monterey Jack cheese

½ cup heavy cream

Cookware needed: skillet, rectangular baking dish or casserole, mixing bowl

Prepare the Veal Scaloppini Picatta recipe on page 121 through cooking the veal in the skillet, and preheat the oven to 375 degrees.

When you place the veal slices in the baking dish, cover each one with a slice of prosciutto and a slice of cheese.

When preparing the sauce, add the heavy cream and stir. Pour over the veal.

Bake for 15 or 20 minutes, until the cheese has melted. Do not cover the baking dish unless you need to hold it longer, in which case, cover the pan and turn off the oven.

PREPARATION TIME: *20 minutes*

TOTAL TIME: *35 to 40 minutes*

Lamb, No Longer Just for Spring

"I LOVE LAMB, but what can you do with it?" I was asked once. It's a good question because lamb usually is served either as chops with mint jelly or, in the spring, as a "leg of lamb."

And, unlike chicken and pork which we like to "dress up" because we serve it so often, lamb is thought of as being a delicacy, an expensive meat that is saved for special occasions.

Further, lamb really does have a distinctive taste, and if you like it, that's what you want—lamb that tastes like lamb.

But no longer is lamb as expensive as it once was, and, as America's taste buds have become more adventuresome, curried lamb and barbequed lamb are being served more frequently.

So if you're looking for a different dish that's very good, try one of the following quickly prepared lamb recipes. You may be surprised at how well received they will be by your family and guests.

Sage Advice

To my way of thinking, lamb is best when it is cooked medium well to well done. There are some people, though, who like rare lamb. So, if you're preparing any of these lamb chop entrées for a small party, you might ask your guests how they like their lamb cooked.

Lamb Chops in Sherry Marinade

IT ONLY TAKES a matter of minutes to mix together this marinade, even if you take the time to press a couple of garlic cloves. Just be sure to bring the chops back to room temperature before grilling. The chops can either be grilled or prepared on the stovetop.

SERVES 4 TO 6

1 teaspoon dry mustard
1 teaspoon salt
½ teaspoon pepper
½ cup dry sherry

¼ teaspoon prepared minced garlic, or ½ teaspoon minced pressed garlic
8 lamb chops
Cookware needed: broiler pan or skillet

Sage Advice

If preparing for real lamb lovers, increase the amount of marinade made and number of lamb chops accordingly.

Combine the mustard, salt, pepper, sherry, and garlic.

Pour the mixture over the lamb chops. Cover them and refrigerate for about 3 hours, turning occasionally.

Forty minutes before broiling time, remove the chops from the refrigerator.

Broil the chops for 4 to 5 minutes on each side, basting with the marinade, or prepare on the stovetop in a heavy skillet (with a tablespoon of oil added) over medium-high heat, using the marinade for basting.

PREPARATION TIME: *5 to 10 minutes, including turning time*
TOTAL TIME: *approximately 20 minutes (plus 3 hours to marinate)*

Barbequed Lamb Chops

PREPARING barbequed lamb chops is as simple as spreading a little of your favorite light barbeque sauce on both sides of the chops, letting them rest for about 30 to 40 minutes, and then either grilling or cooking them on the stovetop as described in the previous recipe.

The
Finishing Touch

To add a finishing touch to barbequed lamb chops, garnish them with very thin lemon slices.

"Thoughtful seasoning may make a good dish into a memorable one. Experiment with various condiment and seasonings, but use them subtly so that the effect is elusive rather than overpowering."

—*THE BOSTON COOKING-SCHOOL COOK BOOK*
BY FANNIE MERRITT FARMER, 1943

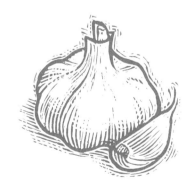

Curried Lamb

*Any experienced cook
will tell you, that there's
more than one way to
cook many dishes.
Oftentimes, time is the
controlling factor. This
is an entrée that can be
prepared with almost
equal ease in the oven or
on the stovetop. It takes
longer to cook in the
oven, but if you prepare it
on the stovetop, you have
to check on it more
frequently to be sure it
isn't cooking too quickly
or drying out.*

*The complement
ary tastes of chutney,
raisins, nuts, chopped
hard-boiled eggs, and
shredded coconut suit
curried lamb and all
curries to a tee.
Serve this dish with a big
bowl of rice and these
condiments offered in
smaller bowls for every-
one to add to their
individual liking.
(See Navy Wives Shrimp
Curry on page 101 for
another curry selection.)*

IF YOU LOVE LAMB STEWS OR CURRIES, and I do, then you've been over-joyed to find that packages of cubed lamb are now available in the meat department of your grocery store. No longer do you have to mess with cutting the meat off the shoulder (a very fatty cut of meat) or the leg. The work has been done for you. All you have to do is make a little curry paste and check on the cooking process every so often.

SERVES 8

½ cup frozen, diced onion
2 tablespoons butter
2 pounds diced lamb
2 tablespoons curry powder
1 teaspoon brown sugar

2 tablespoons distilled white or apple-cider vinegar
¼ cup milk
1 (14-ounce) can chicken broth
Cookware needed: mixing bowl, skillet with lid, baking dish or casserole (optional)

Sauté the onion in the butter.

Add the diced lamb and brown.

Blend together the curry powder, the brown sugar, and the vinegar in a mixing bowl.

Add the mixture to the meat and stir well.

Combine the milk and the chicken broth in the mixing bowl and then pour half into the meat mixture, stirring again to blend all together. Reserve the other half to be added midway through the cooking process.

At this point you can cover the skillet and cook the lamb on the stovetop, simmering for 30 to 40 minutes, or preheat the oven to 325 degrees, put the curried lamb into a baking dish, cover well with aluminum foil, and bake for 1 hour and 15 minutes.

Midway though the cooking time, or when you think it is needed, add the reserved milk and chicken broth mixture and stir well.

PREPARATION TIME: *20 minutes*
TOTAL TIME: *approximately 1 to 2 hours, depending on cooking method*

Mint Jelly Lamb Chops

WHEN I WAS A LITTLE GIRL, I always looked forward to the obligatory Easter leg of lamb—not for the lamb, but for the delicious mint jelly that was served along with it. Several years later, I was delighted when lamb chops smothered in mint jelly were the entrée at a fancy dinner party.

Licking my chops (no pun intended), I begged for the recipe. My gracious hostess produced it on a trusty index card, which I slipped into my pocket and immediately added to my recipe box when I got home. But index cards can be misplaced.

Once when I thought I had lost it, but then found it in some unlikely place, I copied the recipe down in one of my favorite cookbooks so I wouldn't have to panic in the future. But then I couldn't remember which cookbook. Now that it's in this book, I'll know where to find it.

SERVES 4 TO 8

---

1 (10-ounce) jar mint jelly
4 to 8 lamb chops

Garlic salt
Cookware needed: saucepan, broiler pan

Melt 4 or 5 tablespoons of the mint jelly in a saucepan over very low heat, or in the microwave.

Meanwhile, sprinkle the lamb chops with a generous amount of garlic salt and broil them for 4 to 5 minutes on one side.

Turn and broil them for 4 minutes on the other side.

Remove the broiler pan, spoon the melted mint jelly over the lamb chops, and return the pan to the oven and broil the chops for an additional 2 to 3 minutes.

If desired, put some more of the mint jelly on the hot chops. Otherwise, offer the remaining jelly in a bowl at the table.

PREPARATION TIME: *5 minutes*
TOTAL TIME: *20 minutes*

Sage Advice

To my way of thinking, lamb is best when it is cooked medium well to well done. There are people, though, who like rare lamb. So, if you're preparing any of these lamp chop entrées for a small party, you might ask your guests how they like their lamb cooked.

The Finishing Touch

You've figured this one out already, I'm sure. Garnish the mint jelly-glazed lamb chops with a sprig or two of fresh mint, and even a thin lemon slice to add color.

Salads, Vegetables, Potatoes, and Rice

Salads

SEVERAL years ago I read a survey that asked working women what single invention had made their lives easier. Hands down the answer was the microwave. A few years later, I read another such survey, but this time the answer was the food processor.

Today, if someone were to ask me the question, I'd say prewashed, ready-to-serve salads. Even with the help of the handy salad spinner, I have always found it takes a lot of doing to rinse and spin and then layer lettuce leaves between paper towels to soak up that last bit of unwanted moisture.

Thanks to the new cello bags of salad greens—from iceberg lettuce to mesclun—that eliminate those time-consuming steps, today's cooks can create more imaginative salads. Try some of these suggestions, most of which begin with a cello bag of healthy greens.

Lettuce, Orange, and Almond Salad

REMEMBER this deliciously light recipe when the best navel oranges begin arriving in the stores from Florida or California (if you don't live in one of those beautiful states).

Not only is this orange and almond salad a change from the usual, but it goes equally well with chicken, pork, or beef.

SERVES 6 TO 8

1 (3-ounce) package slivered almonds

2 or 3 oranges, navel (seedless) if possible, or 1 (15-ounce) can mandarin oranges

3 tablespoons olive oil

Salt and pepper, to taste

2 tablespoons lemon juice

2 packages shredded lettuce

Crumbled feta cheese, to taste

Cookware needed: mixing/salad bowl

Preheat the oven to 325 degrees.

Roast the almonds for approximately 10 minutes, and cool.

Peel and segment oranges, if using fresh, catching the juices in a bowl. Or, pour the juice from the mandarin segments into a bowl.

Add the olive oil, salt, pepper, and lemon juice to the orange juice.

Place the shredded lettuce in a serving bowl.

Add the olive oil mixture and toss well.

Place the oranges and crumbled feta cheese on top, and garnish with the almonds.

PREPARATION TIME: *10 minutes*
TOTAL TIME: *25 minutes*

Greek Salad

WHEN trying to think of a salad to jazz up an All-in-One-Meal, don't forget this one. It doesn't come in a cello bag because of the ripe olives and pepperoncini (which are, along with the feta cheese, what give Greek Salad its distinctive taste). But it's very easy to assemble once you have the ingredients, so give it a try.

SERVES 4 TO 6

For the salad:
1 small bag lettuce or mixed greens/mesclun
1 small red onion, sliced in rings (this is one time where fresh, not frozen, is necessary)
½ fresh green pepper, diced
10 pitted ripe olives
3 to 5 mild pepperoncini, sliced
1 (4-ounce) package crumbled feta cheese, either plain or one of the herb-flavored varieties

For the dressing:
⅓ cup olive oil
2 tablespoons red wine vinegar
½ teaspoon prepared minced garlic
1 teaspoon fresh oregano, chopped (or ½ teaspoon dried)
Salt and pepper, to taste
Cookware needed: 2 bowls

Combine all the salad ingredients in a bowl.

To make the dressing, whisk together all the ingredients.

Pour the dressing over the salad and toss to coat all the ingredients.

PREPARATION TIME: *10 to 15 minutes*
TOTAL TIME: *10 to 15 minutes*

Bag It!

THERE'S YET another way you can make this simple, but so wonderful modern invention work for you. Instead of dumping the salad out into a bowl and then dousing it with dressing, open the bag carefully so you don't split it down the seam. Then add the allotted amount of dressing to the lettuce in the bag and gently shake.

This trick saves you the chore of washing an extra bowl if you are using individual salad plates or bowls, plus the additional aggravation of strewing lettuce leaves all over the countertop or table while you attempt to distribute the dressing evenly—an almost impossible task in itself.

Pickled Cole Slaw

WORRIED about too much mayonnaise in your diet, or just looking for the freshest, coolest slaw you've ever eaten? This cole slaw has something else going for it too, in addition to not using mayonnaise.

It has a long refrigerator life, and because it's vinegar-based you don't have to worry about it going bad if you take it on a picnic on a hot day.

In fact, I got the recipe from my former husband's aunt's cook, Bird, back in the 1960s. They lived in South Carolina, where it really did get hot in that big, 1850s un-air-conditioned house! Bird, who made the slaw from scratch starting with a head of cabbage from her garden, called it "pickled" cole slaw because of the vinegar—a name that has stuck with me all these years.

Many are the times when I've taken the fifteen minutes required to mix up this slaw the night before (it needs some chilling time for the flavors to blend), and served it the next day along with storebought barbeque (make mine Eastern North Carolina pork barbeque, please) and fried chicken, plus some *From Storebought to Homemade* A Side of Beans (page 281) and Jalapeño Corn Bread (page 230). Then I've sat back and accepted the compliments.

SERVES 6

■·■■■■■■■

1 (14-ounce) package slaw (cabbage-based)

½ cup frozen and defrosted, diced green pepper

½ cup frozen and defrosted, diced red pepper (optional)

½ cup diced celery

½ cup distilled white vinegar

2 tablespoons sugar

1 tablespoon celery seed

Salt and pepper, to taste

Cookware needed: mixing bowl or saucepan

Combine the already shredded slaw, peppers, and diced celery (remember the salad-bar trick).

Either in a saucepan on the stovetop or in a bowl in the microwave, heat the vinegar, sugar, celery seed, and salt and pepper over medium-high for 2 to 3 minutes, until the sugar has dissolved. Stir with a wooden spoon, and do not let the mixture burn.

Pour the warm liquid over the slaw, and refrigerate the salad for several hours. Then enjoy the best cole slaw you ever tasted.

■■■■■■■■

PREPARATION TIME: *10 to 15 minutes*
TOTAL TIME: *at least 6 hours to chill*

Frozen Slaw

A VARIATION on Bird's Pickled Cole Slaw, this Frozen Slaw would be suitable for an indoor buffet, but would hardly work for a picnic. Still, it is novel enough to deserve sharing.

SERVES 6

For the dressing:
2 cups sugar
1 cup distilled white vinegar

½ cup water
1 teaspoon celery seed
Cookware needed: mixing bowl, cake pan

Combine the slaw mixture, green pepper, and celery in a large mixing bowl, as for the earlier recipe. Stir in 1½ tablespoons of salt. Cover the bowl and let the slaw stand for 2 hours, then drain it thoroughly. Transfer the slaw into a metal cake pan. (The metal conducts the cold more quickly.)

Combine all the ingredients in a saucepan and prepare as for the Pickled Slaw.

When the sugar has thoroughly dissolved, pour the dressing over the cabbage mixture, cover, and freeze for several hours. Then slice and serve.

PREPARATION TIME: *15 minutes*
TOTAL TIME: *several hours for chilling and freezing*

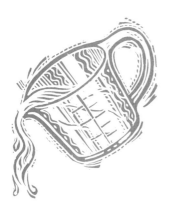

Confetti Beans with Jalapeño

LOOKING for a pretty salad to serve with a steak or chops or even fried chicken? Try this mixture made by opening cans and bags—the amounts of all the contents of which you can adjust to your own likes and tastes.

SERVES 10 TO 12

2 (15-ounce) cans black beans, drained and rinsed

1 (15 ½-ounce) can garbanzo beans, drained and rinsed

1 (10-ounce) bag frozen corn kernels

1 (10-ounce) bag frozen, mixed bell peppers (red, green, and yellow)

3 stalks celery, finely chopped (or about 1 cup if you're buying it from a salad bar)

½ cup diced onions (the frozen variety is fine)

¼ cup diced jalapeño peppers from a can (or to your taste)

1 cup Italian-style salad dressing of your choice (not creamy)

Cookware needed: large mixing bowl

While you are draining the canned beans and preparing the celery, allow the frozen ingredients to thaw on paper towels to absorb the extra moisture.

Then, combine all the vegetable ingredients in a large mixing bowl.

Add the Italian dressing and toss well.

Chill 6 hours before serving.

PREPARATION TIME: *10 minutes*
TOTAL TIME: *10 minutes plus the additional chilling time*

Artichoke, Rice, and Pepper Salad

IF YOU'RE looking for a really unusual salad to pick up an ordinary meal, try this. The multicolored peppers make it as colorful as the Confetti Beans salad, and the curry adds the same element of surprise here that the jalapeños do in that one.

Sage Advice

This salad will hold well in the refrigerator for a day or so.

SERVES 6

1 (6-ounce) package Chicken Vermicelli Rice Mix or another flavored rice

2 (6-ounce) jars marinated artichoke hearts

¼ cup mayonnaise

½ to ¾ teaspoons curry powder

¼ cup frozen, diced onions

¼ cup pimiento-stuffed olives, drained and sliced

¼ cup frozen, diced peppers (red, green, and yellow combination) or strips of peppers if you prefer to use them as a garnish

Cookware needed: saucepan, small bowl, mixing bowl

Cook the rice according to package directions, and while it is cooling, prepare the other ingredients.

Drain the artichokes, reserving the liquid from 1 jar, and slice them into halves or quarters.

Combine the artichoke liquid, mayonnaise, and curry powder.

Combine the rice, artichokes, onion, diced peppers (if using in the salad), and olives in a mixing bowl, toss with the curry mixture, and chill. If diced peppers are omitted, garnish with sliced peppers on top of the salad if it is served in a bowl, or over the individual portions.

PREPARATION TIME: *15 minutes*
TOTAL TIME: *15 minutes, plus the additional time to cook the rice and chill the salad*

Shrimp-Filled Avocado Salad

THIS RICH and delicious salad can be used as an elegant first course for a seated dinner, the main course for a ladies' luncheon, or the perfect accompaniment for a holiday meal when you want something a little different and showy to celebrate the festivity of the season.

It takes literally no time to prepare, but it can't be tossed together in one bowl—unless, that is, you dice the avocado, chop the shrimp, mix in the dressing, sprinkle it extra-well with lemon, and then serve it on a bed of shredded lettuce.

The Finishing Touch

If you love lemon as much as I do, garnish each portion with a slice or even a wedge of lemon that can be squeezed over the salad just before digging in.

SERVES 6

½ cup zesty Italian-style dressing of your choice

⅓ cup mayonnaise

⅛ teaspoon pepper (preferably white, if on hand)

Juice of ½ lemon plus 1 tablespoon

3 pounds medium (not large) cooked shrimp, purchased from the fish section of the grocery store, or bought frozen and thoroughly thawed

3 ripe avocados

Cookware needed: medium mixing bowl

In a medium bowl, combine the dressing, mayonnaise, pepper, and 1 tablespoon lemon juice. Add the shrimp and toss lightly.

Refrigerate overnight.

Just before serving, peel, halve, and pit the avocados.

Place each avocado half on a plate, cavity-side-up, and take a moment to squeeze a few drops of juice from the ½ lemon over each (this keeps the color fresh).

Fill the avocado halves to overflowing with the shrimp mixture.

PREPARATION TIME: *15 to 20 minutes*
TOTAL TIME: *20 minutes, plus overnight refrigeration time*

Grapefruit, Avocado, and Shrimp Salad

IF YOU ARE planning an extra-fancy dinner party where you might be serving beef or chicken, try this super-easy salad that is absolutely delicious, different, and instantly prepared. In fact, the hardest thing about this recipe is deciding which dressing you want to use on it.

**SERVES 8 AS A FIRST COURSE OR
4 AS A MAIN COURSE**

1 cup shrimp, frozen and ready to serve, or from the seafood counter

1 jar grapefruit sections, drained

1 medium avocado, cubed

¼ cup dressing of your choice (see instructions)

1 head "living" (or hydroponic), or Boston lettuce

Cookware needed: mixing bowl

Sage Advice

You can substitute lobster pieces or even the now-popular imitation lobster for the shrimp.

Thaw shrimp, if using frozen, pat them dry, and combine them with the grapefruit sections and cubed avocado.

Decide which dressing you wish to use. A vinaigrette, poppy, light French, or another lightly flavored dressing (not spicy) would be the right choice. Measure the dressing (you do not want to drown this salad in dressing or overpower the light, distinctive flavors of the shrimp, avocado, and grapefruit), add it to the other ingredients, and toss gently.

Cover and refrigerate the salad for 30 to 45 minutes, then spoon it onto the pretty lettuce leaves.

PREPARATION TIME: *10 minutes*
TOTAL TIME: *50 to 60 minutes*

Stalking the Ripe Avocado

"JUST THINKING about shrimp and avocados makes my mouth water," I said to Charlotte Sizer, my trusty assistant. "Trouble is, lots of people don't know how to tell a raw avocado from a ripe one," I added.

"Like the man who stole our avocados," Charlotte

laughed, remembering those days when, as a little girl, she lived in Miami, that semitropical region where people gather bright green key limes, sweet coconuts, juicy mangos, and, yes, ripe avocados from trees growing right in their own yards.

It seems that there was a

particularly large and beautiful avocado tree in Charlotte's family's backyard, which yielded plentiful fruit. Called "alligator pears," those avocados were bumpy and, when ripe, very dark green (almost black), shiny, and soft to the touch.

"There were alleys behind

Avocado and Tomato Salad

TOMATO, mozzarella, and basil salad has become a popular standard. As well it should be. It's delicious. But there's an alternative salad that is just as simple to assemble and will be a change—avocado and tomato salad.

SERVES 6 TO 8

1 to 2 ripe avocados

Juice of ½ lemon

3 to 4 tomatoes

Lettuce leaves (a mixture of romaine and endive, or bagged lettuce)

Light dressing (see *Sage Advice*)

Cookware needed: individual plates

Sage Advice

For the dressing, I recommend a balsamic vinaigrette or one of the fancier tomato vinaigrettes. Catalina is another possibility, but it should be used sparingly so the distinctive avocado taste is not overwhelmed.

Peel the avocado and cut into slices. Sprinkle these with lemon juice to keep them green.

Cut the tomatoes into slices or wedges.

Arrange the avocados and tomatoes on the lettuce and drizzle the salad with a light dressing. If using endive, alternate the leaves with the tomatoes and avocado.

PREPARATION TIME: *10 minutes*
TOTAL TIME: *10 minutes*

the houses in Miami Shores," Charlotte continued, "and one evening, just before dark, I walked into the kitchen, looked out the back window, and saw a pickup truck parked in the corner of the garden under the avocado tree.

"A man was very carefully, so he wouldn't bruise the fruit, picking the bright green avocados off the tree," she explained.

"Rather than calling the police, my mother and I watched him, grateful that we would not have to gather all of the avocados when they ripened, turned black, and fell to the ground—all the while laughing at the surprise the man would get when he discovered that, as beautiful as the green avocados looked, the fruit he was stealing was still raw, gritty,

and unsuitable for eating."

So how *do* you tell a good avocado? Simple.

You go to the grocery story and look for an avocado that is soft to the touch and appears to be on the verge of rotting—dark green to black.

Or you just get the avocado with the little white sticker on it that says "RIPE!"

English Pea and Potato Salad

I STILL remember how delicious this fresh, light, mayonnaise-free potato salad tasted when I had it in England some twenty years ago. There was no way to get the recipe for it, so I picked through my serving—potatoes, celery, peas, and then all those little specks that had to be herbs. It was held together with a wonderful light dressing, something as simple as oil and vinegar.

As soon as I recovered from the inevitable jet lag, I was in the kitchen trying to re-create this English delicacy. Several days had passed since that memorable meal, so my taste buds and memories weren't exactly crystal clear. But this Americanization of the ingredients comes close, and it always receives lots of attention when I serve it, especially in the summer.

Sage Advice

Whole olives or a relish make a nice complement to this salad.

SERVES 8 OR MORE

10 to 12 small new potatoes, unpeeled

1 (8-ounce) bottle Italian-style dressing, regular or zesty, but not creamy

1 (10-ounce) package frozen petite peas

1 cup celery, diced

Salt and pepper, to taste

Cookware needed: saucepan, microwave-safe bowl

The Finishing Touch

Particularly good to serve at a buffet along with mayonnaise-based salads—a nice alternative to pasta salad.

Wash the potatoes, cutting away any bad spots. Dice, put them in a saucepan, and cover them with cold, lightly salted water.

Boil until just soft, or for about 10 minutes.

While the potatoes boil, open the peas into a microwave-safe bowl, add just enough water to barely cover them, and microwave on high for 2 to 3 minutes, or just long enough to thoroughly defrost them.

When the potatoes are done, drain and return them to the saucepan. Then drown, while still warm, with the dressing. Drain the peas and add them to the saucepan followed by the diced celery; toss all the ingredients together, and season to taste.

Transfer all to a serving bowl, and chill before serving.

PREPARATION TIME: *20 minutes*
TOTAL TIME: *2 hours to chill well*

Ham It Up Salad

THIS hearty salad is a great side dish for those times when you're throwing together a simple soup for a trouble-free, but delicious meal. The smoked sausage links make this more substantial than the usual lettuce and tomato salad. The hard-boiled eggs are a plus if you have the time to prepare them, although it is just fine without them.

SERVES 6

6 Roma tomatoes, cut into eighths

2 packages lettuce—Italian, Romaine, or European mix

12 to 18 pitted ripe olives

1 bunch green onions, sliced

1 heaping teaspoon diced pimiento

½ cup vinaigrette or Italian-style dressing (regular, not creamy)

Salt and pepper, to taste

6 to 8 cooked smoked sausage links, sliced or 1 (8-ounce) package of small diced ham bits

4 hard-boiled eggs, quartered (optional)

Cookware needed: mixing/salad bowl

Place lettuce pieces in a salad bowl.

Distribute the tomatoes over the lettuce. Scatter the olives, green onions, and pimiento over all.

Pour the dressing over the salad.

Add a little salt and pepper if you wish.

Garnish the salad with the sausage and eggs, if you are using them.

PREPARATION TIME: *10 minutes*
TOTAL TIME: *10 minutes, or longer if eggs are included*

Sage Advice

You can add to, or subtract from, the number of olives and sausages or ham given in the recipe, according to your preference. Also, so you can plan on how much salad you wish to prepare, this recipe will make 6 ample servings—sometimes more. Experience has taught me that some people like lots of salad, and some, given the choice, take only a couple of lettuce leaves—and then only to be polite.

" It's difficult to think anything but pleasant thoughts while eating a home-grown tomato."

—LEWIS GRIZZARD,
SOUTHERN HUMORIST

Shrimp and Snow Pea Salad

THE RED BELL PEPPER and pink shrimp give this salad a cheerful look. It makes it a great accompaniment for any monochromatic chicken entrée—such as the Champagne Chicken (page 88) or Timeless Chicken (page 97). Feel free to add just a few water chestnuts if you like, and, whatever you do, be sure not to overcook the snow peas.

Sage Advice

Sugar brings soy sauce to life. The addition of just a teaspoon gives the dressing in this recipe an extra-tasty zing.

SERVES 4 TO 6

1 (10-ounce) box frozen snow peas, cooked according to package directions, and cooled

1 tablespoon soy sauce

2 tablespoons lemon juice

1 teaspoon sugar (optional)

3 tablespoons peanut oil

1 small red bell pepper, diced

8 ounces frozen, cooked, and cleaned shrimp, salad size or larger, thoroughly defrosted

1 (4-ounce) can sliced mushrooms, drained

Cookware needed: saucepan, mixing bowl

The Finishing Touch

For serving, mound the salad onto a leaf of Boston lettuce, and sprinkle it with toasted sesame seeds.

Place the snow peas into boiling salted water. Cook for 3 minutes after water returns to a boil. Drain and refresh in cold water. Cool to room temperature.

Combine the soy sauce, lemon juice, sugar if you're using it, and oil in a mixing bowl.

Add the bell pepper, shrimp, mushrooms, and snow peas, and toss to coat all the ingredients with the dressing.

PREPARATION TIME: *10 minutes*
TOTAL TIME: *30 minutes*

Too, Too Tabouli Salad

I WAS introduced to tabouli, or tabuleh, or tabooleh, at a wedding reception. I didn't have a clue what I was eating, but I was hooked. That was long before the convenient boxed varieties became available on our neighborhood grocery shelves. Nevertheless, I was determined to make it, and so I did—spending much time soaking, chopping, and dicing.

Nowadays, I grab a box, follow the directions, and then add a few extra touches left over from those long ago "from-scratch" days. They do involve some chopping and take a little longer, but this is one time I never complain.

If you haven't dared try this Middle Eastern salad, please do. You're missing a delicious and healthy dish if you don't. Even picky eaters go back for extra helpings, once they've tried it.

SERVES 8 TO 10

1 (5.25-ounce) box tabouli

½ cup frozen, diced green pepper, defrosted

1 small cucumber

1 to 2 scallions

5 to 6 mint leaves (optional)

Several sprigs of parsley

1 lemon

Cookware needed: mixing bowl, food processor

Prepare the tabouli according to package directions. Set it aside in the refrigerator.

While the tabouli is chilling, cut the cucumber in half lengthwise and remove and discard the seeds.

Cut the cucumber halves into several chunks. Do the same with the scallions.

Chop both in a food processor to small pieces, about the size of the diced pepper. Transfer these, and the diced pepper, to a small bowl.

Wash and pat dry the parsley, then give it a couple of swirls in the food processor, being careful not to puree it. Add it to the pepper, cucumber, and scallions.

Hand chop the mint leaves. Although these are optional, and they definitely add to the effort, the additional flavor is worth it. Add the mint to the pepper, cucumber, scallions, and parsley.

Squeeze the juice of one lemon over the vegetables, being careful that no seeds slip by. Stir, and then add all to the tabouli.

Chill for at least 1 hour before serving.

PREPARATION TIME: *about 20 minutes*
TOTAL TIME: *1 hour and 20 minutes*

The Finishing Touch

For individual servings, spoon an ample helping into a curled lettuce leaf and garnish the dish with a few small cherry (or grape) tomatoes—sliced, halved, or whole. Or serve the salad in a large bowl without the lettuce leaves, but decorated at the center with thin lemon slices and a sprig of mint leaves or parsley.

Jelled Salads

Although I'm a great fan of today's salads in a bag, they can get monotonous when served week in and week out. When our mothers wanted an easy way to add interest, color, and variety to family meals, they turned to Jell-O—lime, lemon, Bing cherry, even blueberry Jell-O (which seems to have disappeared from the grocery shelves).

To make a jelled salad, you still have to boil the water, or warm the juice drained from the can of fruit to add to the gelatin, and it takes some time for the gelatin to jell. But these salads can always be made ahead of time and pulled out of the fridge at the last minute for lunch or supper.

Here, to add variety to your meals, are some salads that are quickly assembled and awfully good. In fact, because they aren't served as frequently these days as the stand-by green salad, jelled salads are often considered special. And there's more. Sugar free Jello-O works equally well in these recipes.

Apricot Salad

The
Finishing Touch

Sprinkle the salad with chopped nuts, if desired, just before the gelatin has set, to give it a little extra crunch. Serve cold salads—especially jelled salads—on chilled plates, if possible, but never on plates that have gotten warm or hot by being placed on the stove.

THIS TIME, baby food comes to the rescue of the modern cook! A jar of already prepared apricots saves you from having to get out the blender or sieve to prepare the fruit yourself. Another reason to put this recipe on your to-make list is that it can be mixed together all at once, which isn't true of all jelled recipes.

SERVES 8 OR MORE

⅔ cup water

⅔ cup sugar

2 (3-ounce) packages peach or apricot Jell-O

1 (8-ounce) package cream cheese, softened

1 (15-ounce) can crushed

pineapple, drained

1 (4-ounce) jar apricot baby food

1 (12-ounce) container Cool Whip, softened, at room temperature

Cookware needed: saucepan, bowl, mold or muffin tins

Combine the water, sugar, and Jell-O in a saucepan, and bring the liquid to a boil. Remove from the heat and stir in the cream cheese, blending until smooth.

Combine the pineapple, baby food, and Cool Whip, and add to Jell-O mixture.

Pour into a lightly oiled mold or individual muffin tins, and refrigerate until set.

PREPARATION TIME: *10 minutes*
TOTAL TIME: *4 hours to chill thoroughly*

Avocado Aspic

LOOKING for a salad that's a little different? Why not try an avocado aspic?

Mother used to use unflavored gelatin and add lemon juice when she made it, but it's much easier just to use lemon Jell-O instead. This unbelievably easy-to-make salad adds a nice touch to a meal and makes it seem special. Ladies particularly seem to enjoy it.

SERVES 4 TO 6

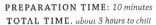

1 (3-ounce) package lemon Jell-O
1 ripe avocado

2 tablespoons mayonnaise
Cookware needed: square baking dish or casserole, mixing bowl

Prepare the Jell-O according to package directions. Transfer it to a square baking dish, and place it in the refrigerator to cool.

Mash the avocado and stir in the mayonnaise to make a smooth paste.

When the Jell-O is partially set, or after about 30 minutes, fold in the avocado mixture and return the mixture to the refrigerator until completely set.

Cut into squares to serve.

PREPARATION TIME: *10 minutes*
TOTAL TIME: *about 3 hours to chill*

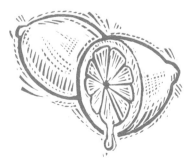

The Finishing Touch

Serve on lettuce leaves with a dollop of mayonnaise on the side, topped with a thin slice of lemon, and, if you wish, a slice of avocado.

" When the salad is served as a separate course, pass with it crackers which have been spread with butter or some tasty cheese, and crisped in the oven. If the buttered crackers are used, serve cream cheese with them."

—*THE BUTTERICK COOK BOOK*, EDITED BY HELENA JUDSON, 1911

Cream Cheese Salad

OF ALL the gelatin recipes, this is my favorite. It's so simple that I used to help Mother prepare it when I was just a little girl in the 1940s. I don't know how, but I had forgotten it until I began looking through her old cookbooks, when I began working on this book.

At the end of the recipe, Mother had written in her well-schooled hand, "Consider the season in selecting flavor for Jell-O and mold used." I'm sure she did, but I only remember it as being green.

And in those days before central air-conditioning, when ladies wore flowered dresses with slips beneath them and glowed, rather than perspired, the pastel-green color and frothy consistency of this salad epitomized summertime to me. It still does, even when I serve it at Christmas. After all, green is a year-round color.

SERVES 6 TO 8

1 (3-ounce) package lime (or other flavor) Jell-O

2 cups hot water

1 (8-ounce) package cream cheese

½ cup chopped pecans

Cookware needed: mixing bowl, mold

The Finishing Touch

Add a few drops of food coloring to deepen the green and serve on Saint Patrick's Day! Add a dollop of whipped cream or Cool Whip, and this can become a dessert salad.

Dissolve the Jell-O in 1 cup of the hot water and the cream cheese in the second cup. Stir both until smooth.

Combine the Jello-O and cream cheese, and refrigerate approximately 30 to 45 minutes, until the mixture begins to set. Then add the chopped pecans.

Pour the "salad" into an oiled mold, and chill until set.

PREPARATION TIME: *10 minutes*
TOTAL TIME: *3 hours or until set*

Lime Yogurt Salad

THE DIFFICULT thing with multilayered jelled salads is getting the timing right. To make some recipes, it takes a battery of alarm clocks to remind you when it's time to add the ingredients or assemble the layers.

In this recipe, both layers reach the right consistency at about the same time. So, though you have to be available when the layers are ready, the job is much easier.

SERVES 8

1 (15-ounce) can sliced pears
2 (3-ounce) packages lime Jell-O
2 cups boiling water

1 (8-ounce) container vanilla-flavored yogurt
Cookware needed: saucepan, 2 mixing bowls, 8-inch square pan or salad mold

Drain the pears, reserving ½ cup of the syrup.

Dissolve the Jell-O in the boiling water, and stir well.

Measure 1 cup of the Jell-O mixture into a mixing bowl. Whisk in the yogurt and pour this mixture into a square baking pan or a lightly oiled mold.

Refrigerate until set but not firm, approximately 45 minutes, or about 10 minutes longer for a deeper mold.

Meanwhile, add the measured syrup to the remaining Jell-O, and chill until the yogurt mixture is ready.

Arrange the pear slices on the yogurt layer, and gently spoon all of the clear lime Jell-O on top. Repeat, *gently*. The Jell-O will very easily tear a hole in the delicate yogurt layer if it is added too hastily.

Return the salad to the refrigerator, and chill until firm, about 3 hours.

Cut the salad into squares, and serve it on individual plates, with or without a lettuce leaf underneath. If using a mold, dip it briefly in warm water, set a serving plate on top of the mold, and flip plate and mold over to release the salad. Place the whole salad on the table or buffet with a pretty serving spoon.

PREPARATION TIME: *15 minutes*
TOTAL TIME: *4 hours*

Sage Advice

Just as the temperatures of ovens vary, so do the temperatures of refrigerators. Further, different parts of a refrigerator can be cooler or warmer than others. This means that the cooling process for any jelled dessert can vary, and the "chilling" times given in recipes must be taken as approximate.

The Finishing Touch

This is another one of those salads that works equally well as a fruit salad or a light dessert. If using it as a salad, serve it on lettuce and accompany it with a little mayonnaise or even yogurt. But if serving it as a dessert, add extra sweetness by topping it with whipped cream or ice cream and a slice or two of lime, or an extra slice or two of pear.

Mango Soufflé

LIGHT, frothy salads are perfect for the summertime. That's a given. But often they are a welcome contrast to a heavy entrée like roast beef or even a cream-based chicken casserole, whatever the time of year.

The perfect solution—mango soufflé.

I was introduced to this Americanized tropical treat in Beaumont, Texas, where it is a real favorite. So much so that I heard about it several times before I actually tasted it!

First, I was told that my hostess would have a light snack, "and mango soufflé" waiting for me when I arrived at her home around 9 PM. When I made an interim stop before getting there, I was reminded that "Martha has some mango soufflé waiting for you."

When I did arrive at her home, Martha Hicks graciously reminded me that she had a light snack waiting, "and mango soufflé." By then my mouth was watering.

Although calling this trouble-free Jell-O salad a soufflé may be a slight exaggeration, its taste will never disappoint.

On the other hand, since a little whipped cream (or Cool Whip) served with this accompaniment immediately transforms it into a dessert, maybe calling it a soufflé is appropriate after all.

The
Finishing Touch

This pretty, apricot-colored salad is particularly lovely when served on a ruffled, red-tipped lettuce leaf. Garnish it with a slice of fresh mango, if available, or a few mandarin orange segments, whether serving it as a salad or a dessert.

SERVES 12

1 (8-ounce) package cream cheese

2 (15-ounce) cans mango

3 (3-ounce) boxes lemon Jell-O

3 cups boiling water

Cookware needed: food processor, mixing bowl

Combine the cream cheese and mango in a food processor (or blender) until perfectly smooth.

Dissolve the Jell-O in the boiling water.

Combine the mango and Jell-O mixtures and refrigerate in an oiled mold until set, approximately 3 to 4 hours.

PREPARATION TIME: *10 minutes*
TOTAL TIME: *3 to 4 hours to chill*

Orange-Pineapple Mold

THE BLENDER does all the work of preparing this simple, but very refreshing and attractive salad. Further, there's no reason to buy a whole package of carrots, then peel and chop them. Buy already sliced carrots in a cello package, or buy just the amount you need from a salad bar.

SERVES 6 TO 8

1 cup hot water

1 (3-ounce) package orange-pineapple flavored Jell-O

1 (20-ounce) can crushed pineapple, drained, juice reserved

½ cup sliced carrots

Cookware needed: blender, 1½-quart mold or ring mold

Place the hot water and Jell-O in a blender. Cover and blend for 25 seconds.

Add the reserved pineapple juice to the Jell-O in the blender. Slowly add the carrots to the mixture and blend until they are finely chopped. Turn blender off and fold in the crushed pineapple.

Pour the mixture into a lightly oiled 1½-quart (ring) mold, or into 6 to 8 individual molds.

Chill until firm, approximately 4 hours.

PREPARATION TIME: *5 minutes*
TOTAL TIME: *approximately 4 hours*

The
Finishing Touch

This is a particularly good salad to have for a luncheon when chicken salad is on the menu. Mound the chicken salad in the middle of the ring mold for a very pretty presentation.

Tangy Tomato Aspic

THERE'S an unspoken rule in the South when it comes to luncheon menus: You can't serve chicken salad without an accompaniment of tomato aspic.

When growing up, I never particularly liked tomato aspic. I preferred a few sliced tomatoes, or a jelled fruit salad. But then Tangy Tomato Aspic appeared on the scene. It's the V-8 juice combined with the lemon-flavored Jell-O that make this such a tangy and refreshing treat. Try it, with or without chicken salad.

SERVES 12

1 envelope unflavored gelatin

¼ cup cold water

6 cups V-8 juice (use the spicy variety if you want real zing)

3 (3-ounce) packages lemon Jell-O

Cookware needed: mixing bowl, saucepan, 9 x 13-inch baking dish

The
Finishing Touch

For even more flavor and a little crunch, try stirring in one (or more) of these additional ingredients about 30 minutes after the aspic has begun to set: diced green pepper, sliced Spanish olives (with, or without, the pimiento), diced celery, diced or grated onion, grated carrot.

In a small bowl, sprinkle the gelatin over the cold water to soften it.

Heat 2 ½ cups of the V-8 juice in a saucepan and stir in the lemon Jell-O until it has dissolved.

Add the unflavored gelatin and stir well.

Add the remaining juice and mix thoroughly.

Pour the mixture into a 9 x 13-inch baking dish, and refrigerate until set, approximately 3 hours.

PREPARATION TIME: *15 minutes*
TOTAL TIME: *3 hours and 15 minutes*

Vegetables and Fruits

Some memories never fade. Like the time my daughter, Joslin, called me for an old family recipe. (Well actually, you'll probably identify this as one of *your* old family recipes, too.)

Seems that she and her husband, Mike, were having friends for dinner, and she wanted to prepare her grandmother's asparagus casserole. "You know, the one we loved so much at Thanksgiving and Christmas. When you find it, give me a call, and I'll write it down," she said.

"I don't need to look it up, and you're not even going to need a pencil and paper for this one, honey," I replied, smiling to myself, remembering when my mother had told me the same thing.

"Just drain three cans of asparagus and mix them with one can of cream of mushroom soup. Toss in lots of slivered almonds. Put it in a baking dish. Top with extra-sharp Cheddar. Bake at 350 for 25 to 30 minutes, and you've got it."

"But it's so good," Joli (as I call her) exclaimed. "I thought it *had* to be complicated."

It's not. And neither are any of the other vegetable dishes included in this section.

While there seems to be an endless supply of quickly made entrée and dessert recipes available in cookbooks, there doesn't seem to be as large a selection of different, really imaginative, vegetable recipes to choose from.

Don't get me wrong. Your grocer's freezer section is filled with vegetables, but they're usually just that...the vegetable in its most basic form—peas, corn, okra, broccoli, carrots, or a mixture.

By occasionally dressing up those vegetables, your family (especially the kids, if they are young) will enjoy them more.

That's what this chapter does. It takes the basic vegetable (whether frozen, canned, or fresh) and combines it with other ingredients to make it special and provide more mealtime variety, the same way our mothers and grandmothers did—quickly and effortlessly.

The results are often so good that they will surprise you.

Artichoke and Spinach Casserole

Sage Advice

Some people prefer to place the artichoke hearts in the baking dish first, and then prepare the cream cheese and spinach mixture to put over it. But this requires an extra mixing bowl, which explains why I like to combine the mixture in the baking dish and then stir in the artichokes. By the way, I sometimes add an extra can of artichoke hearts.

The Finishing Touch

You can top this casserole with a cup of buttered bread crumbs, if you wish.

I'VE MENTIONED in the first chapter that I always stock up on artichokes when Joli is coming home. That's so I can make an Artichoke and Spinach Casserole. She's so crazy about it that, when she was pregnant, this was one of her cravings. Some people include a stick of butter with the ingredients, but frankly, we find it is just as good without it.

SERVES 8 TO 10

3 (10-ounce) packages frozen, chopped spinach

1 tablespoon lemon juice

1 (8-ounce) package cream cheese, softened

1 (14-ounce) can artichoke hearts

1 stick butter (optional)

Cookware needed: saucepan, baking dish or casserole

Preheat the oven to 350 degrees.

In a saucepan, warm the frozen, chopped spinach over low heat just enough to thoroughly defrost it, or defrost in the microwave.

Drain the spinach very well, squeezing it if necessary, and put it into a baking dish.

Squeeze the lemon juice over the spinach, add the cream cheese, and blend well with a fork.

Stir in the artichoke hearts and bake for 30 to 35 minutes.

PREPARATION TIME: *20 minutes*
TOTAL TIME: *approximately 1 hour*

Pureed Artichokes

THIS DELICIOUS and surprising vegetable is an excellent accompaniment to beef tenderloin or a simple chicken dish. You can make it in the blender or food processor without using any additional bowls, and then heat it according to your own schedule—in a saucepan, in a baking dish, or even in the microwave. Furthermore, the dish works equally well for a seated dinner or a buffet.

"It's a little known fact that in 1949, Marilyn Monroe, then just a budding starlet, was crowned Artichoke Queen in Castroville, California."

SERVES 4

2 (7-ounce) cans artichoke bottoms, drained

½ cup whipping cream

1 stick butter, cut in pieces

1 teaspoon salt

½ teaspoon freshly ground pepper

Cookware needed: food processor or blender, baking dish or casserole, saucepan, or microwave-safe bowl

Put the drained artichoke bottoms in a food processor or blender and chop.

Add the remaining ingredients and puree until smooth (this will take only a minute or two), scraping down the sides of the container.

Heat thoroughly (about 20 minutes in the oven at 350 degrees, 10 minutes in a saucepan over low heat, or 2 to 3 minutes in the microwave) and serve.

PREPARATION TIME: *5 minutes*
TOTAL TIME: *approximately 20 minutes*

Asparagus Casserole

IN THE INTRODUCTION to this section, I recounted telling Joli how to make that perennial favorite, Asparagus Casserole. But here it is in "proper" recipe form so you can easily find it for the holidays—or for just any day.

SERVES 6 TO 8

2 to 3 (15-ounce) cans asparagus tips or spears

1 (10-ounce) can cream of mushroom soup

½ cup slivered almonds

1 cup Cheddar cheese, grated

Cookware needed: baking dish or casserole

Preheat the oven to 350 degrees.

Drain the asparagus and put it in a baking dish, add the cream of mushroom soup and almonds, and blend.

Sprinkle the Cheddar cheese on top.

Bake for approximately 30 minutes, or until the cheese has melted and the casserole is bubbling.

PREPARATION TIME: *5 minutes*
TOTAL TIME: *35 minutes*

Thank goodness my children ate their vegetables!

OTHER MOTHERS weren't so lucky, and I still remember watching one good friend, with green beans on a fork, chasing her daughter around the house, all the while begging her to please eat just one green bean for Mr. Green Jeans, a popular TV character.

I usually served our family vegetables tossed in a little butter and salt and pepper in the saucepan while they were cooking.

At mealtime, we may have had barbequed chicken or pork chops prepared with cream of mushroom soup, but the vegetables were served au naturel.

But that doesn't mean I never whipped up a Vidalia Onion Casserole or Tomato Puddin'. I did and I do. But only when serving a simple steak, chops, or fish.

In fact, in my storehouse of memorable meals is a menu from one "fancy" dinner party that totally failed because the hostess served nothing but casseroles. The meat was in a casserole, the potatoes were in a casserole, the green beans were in a casserole, and the broccoli was in a casserole. My entire plate was a puddle of cream-colored, cream-based food that all tasted alike.

So, when planning your meals, remember that simply served vegetables are sometimes the best choice. If you want to dress them up just a little, sprinkle them with toasted sesame seeds or French Fried Onion Bits, or stir in a few toasted almond slivers (almondine), or even crunchy pine nuts.

Broccoli, Dressed-Up with Fried Bread Crumbs

JUST LIKE quiche did a few years ago, broccoli is taking it on the chin these days. I wonder if former President Bush would have been so critical of this nutritious vegetable if he'd been served Broccoli, Dressed-Up with Fried Bread Crumbs.

SERVES 4 TO 8, DEPENDING ON THE AMOUNT OF BROCCOLI USED

1 to 2 (14-ounce) bags frozen broccoli florets (or pieces with stems), thawed

6 tablespoons butter

6 tablespoons dry bread crumbs

1 hard-boiled egg, chopped (optional)

Salt and pepper, to taste

Juice of 1 lemon

Cookware needed: skillet, aluminum pan or heat-resistant bowl

Melt 4 tablespoons of the butter in a skillet, and fry the bread crumbs, stirring until lightly browned.

Transfer the bread crumbs to an aluminum pan (or heat-resistant bowl) and set it on the back of the stove to keep warm. Add the chopped egg (if including) and salt and pepper to taste.

Put the remaining 2 tablespoons of butter in the skillet, add the broccoli, sprinkle it with the lemon juice, and cook until heated through.

Arrange the broccoli on a serving platter and garnish it with the buttery bread crumbs.

PREPARATION TIME: *15 minutes*
TOTAL TIME: *15 minutes*

The
Finishing Touch

Create a sweeter dish by eliminating the bread crumbs and adding ¾ cup raisins (golden or brown) to the broccoli while it is heating. Then garnish the dish with 2 ounces of slivered, toasted almonds.

Broccoli au Gratin

TRY serving the prevous broccoli recipe "au gratin" by putting the vegetable and the bread-crumb mixture in a baking dish after it has heated through, and covering it completely with additional dry bread crumbs, dots of butter, and grated cheese.

Run this under a preheated broiler, 5 inches below the heat for less than 5 minutes, until a glazed, golden crust has formed. Beware of stepping away from the kitchen when you have food under a broiler—it browns very quickly.

Sage Advice

The finished product will be more moist, or "fondant" in texture if you select an American or Cheddar cheese, and drier if you use Parmesan or Romano.

SERVES 8

PREPARATION TIME: *15 minutes*
TOTAL TIME: *20 minutes*

Dressed-Up Broccoli Casserole

YOU CAN create a creamy version of the Broccoli, Dressed-Up with Fried Bread Crumbs (page 153) by adding 1 (10-ounce) can of a cream-based soup [(broccoli, celery, chicken), diluted with enough milk or cream to make it pourable (about ½ cup)], to the broccoli and bread crumbs, and pouring the mixture into a buttered baking dish.

Sprinkle the top with crushed Cornflakes or Ritz crackers and grated cheese and run it under the broiler until golden.

SERVES 8

PREPARATION TIME: *15 minutes*
TOTAL TIME: *20 minutes*

California Casserole

FOR A SLIGHT variation on the Dressed-Up Broccoli Casserole (on the previous page), use the frozen California blend of vegetables. This adds a few more vitamins, and the carrots give it the color your plate may be lacking.

SERVES 6

1 (16-ounce) bag frozen blend of broccoli, carrots, and cauliflower, thawed

1 (5-ounce) can sliced water chestnuts

1 (10-ounce) can cream-based soup (broccoli, celery, chicken)

1 soup can milk or cream

1 (3-ounce) package Parmesan cheese, grated

Cookware needed: baking dish or casserole

Preheat the oven to 325 degrees.

Combine the vegetables with the water chestnuts, and pour the mixture into a greased baking dish.

Combine the soup and milk or cream, and pour this mixture over the vegetables.

Top with Parmesan cheese, and bake for 35 minutes, or until bubbly.

PREPARATION TIME. *10 minutes*
TOTAL TIME: *approximately 45 minutes*

Carrot Surprise

WHAT'S IN A CAKE? Eggs, sugar, flour, vanilla. We know how good that is. Add the natural sweetness of baby carrots and you have an especially tasty combination. One that even the picky vegetable eaters will eat and then ask, What *is* this? That's why my friend Elizabeth Clement calls this recipe her Carrot Surprise.

SERVES 4

" I think people get more tired of vegetables fixed the same way than of anything else about a meal. I am always on the lookout for new and interesting ways to vary the cooking of vegetables to eliminate this monotony."

—VIRGINIA MCDONALD, *HOW I COOK IT*, 1949

1 (1-pound) bag baby carrots
1 stick butter, melted
3 eggs
½ cup sugar

3 tablespoons flour
1 teaspoon baking powder
1½ teaspoons vanilla extract
Cookware needed: blender, baking dish or casserole

Preheat the oven to 350 degrees.

Boil the carrots in water until tender, about 15 minutes. Drain.

Transfer the carrots to a blender, add the butter, and blend for 1 minute.

Add the remaining ingredients, and blend well.

Pour the carrot mixture into a greased baking dish, and bake for 45 minutes.

PREPARATION TIME: *15 minutes*
TOTAL TIME: *60 minutes*

Glazed Carrots

SOME recipes (like tuna casserole) have been around so long that I assume everyone knows them. Not so, as I've discovered while writing this book.

Take glazed carrots, for example. Just the other day, while I was visiting with my daughter and some of her friends, the age-old question, "How *do* you get the kids to eat their veggies?" came up.

Invariably, the recipes started flying—including a couple for glazed carrots. When the pens and scraps of paper came out, I knew what the kids in that neighborhood were going to be eating that night! And I realized that some of the moms were going to be fixing glazed carrots for the first time.

Hopefully, the parents were going to be eating them too. They're tasty and good for you, and a cinch to make in no time at all

SERVES 4

3 tablespoons butter
2 tablespoons brown sugar
1 can Le Seur baby carrots

Cookware needed: saucepan or microwave-safe bowl

Combine the butter and brown sugar in a saucepan, for stovetop cooking, or a microwave safe bowl. Heat over medium-low or in the microwave just long enough to melt and blend the ingredients.

Add the baby carrots, and stir gently. Heat until warm.

PREPARATION TIME: *3 minutes*
TOTAL TIME: *10 minutes*

Glazed Carrots with Onions

FOR MORE adult palates, try this variation.

SERVES 8

3 tablespoons butter

2 tablespoons peanut oil

1 (2-pound) bag baby carrots

½ cup frozen, chopped onion

2 teaspoons fresh thyme

2 tablespoons brown sugar

1 tablespoon water

Salt and pepper, to taste

Cookware needed: skillet with a lid

Heat the butter and oil in a skillet with a lid.

Add the carrots, onion, thyme, brown sugar, and water.

Season with salt and pepper to taste and mix well.

Simmer, covered, for 15 minutes, stirring from time to time.

Remove the cover and cook another 5 minutes on high heat until the liquid is reduced to a syrupy glaze.

The
Finishing Touch

Garnish the finished dish with chopped parsley, if you wish.

PREPARATION TIME: *3 to 5 minutes*
TOTAL TIME: *approximately 25 minutes*

The Great Celery Mystery

FOR THE LIFE OF ME, I can't figure it out, and neither can some of my chef friends.

We can buy frozen seasoning blends and soup starters that have celery in them.

Why, then, can't we buy packages of frozen, diced celery? A tremendous number of recipes, whether they are meat or vegetable casseroles, mixed vegetable dishes prepared on the stovetop in a skillet, or salads, call for diced celery. Frozen, diced onions and peppers (the red, green, and yellow, sweet or bell varieties) are available, *why* not celery?

Celery Casserole

FEW PEOPLE cook a celery casserole, and I know why. It takes too much time to cut, chop, and dice the main ingredients. Sometimes, when I've been really pushed for time but I wanted to serve this vegetable accompaniment, I've raided the chopped-celery bin at the salad bar. (One time, a fellow customer actually asked me what I was going to do with it! I was tempted to say something about rabbits, but I didn't.)

This is actually a very good casserole, and one that I hope will become more popular. I had it the first time at Geri Winstead's house around 1970, and I've never forgotten it.

SERVES 6

3 cups diced celery

¼ cup slivered almonds

1 (5-ounce) can sliced water chestnuts

1 (10-ounce) can cream of chicken soup or 1 (10-ounce) can cream of celery soup (for a vegetarian version)

¾ cup half-and-half

1 (4-ounce) can sliced mushrooms, drained

Salt and pepper, to taste

Dash Worcestershire sauce

½ cup Parmesan cheese, grated

½ cup Ritz cracker crumbs

Cookware needed: small saucepan, 1 ½-quart baking dish or casserole

Preheat the oven to 350 degrees.

Boil the celery until almost tender, approximately 5 minutes. Drain well and put it in the bottom of a baking dish.

Add almonds and water chestnuts to the celery.

Empty the soup into a saucepan, and slowly stir in the half-and-half. Add the mushrooms, salt, pepper, and Worcestershire sauce, and heat over low heat until bubbly.

Pour the soup mixture over the celery, then sprinkle all with the Parmesan and cracker crumbs.

Bake until hot and bubbly, about 25 to 30 minutes.

PREPARATION TIME: *15 minutes, or less if you buy the celery already diced*

TOTAL TIME: *approximately 45 minutes*

Scalloped Corn

WHEN THE SNOW is knee-deep up New Hampshire way and writer Bea Cole is trying to make a newspaper deadline—she also takes care of her three active daughters—she often relies on this trusty, sure-to-please, dinner standby.

SERVES 4 TO 6

1 (15-ounce) can corn kernels

1 cup Cornflakes

¾ cup milk

1 tablespoon butter

Cookware needed: baking dish or casserole, with lid

Preheat the oven to 350 degrees.

Combine the corn, Cornflakes, and milk in a greased baking dish.

Dot the top with the butter.

Cover and bake for 30 minutes, or until milk is absorbed. Stir occasionally.

Serve hot.

PREPARATION TIME: *5 minutes*

TOTAL TIME: *35 minutes*

"It is not elegant to gnaw Indian corn.

The kernels should be scored with a knife,

scraped off into the plate, and then eaten with a

fork. Ladies should be particulary careful how

they manage to ticklish a dainty,

lest the exhibition rub off a little desirable

romance."

—CHARLES DAY, *HINTS ON ETIQUETTE,* 1844

Eggplant Soufflé

THERE'S nothing prettier than unblemished, deep purple eggplants piled high in a basket at the farmer's market. At the height of the summer, eggplant is like squash—so plentiful, it goes begging. That's when I buy twice as much eggplant as we can possibly eat, even if I served it for breakfast—not an appetizing thought.

Then I move on to the baskets of zucchini and crookneck squash and buy double portions of those.

When I get my bounty home, I first arrange a big bowl of the vegetables for the dining room table. What's left over goes into the kitchen.

Though I love fried eggplant, I've usually overstayed at the market, chatting with friends, exchanging recipes, and just enjoying the day. Now I don't have the time or the inclination to stand over a hot skillet and turn each carefully battered eggplant slice at that split second when it reaches golden brown.

It's much easier just to boil some water, get a bag of grated cheese from the refrigerator, take down the canister of storebought bread crumbs, and whip up an eggplant soufflé. It will be ready by the time I've sliced some homegrown tomatoes and put out the baked beans, slaw, and chicken I grabbed from the Colonel on the way home from the market.

SERVES 6 TO 8

2 medium eggplants
½ plus ⅛ teaspoon salt
2 tablespoons butter
2 eggs, lightly beaten
⅓ cup milk

⅛ teaspoon pepper
1 cup Cheddar cheese, grated
1 cup bread crumbs
Paprika
Cookware needed: saucepan, baking dish or casserole

Peel and cube the eggplant.

Place the eggplant in a saucepan and cover it with water to which ½ teaspoon salt has been added. Cook until soft, or about 10 minutes.

Drain the water, and mash the eggplant.

Add the butter, eggs, milk, the remaining salt, and the pepper, and blend well.

Preheat the oven to 350 degrees.

Put a layer of the eggplant mixture in a well-greased baking dish.

Spread a layer of cheese and then a layer of bread crumbs on top.

Repeat these layers, ending with the bread crumbs. Sprinkle the top with paprika.

Bake for 30 to 40 minutes or until set.

PREPARATION TIME: *20 minutes*
TOTAL TIME: *approximately 60 minutes*

ETZ Casserole

(Eggplant, Tomato, Zucchini Casserole)

OK. You bought the eggplant and zucchini at the market, not the grocery store. And the fresh tomatoes may have come from a neighbor's yard, or even your own yard. Not *every* single recipe in this book is made from *all* storebought canned or frozen ingredients. But the cheese and bread crumbs are definitely from the store.

And so, just in case you've gone overboard on the tomatoes, too, here is a quick and sure way to use all three of your fresh ingredients from the market, or from the fresh produce department of the grocery store.

SERVES 6 TO 8

Sage Advice

Our mothers always added "just a pinch" of sugar to any dish with tomatoes in it. Today, most canned tomatoes are already well flavored. But when preparing a casserole or skillet recipe that calls for **fresh tomatoes**, *a pinch of sugar (¼ to ½ teaspoon) helps cut the natural acidity of the tomatoes.*

3 tablespoons olive oil

½ cup frozen, diced combo of onion and green pepper, or some of each

1 clove garlic, minced, or ½ teaspoon prepared garlic

1 medium eggplant, cubed

2 or 3 medium zucchini, sliced

3 or 4 medium tomatoes, peeled and cut into small chunks

½ cup stuffed Spanish olive pieces (not whole)

¼ teaspoon sugar (see *Sage Advice*)

Salt and pepper, to taste

¾ cup unflavored and dry bread crumbs

¾ cup Parmesan cheese, grated

Cookware needed: covered skillet, baking dish or casserole

In a skillet with a lid, heat the olive oil, and sauté the onion, green pepper, and garlic for 2 to 3 minutes.

Add the eggplant and the zucchini, and cook over medium heat until the vegetables are soft, approximately 10 to 15 minutes.

Preheat the oven to 325 degrees.

Add the tomatoes, the olive pieces, and salt and pepper to taste. Cover the skillet and cook the mixture another 10 minutes.

Pour the mixture into a lightly greased baking dish, and top the vegetables with bread crumbs and Parmesan cheese.

Bake for 30 to 40 minutes.

PREPARATION TIME: *15 to 20 minutes*
TOTAL TIME: *approximately 1 hour*

Green Bean Bundles

REMEMBER Goldy Bear's caterer's advice to always use the French name for food? This green bean dish comes to you from the ladies of Beaumont, Texas, who sometimes call it "Paquets de Haricots Verts."

It matters not what you call it, or actually whether you use green beans or flat, Italian pole beans. This a delicious and ingenious way to serve green beans for a large buffet.

SERVES 9 TO 12

15 to 16 strips bacon

1 box plain wooden toothpicks (use as many as you need)

3 (15 ounce) cans whole green beans, or Italian pole beans, drained

1 cup brown sugar

1 cup butter, melted

½ teaspoon garlic salt

Soy sauce, to taste

Cookware needed: mixing bowl, 9 x 13-inch baking dish or casserole

Cut the bacon strips in half lengthwise.

Wrap 9 or 10 green beans in a "bundle" (or stack them if using the pole beans) using the bacon strips to "tie" them, and secure the bundles with toothpicks.

Place the bundles in a baking dish.

Combine the brown sugar, butter, garlic salt, and a splash of soy sauce, and pour the mixture over the bundles.

Refrigerate overnight.

Preheat the oven to 350 degrees.

Bake the beans uncovered for 30 minutes.

PREPARATION TIME: *15 minutes*
TOTAL TIME: *45 minutes*

Sage Advice

Experiment. Be creative. Have fun. That's just as much a part of cooking as the eating to my way of thinking. And that's just what I did when trying to dress up a simple chicken and rice main course for dinner. I really didn't have time to "bundle" the beans in the bacon. Furthermore, I only had turkey bacon on hand. Add to that, Bob is borderline diabetic (inherited, so I avoid dishes requiring lots of sugar). I simply put the contents of 1 (15-ounce) can of whole green beans, drained, between 6 turkey bacon strips in a small round baking dish (3 strips on top; 3 strips on bottom). Instead of preparing the ample amount of brown sugar and butter marinade called for in the recipe, I made a much smaller amount by using a heaping tablespoon of DiabetiSweet™ and an equal amount of Land O Lakes honey butter, plus some soy sauce and garlic salt. It was simple, easy, took no time, and was delicious. Just the right accompaniment.

Green Bean Casserole

Sage Advice

Of course, you can cook the green beans first if you wish, but they will cook perfectly well this way too. Or, if you wish, use 1 (14-ounce) can of French-style string beans and simply drain them before combining them with the mushroom soup.

To the above recipe, add 1/2 package of Lipton's onion soup mix (dry), omit the French fried onions, and spread the top with a thin layer of packaged dry bread crumbs—combined with butter, or Cheddar cheese, if you wish.

Some people like to add one or more of the following ingredients to the green bean and mushroom soup combination: small peas, slivered almonds, sliced green olives, pimientos.

IF YOU'RE flipping through this book looking for new and different recipes, you should keep turning the pages because this green bean casserole has been a standard on almost every American dinner table for decades.

Whenever the Jenkins family held a large get-together or gathered for a holiday meal, Shipley Jenkins, my sister-in-law, offered to bring the green bean casserole. In fact, it got to the point where we'd just call Shipley and say, "Be sure to bring the green bean casserole," because that was what she was going to do anyway.

Since my kids loved Aunt Shipley and her green bean casserole, I was always delighted to know they'd have a favorite vegetable dish for these occasions, no matter what else happened to show up on the table.

The version given below is the simplest of all green bean casserole recipes, but read on to the variations for some additional ideas about how to prepare it.

SERVES 4 TO 6

1 (16-ounce) bag frozen French-style green beans

1 (10-ounce) can cream of mushroom soup

1 (2.8-ounce) can French Fried Onion Bits (a fat-free variety is now available)

Cookware needed: baking dish or casserole

Preheat the oven to 350 degrees.

Allow the string beans to defrost slightly, then combine them with the mushroom soup in a baking dish.

Lavishly sprinkle the top with as many of the onion toppers as you wish (or the ones you have left after nibbling on them while preparing the rest of the casserole).

Bake for 30 minutes or until bubbly.

PREPARATION TIME: *5 minutes*
TOTAL TIME: *35 minutes*

Cheerful Green Beans

ONE HOSTESS who served this colorful and quite delicious green bean dish called it her "Christmas" green beans. But it's too good to have just once a year, so I prefer to call it "Cheerful" green beans.

Incidentally, asparagus or broccoli may be used in place of the green beans if you like.

SERVES 4 TO 6

½ cup frozen red bell pepper strips, or 1 medium fresh pepper, cut in strips

2 tablespoons olive oil

1 teaspoon prepared garlic, or 2 cloves, finely minced

¼ cup balsamic vinegar

Salt and pepper, to taste

1 (16-ounce) bag frozen string beans, thawed (I prefer the very small, whole variety)

Cookware needed: skillet

In a skillet, sauté the pepper strips in the olive oil.

Stir in the garlic, vinegar, salt, and pepper, and add the green beans.

Cook for 3 to 4 minutes, stirring occasionally, or until the beans are thoroughly warmed.

PREPARATION TIME: *approximately 10 minutes, depending on vegetables used*

TOTAL TIME: *approximately 15 minutes, depending on vegetables used (see Sage Advice)*

Sage Advice

If you use the very small and tender string beans, you really don't have to thaw them, although you may if you prefer. If using another variety of frozen beans, you may wish to blanch them, or cook them according to package directions before combining them with the other ingredients.

The
Finishing Touch

A little freshly grated Parmesan cheese on the top is a nice finishing touch.

Vidalia Onion Casserole

GOOD RECIPES travel fast.

I first tasted Vidalia Onion Casserole in Jackson, Mississippi, while touring with my book, *Southern Christmas*. When I begged for the recipe, my hostess, Martha McIntosh, gave me a copy of the newly published Jackson Junior League cookbook, *Come On In!*

The casserole (and the cookbook) became an instant hit in our home, especially with my daughter, Joslin. After graduating from college, when she moved to Richmond, Virginia, and began cooking and entertaining on her own, Joli copied the recipe down on an index card and kept it close at hand.

Like her mother and grandmother before her, Joslin soon began assembling her own collection of cookbooks. One of the first ones she bought was *Virginia Fare*, published by the Junior League of Richmond. You can imagine her delight when she found it included another, ever so slightly different recipe for Vidalia Onion Casserole.

That's the other thing about recipes. Often you can skimp on the milk and go heavy on the eggs, or substitute chicken broth for beef bouillon. You can even use Parmesan or Cheddar cheese. But there are certain main ingredients that should not be changed.

Such was the case with the two Vidalia onion casseroles. Although the secondary ingredients varied, both recipes contained the two magic components that give this casserole its soul—Vidalia onions and buttery crackers.

You can choose from several different brands of cracker (as long as they're buttery). But please. *Only* if Vidalia onions are not in season should you ever consider using a substitute. And then, be sure to use sweet yellow onions. Too pungent an onion taste doesn't work in this recipe.

If you haven't had this casserole, you're in for quite a treat, and I'll wager it will become a favorite in your house as well. Pass it on.

SERVES 8 (WELL, MAYBE ONLY 6—IT'S THAT GOOD!)

2 sticks butter

3 to 4 large Vidalia onions, sliced in rings

40 to 50 buttery crackers, crushed (one package of a 2-pack, 16-ounce box of Ritz or Town House crackers will yield the right amount)

1 (8-ounce) package Cheddar cheese, grated

3 large eggs, beaten

¾ cup milk

⅛ teaspoon paprika

Salt and pepper, to taste

Cookware needed: mixing bowl, baking dish or casserole

Melt one stick of butter in a large skillet.

Sauté the onion rings in the butter until translucent.

Melt the second stick of butter in a microwave-safe mixing bowl, and add the crushed crackers, reserving at least ¼ to use on top of the casserole.

Preheat the oven to 350 degrees.

Grease a baking dish and cover the bottom with some of the buttered crumbs. Place a layer of sautéed onion over the crumbs, followed by some of the cheese. Repeat these layers, ending with the cheese.

Combine the beaten eggs, milk, and paprika, and add a little salt and pepper. Pour the milk mixture over the onions, bread crumbs, and cheese.

Top the casserole with the reserved, unbuttered crumbs.

Bake for 35 to 45 minutes, or until bubbly and golden brown.

PREPARATION TIME: *20 minutes*
TOTAL TIME: *approximately 1 hour*

Sage Advice

There's no short cut around sautéing the onion. But using an already grated Cheddar cheese (I prefer the sharp variety) and crushing the crackers in their wrapping helps to speed the preparation time along.

Peas in a Boat

COLOR, nutrition, style, taste—this vegetable selection has it all. Plus, it's unusual; you won't see it served every day.

Thanks to the availability of canned peas (Le Seur, please), your trusty blender, and already flavored bread crumbs, most of the work required to make this attractive choice has been done for you. It's a wonderful accompaniment to a rotisserie chicken (straight from the store, of course), and a quickly assembled Pecan Rice casserole. It gives the whole meal a "homemade" look and quality.

SERVES 6

6 yellow (crookneck) squash, small and well shaped

1 (6-ounce) can Le Seur baby peas, drained

1 tablespoon butter

Salt and pepper, to taste

1 teaspoon sugar

2 to 3 tablespoons heavy cream

2 heaping tablespoons flavored bread crumbs

2 teaspoons Parmesan or Cheddar cheese, grated

Cookware needed: saucepan, blender, baking dish or casserole

Boil the whole squash until tender, no more than 5 minutes.

Drain, and cut the vegetables in half lengthwise. Scoop out the seeds to make a boat-shaped cavity. (Leave some of the meat on the squash peel, so that you don't scrape down to the outer skin.)

Preheat the oven to 350 degrees.

Combine the peas, butter, salt, pepper, sugar, and cream in a blender and puree until soft but not runny. (Begin with just 2 tablespoons of the cream, and add more only if needed.)

Fill the squash cavities with the pea mixture, and place them in a greased baking dish.

Combine the bread crumbs and cheese, and sprinkle over the squash.

Bake for 12 to 15 minutes.

PREPARATION TIME: *15 to 20 minutes*
TOTAL TIME: *30 to 40 minutes*

Peas in Tomatoes

LOOKING for an even more colorful way to dish up that year-round favorite, green peas? Try serving them in a hollowed-out tomato shell.

Do not purée the peas; simply season them with a little butter, salt, and pepper. It's that simple. But in this instance, frozen petite peas are a better choice than the canned variety.

SERVES 6

6 firm tomatoes

1 (10-ounce) package frozen petite peas

Salt and pepper, to taste

1 to 2 tablespoons butter

Cookware needed: microwave-safe bowl, baking dish or casserole

Preheat the oven to 350 degrees.

Slice the top off each tomato and scoop out the seeds and just enough of the pulp to make room for an ample quantity of the peas.

Put the unfilled tomatoes in a greased baking pan and bake for 12 to 15 minutes.

While the tomatoes are baking, barely cover the petite peas with water and microwave on high for 2 to 4 minutes—just long enough to thaw and warm them.

Season the peas with salt and pepper and add the butter, just as you would if you were going to serve them as is.

Fill the tomatoes with the peas and garnish with a sprig of fresh parsley.

PREPARATION TIME: *15 minutes*
TOTAL TIME: *30 minutes*

Sage Advice

For another variation, slice an acorn squash in half, and scoop out the seeds. Fill a baking pan with enough water to cover the bottom, and turn the squash flesh (flat) side down in the pan. Bake at 325 degrees for about 40 minutes, or until soft. (Or you can microwave them for 10 to 15 minutes.) Turn the squash over, fill with the peas, and season with salt, pepper, and freshly ground nutmeg.

Portobello Deluxe

MARY MURPHY loves to cook. But she seldom does. "Just don't have the time," she says.

I know why she doesn't have the time. When she's not running the family gas station, she's seeing about family members, or she's looking after an orphaned dog or injured bird someone has dropped by the station, or—most likely—she's reading a book. Mary's the most voracious reader I've ever known. But she does find time to fix this easy portobello mushroom dish.

When I asked Mary if she serves this as an entrée, a salad, or an appetizer, she replied, "It's a meal. The mushroom is filling, the cheese is the protein, and the tomato is the vegetable."

Truth is, you can serve this versatile item any number of ways. The availability of both whole and sliced, ready-to-serve portobellos helps too. And if onions are to your liking, try adding a slice or two before finishing the dish with the cheese topping.

Incidentally, if you've been timid about trying portobello mushrooms at home because they seem to be one of those exotic restaurant foods, this recipe will convince you otherwise.

Sage Advice

If the mushrooms and tomatoes are particularly plump and thick, prepare the recipe through the Italian spice stage, and then cook the vegetables under the broiler for 5 to 10 minutes. Then add the grated cheese and continue to broil until the cheese has melted to your liking.

PREPARE 2 HALVES OR 1 WHOLE MUSHROOM PER PERSON

Portobello mushrooms either whole, or halved

Olive oil or cooking spray

Fresh tomatoes (1 slice per mushroom)

Italian spices, to taste

Grated cheese (mozzarella, Cheddar, Monterey Jack, your choice)

Cookware needed: cookie sheet or shallow baking dish or casserole

Brush a little olive oil on each mushroom bottom, or over the slices, or spray with cooking spray.

Slice the tomatoes to conform to the shape of the mushrooms and place them on top.

Sprinkle the tomatoes with a generous helping of Italian spices.

Top with an ample layer of cheese.

Broil for 5 to 10 minutes, or until the cheese is bubbly and melted.

PREPARATION TIME: *10 minutes*
TOTAL TIME: *15 to 20 minutes*

Spinach, Cream Cheese, and Tomato Casserole

IF YOU LIKE spinach and cream cheese, but are not wild about the Artichoke and Spinach Casserole, here's a dish you may like that substitutes tomatoes for artichokes.

SERVES 8 TO 10

- 3 (10-ounce) packages frozen, chopped spinach
- 1 tablespoon lemon juice
- 1 (8-ounce) package cream cheese
- 3 to 4 large, perfectly ripe tomatoes, sliced thick
- 1 cup Parmesan cheese, buttered bread crumbs, or a combination of the two

Cookware needed: saucepan, baking dish or casserole

Preheat the oven to 350 degrees.

In a saucepan, warm the frozen, chopped spinach over low heat just long enough to thoroughly defrost it, or defrost in the microwave.

Drain the spinach very well, squeezing it if necessary, and put it into a baking dish. Squeeze the lemon juice over the spinach, add the cream cheese, and blend well with a fork. Top the spinach mixture with the tomato slices.

Sprinkle with the Parmesan cheese and/or bread crumbs, and bake for 30 to 35 minutes.

PREPARATION TIME: *20 minutes*
TOTAL TIME: *approximately 1 hour*

Very Good Winter Squash

DON'T let the cream, Madeira, and pecans in this recipe mislead you. This squash dish isn't just for company, at least not at our house. You'll find me serving it for dinner even when there are only the two of us.

I like winter squash seasoned with only a little butter and salt and pepper. But when I fix it that way, Bob always leaves his untouched. I wasn't about to give up this nutritious and colorful (how often have I used those words to describe some of my favorites?) vegetable. Time to get out the seasonings.

I think you'll like the results. Bob does. His exact words were, "Say, this stuff is good."

SERVES 6 TO 8

The Finishing Touch

If you wish, you can combine ¼ cup of bread crumbs with 2 tablespoons of melted butter and sprinkle this mixture on top of the squash before baking. Another option is to top it with miniature marshmallows.

2 (12-ounce) packages frozen winter squash, defrosted

2 tablespoons butter, melted

1 ½ cups heavy cream

1 teaspoon cinnamon

¼ to ⅓ cup Madeira or cream sherry

¼ teaspoon salt

Freshly ground pepper, to taste

½ cup chopped pecans

Cookware needed: mixing bowl, baking dish or casserole

Preheat the oven to 350 degrees.

Put the defrosted squash in a well-greased baking pan or baking dish.

Add the melted butter, cream, cinnamon, Madeira or sherry, salt, and pepper, and mix well.

Fold in the pecans.

Bake uncovered for 30 minutes or until bubbling.

PREPARATION TIME: *5 minutes*
TOTAL TIME: *35 to 45 minutes*

Tomato Puddin'

I ALWAYS called the delicious combination of canned tomatoes and stale, crumbled bread, brought to life with a little butter and spices, "stewed tomatoes." But my dear friend Carolista Baum had a much better name for this old-timey dish.

"Tomato Puddin' " she called it, always dropping the final "g" in her soft, Eastern North Carolina accent. Though she prepared it no differently from anyone else, hers was always the best. I'm sure it's because it was "puddin.'"

SERVES 4 TO 6

¼ cup butter, melted

1 (28 ounce) can tomatoes, diced

3 or 4 slices stale bread, broken into quarter-size pieces

½ cup brown sugar

Salt and pepper, to taste

Cookware needed: mixing bowl, baking dish or casserole

Preheat the oven to 350 degrees.

Combine the butter, tomatoes, bread, sugar, and salt and pepper, to taste.

Pour the mixture into a greased baking dish, and bake for 40 to 45 minutes, or until set.

PREPARATION TIME: *10 minutes*
TOTAL TIME: *50 to 60 minutes*

Sage Advice

This is a great way to use up stale bread, especially if you have the tail end of a French or Italian loaf going to waste. The drier the bread, the better the puddin'. And don't even think about using fresh tomatoes. The flavor and texture of the canned ones, combined with the stale bread, butter, and sugar are what make this recipe good.

Gingered Vegetables

AH YOUTH! Many, many years ago, because I was young and didn't know any better, I brazenly asked the waiter at a fancy New York restaurant for a recipe. He told me that the chef wouldn't comply, but I begged so hard that the poor waiter finally must have approached the chef just to get an answer that would shut me up.

You can imagine my fellow diners' amazement when the chef actually appeared at our table.

"Now, which one of you Southerners wants to see me?" he asked in his own Southern drawl.

Obviously, the waiter had said something about the lady with the Southern accent, and *that* had prompted the chef (maybe a little homesick?) to venture into the dining room.

It turns out the chef was from Wilmington, North Carolina, and he gladly shared the ginger sauce recipe I was coveting. His "secret" recipe was so good, I wrote it down in the front cover of four or five different cookbooks so I wouldn't lose it!

When you glance at the recipe, please don't let the long list of sauce ingredients give you pause. You can measure them out in a couple of minutes.

Once that is done, you simply pour the sauce over your favorite blend of frozen vegetables, and you have a spectacular dish—one that will delight a serious vegetarian.

SERVES 12

For the sauce:

4 tablespoons butter

4 tablespoons Chinese oyster sauce

¼ cup sherry vinegar or 4 tablespoons lemon juice

2 tablespoons soy sauce

2 tablespoons freshly grated ginger

1 teaspoon each of the following dried herbs:

Parsley

Chervil

Coriander

Thyme

Oregano

For the vegetables:

1 (2-pound) package frozen vegetable blend that includes snow peas, mushrooms, broccoli, peppers, onions and other Oriental-style vegetables. You may want to mix and match the smaller boxes to make your own combination.

(Other good vegetables include baby corn, carrots, cauliflower. You want to avoid peas, beans, and potatoes.)

Cookware needed: skillet

To make the sauce, melt the butter in a skillet over medium-low heat, and then stir in the liquid ingredients, ginger, and herbs.

Add the vegetables, cover, and cook over medium heat until the vegetables are cooked to your taste—but not so long that they lose their crunch and crispness—for about 8 to 10 minutes.

PREPARATION TIME: *10 minutes*
TOTAL TIME: *approximately 20 minutes*

Curried Fruit

There's a wonderful and true saying: Scratch a cook and you'll get a recipe.

That happened one day when my assistant, good friend, and fabulous cook, Charlotte Sizer, and I began comparing notes on one of our favorite easy-to-make dishes, Curried Fruit. While the ingredients were just about the same, we prepared the dish quite differently. I just mix everything together, but Charlotte uses what I call the "sprinkle and spread" technique.

Following are two variations of the same recipe. You can decide which one you prefer. Charlotte's may be better suited to a party where the food is plated before serving, while mine works well when guests serve themselves.

Whichever way you prepare it, be sure to try this tasty fruit dish. It's colorful, filled with vitamins, combines many different textures, and makes a wonderful accompaniment to either meats or casseroles—and it's a change from the usual vegetables.

Emyl's Mix and Serve Curried Fruit

SERVES 8 OR MORE

1 (15-once) can sliced peaches

1 (15-ounce) can sliced pears

1 (11-ounce) can mandarin oranges

1 (8 ½-ounce) can apricot halves

1 (16 ½-ounce) can dark cherries (or Queen Anne, or maraschino)

1 (15-ounce) can diced pineapple

½ cup light or dark raisins, or a combination of the two for a variety in taste and color

Cookware needed: large saucepan

Reserve the peach and pear juices in a mixing bowl. Drain the remaining fruit, and pour the fruit (at random) into a large, heavy saucepan or pot.

To the reserved juice, add:

½ cup brown sugar

1 tablespoon cinnamon

¼ teaspoon nutmeg (about 5 turns of a nutmeg grinder)

2 tablespoons curry powder

2 tablespoons butter

The
Finishing Touch

This colorful fruit accompaniment looks pretty when served in a heat-tolerant crystal bowl.

Whisk to blend and pour the juice mixture over the fruit. Simmer about 25 minutes, stirring occasionally.

PREPARATION TIME: *5 minutes*
TOTAL TIME: *30 minutes*

Charlotte's Spread and Sprinkle Baked Fruit

SERVES 8

Cookware needed: Bake this version in a shallow, glass oven-to-table baking dish or casserole.

Use the same canned fruits as in the previous recipe, except omit the mandarin oranges and substitute pineapple rings (8 to 10 per 15-ounce can) for the diced pineapple, and halved peaches and pears for the sliced ones. Plan on enough to prepare at least one fruit ring (beginning with a pineapple ring) per person

Preheat the oven to 325 degrees.

Begin by spreading the pineapple rings in a single layer on the bottom of a lightly greased baking dish. Arrange either a halved peach or a pear in the center of each ring, pouring in enough of the canned juices to reach a level of approximately ¼ inch.

Build the dish prettily, placing a cherry in the center of each fruit half. Fill in the bare spots in the baking dish with the raisins and apricots.

Sprinkle the brown sugar, cinnamon, nutmeg, and curry (optional) over the fruit and dot with the butter.

Bake for 35 to 40 minutes. Baste with the pan juices twice during cooking.

PREPARATION TIME: *10 minutes*
TOTAL TIME: *50 minutes*

"The pleasure of preparing and eating good food can only be enhanced by the pleasure of sharing it with friends."

—RUTH MELLINKOFF, *THE UNCOMMON COOK BOOK,* 1968

Sage Advice

If you prefer, flavor your baked fruit with sherry rather than curry. Pour ¼ cup over the fruit before sprinkling it with the spices, or soak 10 prunes in enough sherry to cover for 20 minutes, then add them to the baking dish before baking—delicious!

When buying raisins for baking, not just snacking, the cylindrical container with a plastic top does the best job of keeping the fruit moist and fresh. Light/golden raisins are sweeter and lighter tasting.

Potatoes, Pasta, and Rice

*"Skill in cooking
is as readily shown
in a baked potato
or a johnny-cake,
as in a canvas-back
duck."*

—*THE STAR COOK BOOK,*
BY MRS. GRACE
TOWNSEND, 1895

Potatoes were the standard fare in our home when I was growing up. Baked potatoes, new potatoes, sweet potatoes, boiled potatoes, fried potatoes, smashed potatoes, scalloped potatoes. Then I married.

My husband's family roots sprang from South Carolina, and they ate rice. White rice. Plain white rice.

Over the years, I grew to love rice just as much as potatoes, especially once I learned what you could do to plain white rice to vary it a little.

Today's boxed rices provide a lot of variety, but here are a few additional recipes that are quick, easy, and will give more of that "homemade" feeling at meal time.

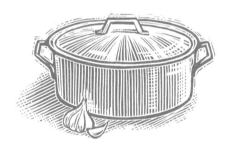

Bouillon Rice

WHEN MY GOOD FRIEND and Southern writer, Sharyn McCrumb, isn't meeting publishing deadlines or traveling to Europe to lecture on her Ballad series of books, she's busy with her three children. And whenever one of the kids has to take a "covered dish" somewhere, off they go to the kitchen to make Bouillon Rice.

SERVES 4 TO 6

1 stick butter
½ cup frozen, diced onion
1 (10-ounce) can beef broth
1 (10-ounce) can beef consommé

2 cups uncooked rice
Cookware needed: skillet, covered baking dish or casserole

Preheat the oven to 350 degrees.

Sauté the onion (or microwave it) in the butter, until lightly browned.

Transfer the onion and butter to a baking dish and add the beef broth and consommé.

Add the rice, cover (using aluminum foil if you do not have a fitted lid), and bake for 1 hour.

PREPARATION TIME: *7 to 8 minutes*
TOTAL TIME: *approximately 1 hour and 10 minutes*

Pecan Rice

IF YOU'RE as wild about pecans as I am, you're always looking for ways to slip their sweet, crunchy taste and texture into your meal time. Bouillon rice becomes a rice and pecan casserole with these simple additions.

1 ½ cups chopped pecans

¾ teaspoon dried thyme

2 tablespoons dried parsley

To this you can also add:

1 heaping teaspoon prepared garlic

1 (4-ounce) can sliced mushrooms, drained

Prepare Bouillon Rice as described in the previous recipe. When putting the rice in the casserole, also add the ingredients above.

PREPARATION TIME: *varies according to selected ingredients*
TOTAL TIME: *a little more than 1 hour*

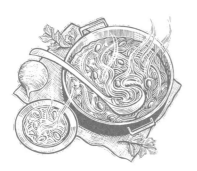

Creamy Rice

REMEMBER RICE AND GRAVY? That one-time favorite seems to have all but disappeared from today's tables. But here's a rice dish that makes its own delicious "gravy" or sauce. You wouldn't want to serve it with a meat or vegetable casserole made with a cream soup, but it is awfully good with grilled meats and a salad.

If the recipe looks familiar, that's because it's another a variation on Bouillon Rice (page 179).

SERVES 4 TO 6

½ cup frozen, diced onion

1 stick butter

1 (10-ounce) can cream of mushroom soup

1 soup can water

1 (10-ounce) can beef consommé

2 cups uncooked rice

Cookware needed: skillet, baking dish or casserole, with a lid

Preheat the oven to 350 degrees.

Sauté the onion (or microwave it) in the butter until brown.

Transfer the onion and butter to a baking dish.

Add the mushroom soup mixed with the water and the consommé.

Add the uncooked rice and stir to blend. Cover the baking dish and bake for 1 hour.

PREPARATION TIME: *7 to 8 minutes*
TOTAL TIME: *approximately 1 hour and 10 minutes*

Easy Oven Rice

LIKE SHARYN MCCRUMB'S Bouillon Rice, the good thing about Joan Sprinkle's Easy Oven Rice is that it cooks in the oven—so that once you've assembled the ingredients you are free to do other things. Even though I'm a great fan of instant rice, you have to be close by to keep the rice from sticking or, as I've been known to do, burning up the pan!

SERVES 4

1 (10-ounce) can French onion soup, undiluted

½ stick margarine, melted

1 (4-ounce) can sliced mushrooms, drained, liquid reserved

1 (8-ounce) can sliced water chestnuts, drained, liquid reserved

1 ⅓ cups liquid (made from the liquids of the mushrooms and water chestnuts, plus added water)

1 cup uncooked long grain rice

Cookware needed: baking dish or casserole

Preheat the oven to 350 degrees.

Combine the soup and margarine and stir well.

Combine all of the ingredients and pour the mixture into a lightly greased 10 x 6 x 2-inch baking dish.

Cover and bake for 1 hour and 10 minutes.

PREPARATION TIME: *10 minutes*
TOTAL TIME: *1 hour and 20 minutes*

Apple Rice

RICE AND PORK CHOPS go together as, well, apples and pork chops. So why not make it easy on yourself and prepare this quick and unusual apple rice. It works very well for brunch too, if you're serving sausage links.

SERVES 8

¼ cup frozen, diced onion
½ cup diced celery
2 tablespoons butter
2 cups uncooked rice
1 cup apple juice
1 cup water

1 teaspoon onion salt
½ teaspoon cinnamon
1 medium apple, cored and finely chopped
Cookware needed: skillet, saucepan and baking dish or casserole

In the skillet, sauté the onion and celery in the butter, until lightly browned.

While the vegetables are cooking, prepare the rice according to package directions, but use 1 cup of apple juice and 1 cup of water, and onion salt rather than regular salt. Add the cinnamon and the apple to the rice mixture and cook.

When the rice is ready, stir in the sautéed celery and onion.

PREPARATION TIME: *10 minutes*
TOTAL TIME: *35 minutes*

FOR ANOTHER sweet rice that goes with simple pork dishes try this variation.

SERVES 8

1 to 2 teaspoons cinnamon
1 cup raisins (golden or brown)

1 (2-ounce) package slivered almonds, toasted is best or 1 (5-ounce) can sliced water chestnuts, drained

To either the basic Bouillon Rice recipe (page 179) or to 4 cups of instant rice (cooked), add the above ingredients.

Stir well and serve.

PREPARATION TIME: *10 minutes*
TOTAL TIME: *20 minutes if using instant rice*
1 hour and 10 minutes if using Bouillon Rice

Sage Advice

If you are going to serve this immediately, pour the cooked rice into a warmed baking dish (just rinsing the dish in hot water will heat it). But if it will be a while before you serve it, pour the rice into a baking dish, cover it with aluminum foil and let it rest in a warm oven, making sure it doesn't get too dry by covering with aluminum foil.

The Finishing Touch

Add a few chopped pecans, and you have an even fancier dish— almost good enough to call a rice pudding and serve for dessert, except for the onions!

No-Fail Potatoes

IT'S EASY to tell when my across-the-street neighbors are at home. There's a steady stream of cars in front of the house. Bobbye Raye Womack is having a baby shower, or a wedding party, or a gathering for out-of-towners who've come for a funeral, or a just-for-fun brunch, or a spur-of-the-moment afternoon tea party. Any occasion or no occasion at all, is her reason to have friends drop in, and there's always a fabulous spread.

This tasty and trouble-free potato dish is a standby she's been using for thirty-plus years. And, she says, when her guests wander back to the kitchen, it's because they want to lick the bowl.

SERVES 6

Sage Advice

Like all experienced cooks, Bobbye Raye gives directions for this recipe in a rather off-hand way. "Well, sometimes I use 4 eggs. And sometimes I'll use a big container of sour cream and a small container of cottage cheese. Sometimes I put cheese in it. Sometimes I cook it plain. Sometimes I put cheese on top. It always tastes good." Take her sage advice and try your own variations on this basic no-fail recipe.

2 cups instant mashed potato flakes

1 (8-ounce) container sour cream

1 (8-ounce) container cottage cheese

2 eggs, well beaten

Salt, pepper, and anything else you want to add, to taste (Suggestions are Cheddar, Parmesan, or other cheese; bacon bits; chives)

Cookware needed: mixing bowl and baking dish or casserole

Preheat the oven to 350 degrees.

Combine the potato flakes, sour cream, cottage cheese, and eggs.

Add salt and pepper to taste, along with any other additions you choose, and pour the mixture into a well-greased baking dish. Bake for 45 minutes.

PREPARATION TIME: *5 to 10 minutes*
TOTAL TIME: *approximately 1 hour*

Party Potatoes

THIS RECIPE is one you might want to use should you have cream cheese but no cottage cheese on hand. Otherwise, Party Potatoes and No-Fail Potatoes are very similar.

SERVES 8

4 cups hot, mashed potatoes, either prepared from a box or ready-to-serve from the refrigerated or hot deli section of the grocery store

⅓ cup butter

1 (8-ounce) package cream cheese, softened

¼ cup sour cream

Salt and pepper, to taste

Paprika, to taste

Cookware needed: 2 mixing bowls, baking dish or casserole

Stir the butter into the hot potatoes.

Whip the cream cheese with the sour cream until smooth and fluffy.

Preheat the oven to 325 degrees.

Stir the cheese mixture into the potatoes. Add salt and pepper, to taste.

Spoon the potatoes into a buttered baking dish, sprinkle with the paprika, and bake for 30 minutes.

PREPARATION TIME: *5 to 10 minutes*
TOTAL TIME: *approximately 1 hour*

Potato Mushroom Casserole

READY-TO-COOK frozen French fries were one of the first "quick" foods I remember using. No longer was it necessary to scrub and slice the spuds. Soon thereafter, stuffed, twice-baked, hash-brown, and fancy crinkled, and shoestring potatoes were available in the freezer section.

This casserole, which once required the obligatory scrubbing and slicing, can now be made in a snap, thanks to yet another, new potato product—frozen, herbed potato wedges.

SERVES 6 TO 8

1 (2-pound) package frozen, herbed potato wedges

1 (8-ounce) can sliced mushrooms, drained

1 cup Swiss cheese, grated

1 cup whipping cream

Cookware needed: rectangular baking dish or casserole

Preheat the oven to 375 degrees.

Layer the potato wedges and mushrooms in a rectangular baking dish.

Combine the cheese and whipping cream and pour the mixture over the potatoes and mushrooms.

Bake for about 30 minutes or until bubbly.

PREPARATION TIME: *10 minutes*
TOTAL TIME: *40 minutes*

Mama Mia Potatoes

USE ITALIAN CHEESES and herbs to give mashed potatoes a bit of pizzazz and make them exceptionally flavorful.

SERVES 8

4 cups hot, mashed potatoes, either prepared from a box or ready-to-serve from the refrigerated or hot deli section of the supermarket

Butter, salt and pepper, to taste

½ cup Parmesan cheese, grated

8 ounces mozzarella cheese, sliced

⅓ to 1 cup Italian-style bread crumbs

Cookware needed: mixing bowls, baking dish or casserole

Preheat the oven to 350 degrees.

Flavor the potatoes with butter, salt, and pepper, to taste.

Spread half the potatoes in a baking dish and sprinkle them with half the Parmesan cheese.

Layer the mozzarella cheese slices over the Parmesan, saving a few slices for the top.

Spread the remaining potatoes over the cheese layer, add more Parmesan and end with the remaining mozzarella slices.

Sprinkle the flavored bread crumbs on top and bake for about 15 minutes, or until the mozzarella cheese has melted.

PREPARATION TIME: *10 minutes*
TOTAL TIME: *approximately 30 minutes*

Sherried Sweet Potatoes

SPEAKING OF the new products that are showing up on grocery shelves these days, I distinctly remember watching one Thanksgiving-eve shopper down on her hands and knees reaching to the back of the bottom shelf, hoping to retrieve a can or two of orange-pineapple sweet potatoes.

No reason for me to follow suit. She got the last ones. I waited until after Thanksgiving, then helped myself to a couple of cans from the newly stocked shelves. They sure do make this next casserole easy to assemble!

SERVES 10

Sage Advice

If you wish, you can add orange juice to taste to the can juices, or even a little orange zest. If you can't find the orange-pineapple variety of sweet potatoes, use candied yams and add a cup of orange juice to the can juices.

3 (15-ounce) cans orange-pineapple sweet potatoes

6 tablespoons butter, either melted or cut into small pieces

¼ cup chopped walnuts

½ cup raisins

⅓ cup dry sherry

Cookware needed: baking dish or casserole

Preheat the oven to 325 degrees.

Scoop the sweet potatoes out of the cans one by one and transfer them to a baking dish, slicing them as you go. (This technique keeps you from having to dirty another bowl.)

Combine the juices from the potato cans into one can, add the butter, walnuts, raisins, and sherry, and pour the mixture over the potatoes.

Bake for about 30 minutes, basting occasionally, until the potatoes are well glazed.

PREPARATION TIME: *10 minutes*
TOTAL TIME: *40 minutes*

Dressed-Up Noodles

TIRED OF serving rice or potatoes with beef or pork? How about dressing up some egg noodles? That's what Mother used to do. These days Italian pastas seem to dominate the family dinner plate. That's what makes this dish a pleasant change.

SERVES 4

1 (8-ounce) box egg noodles
½ stick butter, cut up
Lots of freshly ground pepper
Salt, to taste

¼ to ½ cup finely chopped parsley
Cookware needed: large saucepan

Prepare the egg noodles according to package directions.

To the cooked and drained noodles, add all the remaining ingredients. Stir gently to combine without breaking up the noodles.

PREPARATION TIME: *5 minutes*
TOTAL TIME: *10 to 15 minutes,*
depending on your desired tenderness
for the noodles

You-Take-the-Credit Caramelized Onion and Blue Cheese Rissoni

WHEN FRIENDS of mine told friends of theirs about *From Storebought to Homemade* wonderful recipes began flooding in from folks I'd never even met. Caramelized Onion and Blue Cheese Rissoni is one of those.

I read through it (my mouth began watering) and got to the end. There, quite unexpectedly, a note was tacked on: "If there are any mistakes, they are Eric's fault. Otherwise, the credit is all mine! Linda." I didn't have a clue who Eric or Linda were!

That's the wonderful thing about great food. We love to share it, and when it's really good, to take all the credit.

There were no mistakes, so Linda is clear to take all the credit. Now it's your turn to take credit for this unusual, and unusually good, recipe.

SERVES 8

1 (1-pound) package rissoni, or other short soup pasta

1 tablespoon butter

3 tablespoons olive oil

4 onions, sliced

1 (6-ounce) package blue cheese

3 ½ ounces mascarpone

2 cups packaged shredded English spinach leaves, or baby spinach leaves

Salt and pepper, to taste

Cookware needed: large pot, large skillet, mixing bowl

Cook the rissoni in rapidly boiling salted water until al dente, about 5 minutes.

While the pasta is cooking, heat the butter and olive oil in a large heavy-bottomed skillet. Add the sliced onion and cook over low heat for about 20 to 30 minutes, until golden brown and caramelized. Remove the onion from the pan with a slotted spoon and drain it on paper towels.

Drain the rissoni well and return it to the pot.

Combine the blue cheese, mascarpone, and onion in a bowl and then add the mixture to the rissoni.

Add the spinach and toss thoroughly. Season to taste with salt and freshly ground black pepper before serving.

PREPARATION TIME: *20 minutes*

TOTAL TIME: *35 minutes*

Grits, No Longer Just for Southerners

Never, in all my memories, can I recall seeing my Massachusetts-born-and-bred father eat grits. Other than creamed onions, grits were the only dish I think he ever refused.

Of course, my Southern mother loved grits and served them often. But she never dressed them up the way we do these days. A little butter and salt and pepper were the only flavorings she added to that most Southern of dishes.

These days everyone loves grits, but that's because they've changed the flavor by adding lots of cheese to them. If Daddy had ever eaten cheese grits, I think he would have liked them. I prefer cheese grits too—I guess it's my "Yankee" half coming through.

Try these two "dressed-up" cheesy grits recipes. They are delicious served as a side dish in place of potatoes, pasta, or rice, with beef, pork, chicken, and even grilled fish. You'll be pleasantly surprised at how good they are. Even my young grandson, Benjamin, whose father is from Pennsylvania, smacks his lips and asks for more when I fix them for him.

Cheese Garlic Grits

SERVES 6

By using garlic salt and cheese sauce, you can make this delicious accompaniment more or less garlicky or cheesy as you prefer. An alternative way to make Garlic Cheese Grits is to use a garlic cheese roll, which can be found in the cheese section of your grocery store. Use it in place of the cheese sauce and garlic sauce.

2 cups quick grits, cooked according to package directions, piping hot

½ to ¾ cup prepared Cheddar cheese sauce

2 to 3 tablespoons garlic salt

¼ to ½ cup cream

½ stick butter

Salt and pepper, to taste

Cookware needed: pot

Add the cheese sauce, garlic salt, cream (more or less, depending on how creamy you like your grits), and butter to the piping hot grits. Mix thoroughly and season with salt and pepper.

PREPARATION TIME: *5 to 10 minutes*

TOTAL TIME: *approximately 20 minutes*

The Finishing Touch

If you wish to serve this recipe as a casserole, the addition of 2 well-beaten eggs makes the mixture richer and more "solid." Add the eggs to the mixture at the end, then simply pour the grits into a well-greased baking dish or casserole and bake at 350 degrees for 30 to 40 minutes. You can also top the grits with French Fried Onion bits before baking—to add that finishing touch.

Swiss Grits

SERVES 6

2 cups quick grits, cooked according to package directions, piping hot

½ to ¾ cup Swiss cheese, grated

⅓ to ½ cup Parmesan cheese, grated

1 teaspoon salt

⅛ teaspoon pepper

½ stick butter

Cookware needed: saucepan, baking dish or casserole

Preheat the oven to 350 degrees.

To the piping hot grits, add the two cheeses, salt, pepper, and butter and mix thoroughly. Adjust the flavoring to your taste.

Pour the grits into a well-greased baking dish, and bake at for 45 to 60 minutes.

PREPARATION TIME: *5 to 10 minutes*
TOTAL TIME: *60 minutes*

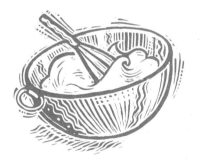

All-in-One Meals

"**WHAT'S** the absolute *easiest* meal-in-one dish you're putting in your book," a young bride asked me. "Easiest, *and* best," she quickly added, no doubt thinking about her new groom.

I couldn't answer. Easiest *and* best? I pondered.

The Brunswick Stew recipe is a long-standing favorite. But then, the Mexican Chicken Casserole is newer, and equally mouthwatering to my way of thinking.

Quickly Assembled Chicken requires only 4 ingredients, plus some peppercorns. And when you sprinkle condiments over Navy Wives Shrimp Curry you're topping a scrumptious dish with its own salad! (Salads are often served with one-dish meals.) Thinking it over, even some of the selections that need extra cooking time are extremely easy to assemble.

And speaking of assembly....There's always the matter of pots and pans when you step into the kitchen. But if you can mix an All-in-One-Meal in its own baking dish, or prepare it in a skillet on top of the stove, you've saved time and effort.

But back to the question at hand.

Easiest? Best? Easiest and best? When *you* decide, let me know!

Meanwhile, to put the whole matter into perspective, and to give credence to how storebought ingredients have changed our cooking habits, read about Country Captain Chicken, and smile!

Have You Had All Your Vitamins Today?

GREEN salads have become so much a part of almost every meal that even old-fashioned tomato-based beef stews with carrots, celery, and potatoes are served with a salad on the side.

There's absolutely nothing wrong with this—especially since the cello-bagged salads have taken all the work out of the process. These packaged salads are so easy, in fact, that they give you more options when preparing an All-in-One Meal. No longer must you be sure that your dinner includes the vegetables necessary to provide your family members with their full share of vitamins.

So fix the Chinese Tuna Casserole for a family meal and don't worry if the kids pick the celery pieces out of it—as long as they eat the Romaine lettuce and shredded carrots on their salad plates.

Country Captain Chicken

THERE are many reasons why chicken is so popular, not least of which is its versatility. The new, already cooked, ready-to-serve chicken products are the answer to many a hurried cook's prayers. They've made it a cinch to prepare everything from Queenly Chicken Salad (page 294) to Chicken Stew (page 205). How easy?

Just for fun, I recently pulled out the recipe for Country Captain Chicken that I used for years to make one of my favorite do-ahead company dishes and compared it with the recipe I've developed by using every convenience food available to me. Read them both and you'll become a convert.

The ingredients are basically the same. But numerous steps have been eliminated and you've cut thirty minutes off the preparation time and an hour off the cooking time.

What remains the same is a delicious dish that can be prepared ahead of time and never fails to delight.

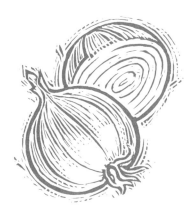

Country Captain Chicken the "old way"

SERVES 8

1 fresh fryer chicken

1 cup flour

1 teaspoon salt

½ teaspoon pepper

1 teaspoon dried thyme

½ teaspoon dried savory

½ teaspoon dried basil

¼ cup butter

½ cup diced onions

½ cup diced green pepper

1 to 2 cloves garlic, minced

1 ½ to 2 teaspoons curry powder

2 cups stewed tomatoes

3 tablespoons currants

6 cups cooked rice

¼ cup slivered almonds, toasted

Cookware needed: a deep, 10-inch skillet, with a lid, a baking dish or casserole, plus a 2-quart saucepan for the rice

Cut up the fryer.

Combine the flour, salt and pepper, ½ teaspoon thyme, the savory, and the basil. Coat each piece of chicken well with this mixture.

Brown the chicken pieces in the butter. Remove, drain, and place the chicken in a baking dish.

To the pan drippings in the skillet, add the onion, green pepper, garlic, curry powder, and remaining thyme and cook, stirring gently, until golden. Add the stewed tomatoes, stir, and simmer for 45 minutes.

Preheat the oven to 350 degrees.

Pour this mixture over the chicken and bake uncovered for 30 minutes.

Add the currants during the last 5 minutes of cooking.

Serve over the rice, garnished with the toasted slivered almonds.

PREPARATION TIME: *40 minutes*
TOTAL TIME: 1 ½ *hours*

Country Captain Chicken the "new way"

I CAN'T believe I ever cut up a fryer chicken, but I did. That step alone took a good 10 to 15 minutes and created quite a mess. Later, I simply bought the cut-up chicken, which saved time and made less mess.

These days I use breaded or already flavored chicken strips and make the dish in no time.

Try this *From Storebought to Homemade* version of the same recipe. The total time it takes is less than the basic preparation time of the old way. I think you'll agree, we've come a long way, baby!

SERVES 8

1 tablespoon olive oil

1 to 2 tablespoons prepared garlic

½ cup combo of frozen, diced onion and green pepper

3 (15-ounce) cans Italian-style stewed tomatoes

1 ½ to 2 teaspoons curry powder

½ teaspoon dried thyme

2 (10-ounce) packages fully cooked breaded or herbed chicken strips

3 tablespoons currants

4 cups instant rice, cooked

¼ cup slivered almonds, toasted

Cookware needed: a deep, 10-inch skillet, with a lid, plus a 2-quart saucepan for the rice

Heat olive oil over medium-high heat in a deep, 10-inch skillet, with a lid.

Add garlic and green pepper and cook approximately 3 minutes to allow the flavors to blend.

To this, add the tomatoes, curry powder, and dried thyme.

Cover and simmer on low heat for 20 minutes.

Add the fully cooked chicken and currants and cook another 10 to 15 minutes.

During these last 10 minutes, prepare the instant rice according to package directions.

Serve the chicken over the rice, garnished with the almonds.

PREPARATION TIME: *10 minutes*
TOTAL TIME: *35 to 45 minutes*

Mexican Chicken Casserole

MEXICAN Chicken Casserole is a "new" cream of mushroom soup-based casserole that everyone is fixing these days. I must have been given ten recipes—each slightly different, but all good.

Of course it's popular. The cook can stir it up in 15 minutes. Kids will ask for seconds. And best of all, you can add to, take from, or substitute the ingredients—according to what you like and what you have on hand.

So, think of this recipe as a guide. Read over the alternative and additional ingredients and let your imagination be your guide.

SERVES 6

Vegetable oil cooking spray

1 (9-ounce) package baked tortilla chips, as many as needed

2 (10-ounce) packages fully cooked chicken slices or pieces, fajita flavored if you wish

1 (10-ounce) can cream of mushroom soup

1 (10-ounce) can cream of chicken soup

1 (10 to 14-ounce) can diced tomatoes and hot peppers, mild, medium, or hot, to your taste

½ cup frozen, diced green peppers

1 cup frozen corn

1 (14-ounce) can black beans, drained and rinsed

1 cup Cheddar cheese, grated

Alternative or additional ingredients:

3 to 4 boneless frozen or fresh chicken breasts, cooked and cubed, may be used in place of the already cooked chicken strips or pieces

1 cup of frozen vegetable gumbo mix (okra, corn, onions, celery, and red peppers) can be used in place of the corn

Sliced ripe or Spanish olives can be added to the mixture or sprinkled on top

Cookware needed: 9 x 13-inch baking dish or casserole, mixing bowl

Preheat the oven to 350 degrees.

Spray the inside of a 9 x 13-inch baking dish with vegetable oil cooking spray and crumble the tortilla chips in the bottom. Lay half the chicken over the chips.

Combine the soups, tomatoes and pepper, and the vegetables and beans in a mixing bowl. Pour half the soup mixture over the chicken.

Repeat the layering of tortilla chips, chicken, and soup mixture.

Crumble a few more tortilla chips over the final layer and sprinkle the Cheddar cheese on top.

Bake for about 30 minutes, or until the casserole is thoroughly hot and the cheese has melted.

PREPARATION TIME: *10 to 15 minutes*
TOTAL TIME: *approximately 30 to 40 minutes*

Sage Advice

If you use fresh or frozen chicken breasts, try this quick-cook method. Chop the breasts into small pieces, place them in a microwave-safe bowl, cover them with water, and microwave until done, approximately 5 to 10 minutes. Or, you can simply toss the chicken into some water in a saucepan, bring it to a boil, and cook over medium heat for about 15 minutes, until the chicken is no longer pink in the middle.

Old-Timey Tuna Casserole

I **PROMISED** to tickle your nostalgic taste buds. My generation's Mexican Chicken Casserole was the tuna casserole. I thought everyone still made it.

Then at a meeting of women ranging from their mid-30s to early-70s, I learned that some of the younger women had never had it, and some of the older ones had lost their old recipes. So here it is.

But like the Mexican Chicken Casserole, there are countless variations of tuna casserole. Garrison Keillor even gave his rendition of the recipe on a *News from Lake Wobegone* broadcast when telling a story about a city fellow who longed to return to his mom's kitchen for her "tuna hot dish" made from macaroni, tuna "out of cans," peas, and "cream of mushroom soup for sauce, and Lipton's dried onion soup for spice, and crunched potato chips on top for crunch."

That's why, I've listed some alternative or additional ingredients.

SERVES 8

1 (12-ounce) package egg noodles, wide or thin

1 (14-ounce) can cream of mushroom soup

1 (8-ounce) can Le Seur petite peas, or 1 cup frozen petite peas

1 or 2 (12-ounce) cans tuna, water-packed, of course, and well drained

½ to 1 cup milk

1 cup Cheddar cheese, grated

Pepper, to taste

Alternative or additional ingredients:

Additional cheese, either grated or a bottled type like Cheese Whiz or Velveeta can be stirred into the casserole mixture

½ cup (or more) slivered almonds or cashews can be added to the casserole mixture

Lipton's dried onion soup mix (à la Keillor)

Crumbled potato chips can be added to the grated cheese for a crunchy topping

Cookware needed: 8-quart pot, baking dish or casserole

Cook the egg noodles according to package directions.

Preheat the oven to 350 degrees.

When the noodles are done, drain them and combine them in a large baking dish with the cream of mushroom soup, peas, and tuna. Add the milk according to your preference for a creamier or drier casserole. Add pepper, to taste.

Top with the cheese, cover loosely with aluminum foil, and bake for 45 minutes, or until bubbly. You can remove the foil for the last few minutes to brown the top, if you wish.

PREPARATION TIME: *10 to 15 minutes*
TOTAL TIME: *approximately 60 minutes*

Chinese Tuna Casserole

ANOTHER version of tuna casserole that circulated back in the 1960s and early '70s was this "misnamed" recipe.

Obviously there's nothing "Chinese" about it, except the chow mein noodles. One night I decided to "dress it up" a little. I took a hint from the name and added some sliced water chestnuts. I have never heard the end of that fateful error.

My son, Langdon, really dislikes water chestnuts...a fact that seemed to have eluded me. To this day, he reminds me that I took a perfectly good recipe and (according to him) deliberately ruined it.

I beg to disagree. Still, you'll notice that I have not included any water chestnuts in the list of ingredients below. But you can!

SERVES 8

1 (8-ounce) can chow mein noodles

2 (10-ounce) cans cream of mushroom soup

½ cup milk

1 (12-ounce) can water-packed tuna, drained

½ cup chopped cashews

1 to 2 cups diced or sliced celery

½ cup frozen, diced onion

Salt and pepper, to taste

Cookware needed: baking dish or casserole

Preheat the oven to 350 degrees.

Combine all of the ingredients, except for ¾ cup of the chow mein noodles, in a baking dish.

After the ingredients are well mixed, top the casserole with the remaining noodles.

Cook for 30 to 35 minutes.

PREPARATION TIME: *10 minutes*
TOTAL TIME: *approximately 40 to 45 minutes*

Company All-in-One Tuna-and-Shrimp Casserole

IF YOU really like canned tuna, and I do, you may be looking for new and different ways to use it. This tuna and shrimp All-in-One Meal may surprise you—with its ingredients and its flavor.

Don't let the longer-than-usual list of ingredients frighten you away. They are mostly items you'll take straight from the freezer or shake from the spice jar.

Sage Advice

If you decide to prepare this really delicious casserole at the last minute, and you have everything except the biscuits, never fear. You can serve this over rice, on top of toasted English muffins, or even on waffles. Another note: I suggested using 2 or 3 cans of artichoke hearts. You can guess that I always make it three. I find that the slightly tart taste of the artichoke hearts adds tremendously to the flavor. Just as I take this liberty, so may you adjust the recipe as you wish. If you don't like artichoke hearts, omit them altogether, add a package of peas or broccoli, and toss in some capers. After all, cooking is supposed to be fun, and you should prepare food to your own liking.

SERVES 8

3 tablespoons butter

1 (10-ounce) package Picksweet seasoning blend, or a frozen, diced combination of onion and green pepper, and celery

1 (10-ounce) bag shelled and cleaned frozen shrimp

½ teaspoon dried tarragon

1 tablespoon dried thyme

1 (16-ounce) jar Ragú® Classic Alfredo or Roasted Parmesan Cheese Sauce

1 (12-ounce) can water-packed tuna, drained

1 (4- to 6-ounce) can sliced mushrooms, drained

2 or 3 (14-ounce) cans artichoke hearts, drained and quartered

1 tablespoon lemon juice

Salt and pepper, to taste

1 (8-ounce) package refrigerator biscuits

Cookware needed: skillet, baking dish or casserole

Preheat the oven to 375 degrees.

Melt the butter in a skillet and sauté the onion, pepper, and celery for about 3 minutes.

Toss in the shrimp, tarragon, and thyme and cook another 2 to 3 minutes.

In a large casserole or baking dish combine the Ragú® sauce, drained tuna, mushrooms, artichoke hearts, lemon juice, salt, and pepper; stir, and then add shrimp mixture and combine.

Arrange the biscuits on top of the casserole so they are not quite touching, to allow space to spoon out each serving.

Bake for 25 to 30 minutes, or until the biscuits are browned and the mixture is bubbling hot.

PREPARATION TIME: *10 to 15 minutes*
TOTAL TIME: *45 to 50 minutes*

Quickly Assembled Chicken Meal-in-One

SOME recipes are so simple that all you are doing is assembling them. There's no stirring, mixing, or basting required. They can even be put together in a baking dish. Those are the ones I *really* like. Especially when they're yummy.

This quickly assembled chicken meal-in-one fits all of the above requirements. Mother fixed it regularly when I was in high school, and she was teaching school, so she had little time to prepare an evening meal. (This was way before the dawning of fast-food restaurants or the eating-out craze.) I, in turn, served it to my children every two or three weeks. My daughter now throws it together for her two young sons. It's become a three-generational family favorite.

The directions for making this recipe are really simple. The only decisions you'll have to make are how many chicken pieces to use and whether to go light or heavy on the whole peppercorns.

Sage Advice

Young children in the finger-food stage really love this dish. All Mom or Dad has to do is to cut the chicken and potatoes into smaller pieces. And, oh, remember to pick out the peppercorns!

SERVES 8

Chicken parts: fresh or frozen chicken breasts, thighs, legs, whatever your family likes (enough for 8 servings)

2 (14-ounce) cans small, whole white potatoes, drained

1 (14-ounce) can sliced carrots, drained

2 (14-ounce) cans French-style green beans, with their liquid

Whole peppercorns, to taste

Cookware needed: rectangular baking dish or casserole

Preheat the oven to 375 degrees.

Assemble by putting the chicken pieces in the baking dish and then spreading the drained potatoes and carrots around them.

Last, add the French-style green beans with their liquid. Toss on a few (10 or 12), or a full handful of, whole peppercorns.

Cover the pan with aluminum foil and bake for 35 to 45 minutes, or until the chicken is done, or white all the way through.

PREPARATION TIME: *8 to 10 minutes*
TOTAL TIME: *50 to 60 minutes*

Quick Chicken Pie

WHEN you get a *From Storebought to Homemade* recipe from a real chef, you know you're on the right track!

Margaret Mullen Breison worked as a *sous*-chef in Atlanta before becoming the head cook for her husband and sons in Thomasville, Georgia. To keep her hand in, she comes up with quick ways to provide dishes with that "home-cooked" flavor.

This quick chicken pot pie is a Breison family favorite that is so good you can serve it to guests by following the hint in *The Finishing Touch!*

Sage Advice
Margaret says that
this dish freezes well.

SERVES 4 TO 6

1 (9-inch) frozen pie crust

1 rotisserie chicken, skinned, meat removed from the bones

either

2 tablespoons butter

2 tablespoons flour

1 cup chicken broth, plus extra to adjust

1 cup half-and-half or milk

Salt and pepper, to taste

or

½ cup chicken broth

1 cup white or Alfredo sauce (this is how I make it)

1 cup peas and carrots, frozen, or other frozen vegetable mixture that includes diced potatoes and/or corn (optional),

1 egg, beaten

Cookware needed: mixing bowl, saucepan (optional), baking dish or casserole

The
Finishing Touch

A friend tells me that one time when she dined at Oscar's, the famed restaurant at the Waldorf, she ordered a meat pie. When it was served, the crust was popped off and placed on her plate first; then the succulent pie was dished out on top of it. Try this technique for a small casual company dinner.

Set the pie crust out to thaw.

Cut or tear the chicken meat into small pieces, and place in a mixing bowl.

Preheat the oven to 325 degrees.

If you wish to make your own white sauce: melt the butter over medium-high heat. Add the flour and cook, stirring, until it is golden, approximately 3 minutes.

Add the broth and milk and cook, stirring, until thickened, usually about 5 minutes. Season the sauce with salt and pepper and pour it over the chicken. Add more broth if it seems too thick.

To make it "my way," simply add ½ cup of chicken broth to 1 cup of already made Alfredo sauce and blend well.

Combine the chicken and sauce (and vegetables, if desired), stir, and pour the mixture into a baking dish.

Top with the pie crust, sealing edges well. Cut a few vent holes in the top with a sharp knife.

Brush the crust with the beaten egg, and bake for 20 to 30 minutes, or until the crust is golden brown.

PREPARATION TIME: *20 minutes*
TOTAL TIME: *50 to 60 minutes*

Chicken Stew

REMEMBER those stories your grandmother used to tell about how everyone looked forward to having chicken for Sunday dinner? Images of Norman Rockwell's family-meal paintings flashed before my eyes when I came upon another of my mother's recipes—this time, one for chicken stew.

Taking a lesson from Margaret Breison's homemade (well, almost) Quick Chicken Pie, I decided to adapt Mother's recipe by using a rotisserie chicken, which would be juicy and have that home-roasted flavor. It works beautifully, and I highly recommend that you try it.

SERVES 6

2 (10-ounce) cans cream of chicken soup (or use 1 can cream of chicken and 1 can cream of mushroom soup)

1 cup thickly sliced celery (this is one time when you may not have to dice the celery pieces you buy from the salad bar!)

1 (1-pound) package frozen stew vegetable mix that includes potatoes, carrots, and onions

2 teaspoons dried ground sage

¼ teaspoon freshly ground pepper

1 rotisserie chicken, skinned, meat removed from the bones

Cookware needed: large saucepan or pot, with lid

The
Finishing Touch

To complete the Norman Rockwell scene around your own table, pass a bread basket filled with piping-hot, buttered biscuits. You can even pour the stew over an opened biscuit the way your great-grandfather used to do!

Pour the soup into a large heavy saucepan or pot and add the vegetables, dried sage, and pepper. Cook over medium or medium-low heat until the liquid is bubbly. Do not let the mixture stick or burn.

Meanwhile, tear or cut the chicken into small pieces. Stir the chicken into the vegetable soup mixture.

Continue to cook until the vegetables are cooked through, about 30 minutes, and adjust the seasoning to your taste.

PREPARATION TIME: *15 minutes*
TOTAL TIME: *approximately 45 minutes*

Sunday-Night Shrimp Casserole

I HAD FORGOTTEN about this simple dish Mother used to fix for Sunday-night supper, until I found it among her recipes. It was handwritten and included a note from her brother, Kenlon: "Hope you'll enjoy this as much as I have." These days, my son-in-law, Mike, is as crazy about the dish as Uncle Kenlon was.

It was easy to prepare in the 1960s, and is even easier to make today. With a little ahead-of-time grocery planning (I usually have either a package of frozen shrimp, *or* the slivered almonds on hand...but seldom both), this dish is a delicious family treat that's also suitable for a casual, relaxed company dinner any night of the week.

By the way, the almonds add an unexpected crunch, so do be sure to include them.

SERVES 6 TO 8

1 (1-pound) bag frozen, cooked medium-size shrimp (add some scallops or imitation lobster **for additional flavor, if you wish,** or substitute already cooked, diced chicken if seafood isn't to your liking)

1 (6- to 8-ounce) can sliced mushrooms, drained

½ cup frozen, diced combo of **onion and green pepper**

½ cup (or more) slivered almonds

1 ½ cups Ragú® Roasted Garlic Parmesan pasta sauce

½ cup sherry

1 cello package Ritz or other cheesy crackers, crumbled (approximately 30)

1 cup Parmesan cheese, grated

3 to 4 cups cooked rice

Cookware needed: baking dish or casserole

Preheat the oven to 350 degrees.

In a buttered baking dish, alternate layers of shrimp (or chicken), mushrooms, onion and green pepper (or only onion, if you prefer), slivered almonds, and sauce.

Repeat until all the ingredients are used.

Top with the crumbled Ritz crackers and sprinkle with the Parmesan cheese.

Bake for approximately 35 to 40 minutes, or until thoroughly bubbling.

Serve over hot rice.

PREPARATION TIME: *15 minutes*
TOTAL TIME: *50 to 60 minutes*

Reuben Casserole

ALTHOUGH cooking is one of Joan Sprinkle's favorite pastimes, she had to get used to serving her physician husband, Jim, and their four children when she, and they, were on the run. Plus, there just was not enough time in the day to garden, play tennis, sew, *and* cook.

Joan began fixing this great Reuben Casserole when Jim was in his medical residency. She continued making it through the kids' growing up years, and now she makes it when they come home—with grandchildren in tow.

This is one of those assemble-in-its-baking-dish meals that should be at the top of the list for anyone who has limited cooking space and who dislikes clean-up time.

SERVES 6 TO 8

2 (10-ounce) cans sauerkraut, drained

2 medium tomatoes, sliced

½ cup Thousand Island dressing (if not on hand, combine mayonnaise, ketchup, and pickle relish to equal this amount—until it looks right, a nice dark pink)

2 tablespoons butter

8 ounces corned beef from the deli, sliced very thin

1 (8-ounce) package Swiss cheese, grated

1 (8-ounce) can flaky buttermilk biscuits

8 crisp rye crackers, crushed

1 teaspoon caraway seeds

Cookware needed: baking dish or casserole

Preheat the oven to 425 degrees.

Spread the sauerkraut in the bottom of an 8-inch baking dish.

Top with the tomato slices and dot with the dressing and butter.

Cover with the corned beef and sprinkle with the cheese.

Bake for 15 minutes.

Remove from oven.

Separate each biscuit into 3 layers and slightly overlap the biscuit layers on top of the casserole to form three rows. Sprinkle with the crackers and caraway seeds.

Bake 15 to 20 minutes, or until the biscuit topping is golden brown.

PREPARATION TIME: *15 minutes*
TOTAL TIME: *approximately 45 minutes*

Quick Ham and Cheese Bake

Sage Advice

I prefer slightly crunchy Brussels sprouts, but Mike likes his more thoroughly cooked. According to your taste (and their size), you may want to add the Brussels sprouts a little later in the baking process.

MY PENNSYLVANIA son-in-law, Mike Hultzapple, loves Brussels sprouts. So do I. But we're the only two in the family who do. Sometimes I cook them just for the two of us. Other times I simply slip those "little cabbages" into this casserole, then give everyone else one Brussels sprout, while piling the remainder on Mike's plate and mine.

SERVES 6 TO 8

1 (10-ounce) can cream of celery soup

½ cup milk

½ cup frozen, diced onion

1 cup diced potatoes (I take them from the frozen, hash-brown potato bag)

1 cup Cheddar cheese, grated

1 (2-ounce) jar pimiento, drained (optional)

1 (10-ounce) package frozen Brussels sprouts

2 cups diced and cooked ham

Cookware needed: baking dish or casserole, with lid

Preheat the oven to 350 degrees.

Combine all the ingredients in a large baking dish, cover, bake for 30 minutes. Remove the cover and continue to cook uncovered 10 to 15 minutes longer, until bubbly.

PREPARATION TIME: *10 minutes*
TOTAL TIME: *approximately 45 to 50 minutes*

The Picky Eater's Beef Stew

I KNOW all about picky eaters.

If a contest were held, my husband, Bob, would be among the finalists. He's getting better, gradually. Meanwhile, though, I moan, groan, and complain as I try to accommodate the few foods he loves to my see-food (if I see food, I'll try it, well, almost always) ways.

This later-life experience of living with a picky eater (Bob and I were married in 1996) has made me sympathetic toward cooks who have to try to please the limited preferences of others.

But what happens when the picky eater is the cook? That's what young Maggie Forgèt admitted when she gave me her recipe for beef stew.

"Since I'm not a big vegetable fan, this is how I make it—beef and juices—and just serve it over rice," Maggie apologized. "But, you *could* add veggies," she conceded.

So here's a veggie-free beef stew that's ready to serve with a side salad, unless the veggie-free eaters dislike salad too.

The mushroom gravy mix provides all the flavorful spices you'll need. That's a boon to today's cook, who wants to use fresh beef but doesn't want to spend the time gathering and preparing the onions and other spices we used to include when we fixed beef stew (also without the veggies), served it over rice, and gave it the fancy name, Boeuf à la Bourguignon. The rich, dark color of the gravy even makes it unnecessary to brown the meat first.

SERVES 6

1 (10-ounce) can cream of mushroom soup

1 package Knorr's mushroom gravy mix (formerly called Hunter's Sauce)

2 pounds cubed stewing beef

1 cup red wine

Cookware needed: large pot, or Crock-Pot

Combine the mushroom soup and gravy mix in the cooking pot.

Add the meat. If using a Crock-Pot, cook on high for 7 to 9 hours. If cooking on top of the stove, simmer gently for 3 to 4 hours.

Stir in the wine approximately 1 hour before serving

PREPARATION TIME: *5 minutes*
TOTAL TIME: *3 to 9 hours*

Sage Advice

These words come from Maggie, a busy young wife and mother. "Be sure to buy stew beef that has already been cut into small cubes. These will be much more tender than the large stew beef pieces."

Quick-Quick Brunswick Stew

"IS YOUR Brunswick Stew as good as your mother's?" my long-time family friend Adele Clement asked me. "We couldn't have a church bazaar without your mother's Brunswick Stew."

After a thirty-eight-year absence, I had returned to Danville, Virginia, the town where I grew up, and before I could even unpack my pots and pans, my culinary talents were being challenged!

Adele's question brought back fond memories of hours Mother and I had spent together in the kitchen, talking all the time we boiled the hens and peeled and chopped the onions and potatoes. If it was summertime, we even shelled fresh lima beans and cut corn off the cob to make this Southern delicacy.

Then we stirred the stew for hours on end, careful to keep it from sticking to the bottom of the pan. And, oh yes, there was the constant tasting of the concoction throughout the stirring time to add exactly the right amount of flavoring—our favorite part, of course.

But Adele's question also put me on the spot, because it had been years since I'd made Brunswick Stew from scratch.

"You'll have to taste mine to decide for yourself," I told her—not wanting to reveal my secret.

Several days later, once I had found my trusty can opener and unpacked my heaviest 8-quart pot, I went to work. In just a matter of minutes, I whipped up a big mess (as we call it in the South) of Brunswick Stew and ran it by Adele's house. (Neither my house, nor I, was ready for dinner guests.)

"You have your mother's touch," she raved, after tasting it. "Now, about the church bazaar..."

You too can have delicious "homemade Brunswick Stew" that everyone will rave about—thanks to Mrs. Fearnow's canned product, which provides the perfect chicken base to which you add your homemade touch.

Sage Advice

If you like larger pieces of tomato, you will want to use the stewed tomatoes. On the other hand, if you prefer your stew to have a soupier consistency, you'll reach for a can of crushed tomatoes.

SERVES 12

1 (14-ounce) can chicken broth

1 cup frozen lima beans (any variety from small to Fordhook will do)

1 cup frozen corn (traditionally yellow, but a mix of yellow and white will work)

1 (14-ounce) can crushed or stewed tomatoes (either works perfectly well—see *Sage Advice*)

1 to 2 cans tomato and jalapeño mix (either 10-ounce Rotel, or 14-ounce house brand)—see the recipe directions below

2 (40-ounce) cans Mrs. Fearnow's Brunswick Stew

Cookware needed: large 8-quart pot with lid

Bring the chicken broth to a boil and add the lima beans and corn. Cover, reduce the heat to a simmer, and cook for 5 to 10 minutes. (Note: Fordhook limas are large and will take longer to cook.)

Add the crushed or stewed tomatoes and one can of the tomato and jalapeño mix, stir, and cook for about 5 minutes to blend the flavors.

Add the already prepared Brunswick Stew, stir well, and cook on medium-low heat for 15 to 20 minutes.

At this point, do what Mother and I always did. Taste it. If you want a spicier stew, open another can of the tomato and jalapeño mix and add more to taste, always allowing a couple of minutes for the flavors to blend before making your final judgment as to whether to add more.

PREPARATION TIME: *15 to 20 minutes*
TOTAL TIME: *35 to 45 minutes, but it will hold on low heat until you are ready to serve it*

The
Finishing Touch

Brunswick Stew is one of my favorite foods. In the South, we serve it with piping-hot ham biscuits any time of day and call it dinner. But you may wish to add a salad to your menu. This is the perfect dish for a casual get-together, especially if you have an attractive pot to serve it from— whether in the kitchen or in the dining room. And if you don't have ham biscuits, don't fret. A good storebought cheese bread, or one of the Jiffy mix corn breads (see pages 228–230) will be just as tasty.

Quick Brunswick Stew

UNFORTUNATELY, Mrs. Fearnow's Brunswick Stew is not available through-out the country. But it can be ordered, either by e-mail (www.snows.com/lov-stew/mailorder.html) or by phone (1-800-222-7839).

For those who love this Southern delicacy, but not the making of it (and if you can't get the canned product to use as a base), here's a short-cut recipe that begins with a rotisserie chicken instead of a raw fryer.

SERVES 12

4 (15-ounce) cans chicken broth

4 cups water

6 medium potatoes, peeled and diced, or a package of the ready-to-cook variety for hash-brown potatoes

1 (32-ounce) bag frozen lima beans (any variety from small to Fordhook will do)

1 (32-ounce) bag frozen corn (traditionally yellow, but shoepeg is good)

2 whole rotisserie chickens, skinned, meat removed from the bones

1 cup frozen, diced onion, thawed

3 (15-ounce) cans crushed or stewed tomatoes (either works perfectly well—see *Sage Advice* on page 210)

1 to 2 cans tomato and jalapeño mix (either 10-ounce Rotel, or 14-ounce house brand)—see the recipe directions below

1 (6-ounce) can tomato paste (optional)

Cookware needed: large 8-quart pot with lid

Bring the chicken broth and water to a boil and add the potatoes. Cook 5 min-utes, then add the lima beans, corn, and onion. Cover, reduce the heat to a sim-mer, and cook for another 15 minutes, or until the lima beans are tender.

Tear or cut the chicken meat into small pieces.

To the pot, add the chicken, the crushed or stewed tomatoes, and the tomato and jalapeño mix. Stir, and cook on medium-low heat for about 30 minutes to blend the flavors and until the mixture begins to thicken.

Now adjust the seasoning and the consistency to your liking by adding another can of the tomato and jalapeño mix and/or a can of tomato paste.

PREPARATION TIME: *30 minutes*
TOTAL TIME: *about 1 hour, but it will hold on low heat until you are ready to serve it*

Baked Pasta

"**WHERE DO YOU** get all your recipes from?" I'm often asked.

By now you've figured out that, like your recipes, mine come from all over—from friends, strangers in airports, family, old cookbooks and magazines, my kids, out of my own head, and often a combination of all the above. These days you can add yet another source to the list—the Internet.

Almost every food company has a score of recipes posted on their Web pages. But who has the time, or who wants to, spend hours surfing the Net looking for a timesaving recipe. (Sounds self-defeating to me!)

Still, these companies' kitchens offer excellent recipes, like this 10-Minute Baked Ziti recipe from Ragú/Lipton, which really exemplifies the concept of *From Storebought to Homemade*. I became familiar with it when I became good phone friends with some of the Ragú folks after discovering Ragú's line of Cheese Creation sauces.

These sauces are delicious, great time-savers, and give a real pick-me-up to many casseroles and entrées. In fact, they have become as much a staple in my kitchen as Campbell's cream soups were in my mother's. For example, I use Ragú's Roasted Garlic Parmesan Cheese sauce instead of the usual cream of mushroom soup in several of my older chicken and shrimp dishes.

But most people associate Ragú with pasta, and here, to save you the time of turning on your computer, are a couple of quick *From Storebought to Homemade* dishes to serve in your home, courtesy of my new-made friends.

"The conscientious housewife of yesteryear rolled out her noodle dough every morning and hung it up to dry in sheets behind the stove. There are still a few old-fashioned wives who make noodles in the old manner, but most people think the manufactured noodle of today is as good as its hand-made ancestor."

—SILAS SPITZER, "EVERYBODY LOVES SPAGHETTI," 1951

10-Minute Baked Ziti

SERVES 8

1 (26-ounce) jar Ragú® Pasta Sauce (your favorite tomato-based flavor)

1 ½ cups water

1 (15-ounce) container ricotta cheese

¼ cup Parmesan cheese, grated

1 (8-ounce) package mozzarella cheese, grated

1 (8-ounce) box ziti

Cookware needed: 9 x 13-inch baking dish or casserole, mixing bowl

Preheat the oven to 400 degrees.

Combine the sauce and water in a mixing bowl.

Stir in the ricotta, Parmesan, and ½ the mozzarella cheese, then the uncooked ziti.

Spoon the mixture into a 9 x 13-inch baking dish and cover it with foil.

Bake for 55 minutes.

Remove the foil, sprinkle with the remaining mozzarella, and bake uncovered for an additional 5 minutes.

PREPARATION TIME *10 minutes*
TOTAL TIME: *1 hour and 10 minutes*

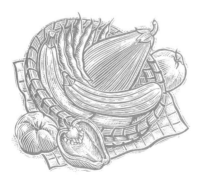

IF YOU'RE looking for an alternative to the tomato-based ziti, try this variation which uses Ragú's® Cheese Creations!™ Parmesan and Mozzarella Sauce. My assistant, Charlotte, suggests that you try other types of quick-cooking pasta, such as curly rotini, bow ties, or angel hair—even some of the tri-colored varieties of these pastas—to vary the look of this meat-free, but very satisfying All-in-One Meal. It's good served with a salad.

SERVES 8

1 ½ (16-ounce) jars Ragú®
Parmesan and Mozzarella
Sauce

1 cup water

1 (15-ounce) container ricotta
cheese

¼ cup Parmesan cheese, grated

1 (8-ounce) package mozzarella
cheese, grated

1 (8-ounce) box ziti, or one of the
other pastas mentioned above

2 eggs beaten

Cookware needed: 9 x 13 inch
baking dish or casserole,
mixing bowl

Sage Advice
*When preparing this
dish, you can add more
sauce if you so wish.*

Preheat the oven to 400 degrees.

Combine the sauce and water in a mixing bowl.

Stir in the ricotta, Parmesan, and ½ the mozzarella cheese, then follow with the uncooked ziti, or other pasta.

Spoon the mixture into a baking dish and cover it with foil.

Bake for 55 minutes.

Remove the foil, sprinkle with the remaining mozzarella, and bake uncovered for an additional 5 minutes.

PREPARATION TIME: *10 minutes*
TOTAL TIME: *1 hour and 10 minutes*

3-Cheese Spaghetti Pizza

AND HERE, especially for when the kids in the house are clamoring for pizza, but you are determined not to call for home delivery one more time this week, is a 3-Cheese Spaghetti Pizza. If you like this recipe, refer to the Hot Cheese Pie on page 52, which also becomes a "pizza," thanks to the cheese and eggs that cook into a crust.

Just as I suggested you could add some meat to that recipe, you can try the same with this one.

SERVES 6 TO 8

1 (8 ounce) box spaghetti

1 (15-ounce) container ricotta cheese

2 eggs, slightly beaten

Salt and freshly ground pepper, to taste

1 (16-ounce) jar Ragú® Parmesan and Mozzarella Sauce

¼ cup Parmesan cheese, grated

Cookware needed: mixing bowl, 10-inch pizza pan

Preheat the oven to 375 degrees.

Cook the spaghetti according to the package directions.

Combine the spaghetti, ricotta, and eggs in a large bowl. Add the salt and pepper, to taste.

Spread this mixture evenly in a greased 10-inch pizza pan.

Spread the Ragú® Parmesan and Mozzarella Cheese Sauce evenly on top.

Bake for 30 minutes or until bubbling.

Let stand 5 minutes before serving.

PREPARATION TIME: *10 minutes*
TOTAL TIME: *40 to 45 minutes*

Lazy Boy Lasagna

THERE are those times when you open the freezer and find you don't have the ready-to-serve meal you thought you had. That's when you turn to the pantry and the refrigerator.

Among the items usually in my pantry is a package of lasagna noodles...the regular pasta that has been available for years. Nowadays, "no boil" lasagna noodles can be found on the shelves of every supermarket. But my son, Langdon, discovered this "no boil" trick years ago when he didn't have the time, or the patience (or probably both) to boil the lasagna noodles first.

He just started layering the ingredients in the baking dish, and when he finished assembling it all, he stuck it in the oven. To his amazement, it worked. He hasn't boiled a lasagna noodle since.

SERVES 10 TO 12

1 teaspoon olive oil

3 to 4 cloves garlic

½ cup frozen, diced onion

1 pound lean ground beef

approximately 48 ounces Ragú® Pasta Sauce (your favorite flavor)

2 (15-ounce) containers ricotta cheese

1 (8-ounce) package mozzarella cheese, grated

10 to 12 lasagna noodles/regular

¼ cup Parmesan Cheese, grated

Cookware needed: skillet, baking dish or casserole

Heat the oil, add the garlic, and sauté briefly to release the flavor and aroma.

Add the onion and ground beef and brown. Drain and set aside.

Preheat the oven to 350 degrees.

Spread a thin layer of the sauce in a baking dish, followed by layers of lasagna noodles, ricotta cheese, meat, a sprinkling of the mozzarella cheese, and more sauce.

Repeat the layering twice more, ending with the noodles and sauce.

Cover the pan with foil and bake the lasagna for 45 minutes.

Remove the foil, add the remaining mozzarella and Parmesan cheese, and bake about 10 to 15 minutes longer, or until the top cheese has melted.

PREPARATION TIME: *15 minutes*
TOTAL TIME: *1 hour and 10 to 15 minutes*

Sage Advice

Langdon says that cooking is like chemistry. You take the ingredients you have, mix them together, and see what happens. So if he doesn't have enough Parmesan cheese for the top, he uses grated Romano. And as far as the specific number of lasagna noodles goes, he says, "however many fit in the baking dish. Break them up, if need be." And, of course, sometimes he uses more or less sauce. So it comes as no surprise that his sage advice is this: "Read the recipe first, check the ingredients you have on hand, and then relax, use what you have, and have fun." Incidentally, by following his directions for assembling the lasagna, you only dirty one skillet and the baking pan. You spoon the rest of the ingredients directly from their containers.

Zippy Breads

"*OUR SUPPER was very good: only bread was lacking; but inquiring of us what sort we wanted, in an hour's time they served us what we had asked for.*"

—The Marquis de Chastellux, traveling in America in the 1780s

How well I remember the hours I spent kneading and rolling, punching down and pinching off bits of dough, in those long-ago days when I thought it was necessary to make homemade bread.

Occasionally, those hours were well spent and generously rewarded when I turned out the perfect loaf. But more often my time was wasted when, for some unknown reason, the bread rose on one side only, or was sad in the middle, or didn't rise at all.

I never thought about it at the time, but I was doing something our ancestors had done since time immemorial—trusting my hard-spent labor to external conditions (heat and humidity) that were out of my control and could, in turn, cause that carefully blended flour and yeast and water to flop in the twinkling of an eye. All of which is why the first real convenience food has to have been bakery-baked bread.

What housewife, after all, had the time to man the special oven required for baking bread in ancient days? (If she had one, that is.) That is why there were *bakeries* in ancient Greece (first) and Rome (by the second century B.C.). A tradition that continues today.

Truth be told, in most homes, homemade bread is a recent indulgence—thanks to the newfangled bread machines!

So, under the circumstances, I choose to buy loaves of bread from the store. But I do thoroughly enjoy mixing up a quick batch of muffins or corn bread or even cheese biscuits.

That's why I'm including only a few recipes for breads. But the ones that are here will add zip to your entire meal and, when served, will make everyone think you could always bake bread...if you wanted to!

"Everybody is always out of bread," Mrs. Grace Townsend

wrote in The Star Cook Book *back in 1895.*

"Prevent it if you can."

A well-stocked traditional breadbasket fills the bill, and one with a loop handle makes for easy passing. A simple rattan or straw-type basket with a checkered or colorful napkin liner is great for informal meals and buffets, but for more formal occasions, a silver or brass basket lined with a damask napkin adds real pizzazz to the table.

Sage Advice

In one of mother's dog-eared cookbooks, there were numerous newspaper clippings with all kinds of kitchen advice. Most of them would be worthless to today's cook, who uses a microwave and food processor as a matter of course. But this one on how to grease a loaf pan or muffin tin is as relevant today as ever. "Margarine and oil can be absorbed into the dough or batter and even make the bread stick to the pan. Always use shortening to grease pans."

Beer Bread

FOOD historians have long pondered the question, which came first—the bread or the brew?

Historians believe that prehistoric man heated water to boiling and then added grain kernels to make an early version of gruel or mash. But, if left alone in the water—which eventually cooled down—the grain fermented, making brew.

Beer bread combines grain and beer in a quick-and-easy loaf that even I can make! The result—-great aroma from the kitchen, a true *From Storebought to Homemade* bread, and raves from the table.

MAKES 1 LOAF

½ cup sugar

2 cups self-rising flour

12 ounces beer (not light)

1 stick butter, melted

Cookware needed: loaf pan

Preheat the oven to 350 degrees.

Combine the sugar, flour, and beer, and transfer the dough to a greased loaf pan.

Allow the dough to stand for about 10 minutes (this can be while the stove preheats).

Bake for 50 minutes.

Pour the melted butter over the top of the bread as soon as it comes out of the oven.

PREPARATION TIME: *5 minutes*
TOTAL TIME: *approximately 60 minutes*

Sage Advice

This is a sweet, moist bread that should be eaten immediately after cooking. For a less sweet bread, use as little as 3 tablespoons of sugar, or for a really sweet bread, use up to a full cup.

Ice Cream Muffins

THIS IS ONE RECIPE you aren't going to believe.

Meredith Maynard Chase, one of the authors of *Caterin' to Charleston*, shared it with me in the mid-1980s when I was living in Raleigh and my former husband was president of Saint Mary's College.

Read the recipe, and then there's more.

MAKES 12 MUFFINS

2 cups self-rising flour or
  Bisquick
2 cups softened vanilla ice cream

Cookware needed: mixing bowl,
  12-cup muffin tin

Preheat the oven to 425 degrees.

Combine the flour and ice cream until smooth. Add a little more ice cream, if necessary to make it creamy.

Grease the bottoms of 12 muffin cups and then fill ¾ full with the batter. Bake for 25 minutes, or until golden.

That's it! Meredith actually recommended sprinkling the muffins with cinnamon and sugar before serving, but that's not necessary.

This recipe isn't just easy. It also has endless possibilities.

When my grandson, Benjamin, was going through his two-or-more-bananas-a-day stage, I made banana-nut bread muffins. Other times I have turned the recipe into strawberry bread muffins, and even rum-raisin muffins.

The secret is to use the best, richest, creamiest ice cream you can find. For the banana-nut bread muffins I used Breyer's Homestyle Butter Pecan ice cream and Bisquick, to which I added ½ cup chopped pecans and three overripe bananas. Benjamin and I ate them for breakfast, lunch, supper, and snacks.

PREPARATION TIME: *5 minutes*
TOTAL TIME: *25 minutes*

Marmalade Muffins

ARE YOU ONE of those folks who loves ketchup, but doesn't like tomatoes?

I'm one who loves oranges but will usually pass up marmalade, if I have the choice between a berry preserve (usually strawberry or raspberry, but even blackberry or gooseberry) *or* marmalade.

That's why I particularly enjoy these quick and delicious marmalade muffins. There's no "berry" choice to compete with their delicious orange flavor. Further, these slightly sweet muffins are a great addition to that special breakfast, or even dinner when chicken, ham, or pork is being served.

MAKES 12 MUFFINS

2 cups Bisquick
2 tablespoons butter, melted
3 heaping tablespoons sugar
½ cup orange juice

2 eggs, lightly beaten
½ cup orange (or lemon) marmalade
Cookware needed: mixing bowl 12-cup muffin tin

The
Finishing Touch

Consider baking these sweet muffins in miniature muffin tins. These minimuffins are delicious with afternoon tea. If you do this, they will bake a little more quickly, in approximately 12 or 15 minutes, and will yield 24 muffins.

Preheat the oven to 400 degrees.

Grease or spray the bottoms of 12-muffin cups.

Measure 1 cup of the Bisquick into a mixing bowl.

Combine the melted butter with the sugar and stir the mixture into the Bisquick.

Add the orange juice and the eggs and stir.

Now add the rest of the Bisquick and mix just enough to moisten.

Lightly stir in the marmalade.

Fill the muffin cups ⅔ full, and bake for 15 to 20 minutes, or until golden brown.

PREPARATION TIME: *10 minutes*
TOTAL TIME: *30 minutes*

Miniature Pineapple Cupcakes

FOR ANOTHER SWEET, dainty treat, try these pineapple muffins that are so sweet you can even call them cupcakes.

MAKES 48 MINIATURE MUFFINS

1 box orange or yellow cake mix

4 eggs

1 (15-ounce) can crushed pineapple

Cookware needed: mixing bowl, 2 24-cup miniature muffin tins

Preheat the oven to 325 degrees.

Combine all the ingredients.

Fill 48 greased miniature muffin cups ⅔ full, and bake 12 to 15 minutes, or until brown.

PREPARATION TIME: *10 minutes*
TOTAL TIME: *approximately 25 minutes*

The
Finishing Touch

To turn these into real "tea" muffins, shake powdered sugar over them when they are cool.

"Do you remember the mouth-watering aroma of homemade bread baking over a slow fire—the memorable sight of steaming bread fresh from the oven—the exquisite taste of each delicious slice...the kind you haven't had since grandmother's day?"

—A NOTE FROM MARGARET RUDKIN OF PEPPERIDGE FARM, 1962

Incredibly Quick Cheese Biscuits

USED to be that no Southern lady could have a party without serving paper-thin, crispy cheese straws. If she made them herself, she would have practiced for years to perfect the technique of pushing them through a cookie press with just the right pressure and to just the right length. Otherwise, she had to buy them (for a pretty penny) from other enterprising ladies who had learned that these delicacies were essential party fare.

These incredibly quick miniature cheese biscuits are a great substitute for those labor-intensive cheese straws, and they're so easy to make that you will want to serve them to your family, not just to the ladies.

Sage Advice

If you're going to be pressed for time, mix the batter the day before and store it overnight in the refrigerator.

MAKES 48 BISCUITS

1 (8-ounce) package sharp
   Cheddar cheese, grated

2 sticks butter, melted

1 (8-ounce) container sour cream

2 cups self-rising flour

½ teaspoon cayenne pepper or
   garlic powder (optional)

Cookware needed: mixing bowl, 2
24-cup miniature muffin tins

Preheat the oven to 350 degrees.

Combine the cheese and melted butter. Cool for 2 minutes, then add the sour cream and mix well. Stir in the flour.

For variety, add ½ teaspoon cayenne pepper or ½ teaspoon garlic powder to the flour before it is added to the cheese, butter, and sour cream mixture.

Fill 48 greased miniature muffin cups ⅔ full.

Bake for 18 to 22 minutes.

PREPARATION TIME: *10 minutes*
TOTAL TIME: *approximately 30 minutes*

Blue Cheese Nibbles

THE FOLLOWING is one of those recipes that made me ponder, "Where should I put it?"

The Blue Cheese Nibbles that Shirley Duncan was kind enough to share with all of us work equally well as a cocktail party treat, an unexpected and delicious indulgence served with soup at lunch, or as a bread passed at a dinner party. With so many options, I concluded they belong under Zippy Breads.

MAKES 32 NIBBLES

1 (8-ounce) can refrigerator biscuits, cut into quarters

½ stick butter (not margarine)

¼ cup blue cheese, crumbled

1 teaspoon Worcestershire sauce

Cookware needed: 9 x 13-inch cake pan, small saucepan or microwave-safe bowl

Preheat the oven to 400 degrees.

Arrange the biscuits in a 9 x 13-inch cake pan so they touch each other.

In a small saucepan or microwave-safe bowl, melt the butter and cheese together.

Add the Worcestershire sauce, and mix well.

Pour the cheese mixture over the biscuits.

Bake for 12 to 15 minutes or until golden brown.

Serve hot.

PREPARATION TIME: *5 minutes*
TOTAL TIME: *20 minutes*

No-Mess Quick Biscuits

"You know you can't write a cookbook without including biscuits in it," a neighbor said, chastising me.
"Biscuits!" another friend, who was along with us, moaned.
"I'm tired of getting flour all over my kitchen."
"You won't if you make those quick biscuits made with mayonnaise," another friend chimed in.
"Or the ones made with sour cream," said yet another.

If you, and your friends and neighbors, are still making biscuits the old-fashioned way…

Or, if you depend on some of the delicious frozen biscuits now available, but have that urge to mix and stir up a batch of homemade biscuits…

Try one of the following three-ingredient, no-mess recipes.

Mayonnaise Biscuits

MAKES 12 BISCUITS

1 cup Bisquick or self-rising flour
½ cup milk
3 tablespoons mayonnaise

Cookware needed: mixing bowl, 12-cup muffin tin

Preheat the oven to 400 degrees.

Combine the three ingredients until smooth.

Spoon the batter into 12 greased muffin cups, filling them about ½ full.

Bake for about 10 to 12 minutes.

PREPARATION TIME: *10 minutes*
TOTAL TIME: *approximately 20 minutes*

Sour Cream Biscuits

MAKES 24 BISCUITS

½ stick butter

1 cup Bisquick

½ (8-ounce) carton sour cream

Cookware needed: mixing bowl, 24-cup miniature muffin tin

Preheat the oven to 425 degrees.

Melt the butter in the microwave or over very low heat.

Stir in the Bisquick and sour cream and mix thoroughly.

Fill 24 miniature muffin cups half to ⅔ full.

Bake for 10 to 12 minutes, or until the tops are well browned.

PREPARATION TIME: *10 minutes*
TOTAL TIME: *approximately 20 to 25 minutes*

Bread should be broken, never cut.

Pastry should be broken and eaten with a fork.

Fish must be eaten with the fork.

Peas and beans require the fork only.

Potatoes, if mashed should be mashed with the fork.

Green corn should be eaten from the cob,

held with a single hand only.

Eat slowly for both health and manners.

Never eat all there is on your plate, nor attempt to do so.

—TABLE ETIQUETTE, FROM *THE STAR COOK BOOK*,
BY MRS. GRACE TOWNSEND, 1895

Cornmeal Biscuits

Oh, and just in case you find those recipes too much trouble, but you're determined to bring a *From Storebought to Homemade* biscuit to your table, try this trick: Separate the biscuits from a can of refrigerator biscuits and roll them in cornmeal, then bake them according to the package directions.

Corny Corn Bread

Being a Southerner, I like my corn bread made from coarse-ground yellow cornmeal, water, eggs, and a little "grease"—be it butter or bacon fat or shortening. But I'm in the minority these days.

My kids like corn added to their cornbread. If that's what you like, you'll want to try these three updated versions of an old-timey favorite.

Sage Advice

Charlotte Sizer, my trusty assistant, says that Jiffy corn bread mix is always dependable.

Corn Bread Plus

SERVES APPROXIMATELY 8

1 (8-ounce) box Jiffy corn bread mix

1 (15-ounce) can whole kernel corn, drained

3 tablespoons butter or, if you have it on hand, bacon grease

Cookware needed: square baking dish

The Finishing Touch

You can dot the bread with pats of butter when you remove the pan from the oven. The butter will melt while you cut the bread into squares to serve immediately.

Preheat the oven to 400 degrees.

Prepare the corn bread mix according to the directions on the package.

Stir in the corn.

Melt the butter or bacon grease in square baking dish over very low heat and spread it all around.

Pour the corn bread mixture on top and bake for 40 minutes or until brown.

PREPARATION TIME: *5 to 6 minutes*
TOTAL TIME: *approximately 45 to 50 minutes*

Sweet Pepper Corn Bread

SERVES APPROXIMATELY 8

1 (8-ounce) package Jiffy corn bread mix

1 (15-ounce) can whole kernel corn with sweet peppers, drained

¼ cup frozen, diced combo of onion and green pepper

3 tablespoons butter or, if you have it on hand, bacon grease

Cookware needed: square baking dish or casserole

Preheat the oven to 400 degrees.

Prepare the corn bread mix according to package directions.

Add the corn and the onion and green pepper combo.

Melt the butter or bacon grease in the square baking dish over very low heat and spread it all around.

Pour the corn bread mixture into the baking dish and bake for 40 minutes or until brown.

PREPARATION TIME: *5 to 6 minutes*
TOTAL TIME: *45 to 50 minutes*

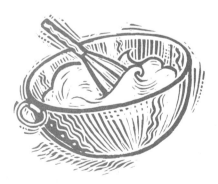

Jalapeño Corn Bread

HERE we go again! Just start with the Jiffy corn bread mix and add ingredients to your taste buds' delight. What makes this bread different from the previous two is that it is more like a spoon bread that you dish out at the table than a bread you cut ahead of time and serve in the traditional "pass the bread" way.

By the way, my son, Langdon, says this is his "pick" of these recipes. He is crazy about it. It can even take the place of a potato, rice, or pasta dish.

Sage Advice

When you add the meat, this bread becomes almost a meal in itself, albeit a very rich one. It's delicious when served with a taco salad and refried beans. I like to prepare it without the meat when I'm having guests in for a casual chili and salad buffet.

SERVES 10 TO 12

1 (8-ounce) package Jiffy corn bread mix

¼ cup melted butter or bacon drippings

1 (8-ounce) can cream-style corn

½ cup frozen, diced combo of onion and green pepper

½ cup Cheddar cheese, grated (or one of the cello-pack cheese mixtures that you have on hand)

1 to 3 tablespoons diced canned jalapeño peppers

½ to 1 pound ground meat, either mild sausage or hamburger, cooked and drained (optional)

Cookware needed: 2-quart baking dish or casserole

Preheat the oven to 400 degrees.

Prepare the corn bread mix according to package directions.

Pour a little of the melted butter or drippings into the bottom of the 2-quart baking dish to grease it.

Add the remaining butter or drippings to the corn bread mix along with all the other ingredients, and pour the batter into the baking dish.

Bake for 45 to 50 minutes, or until set and brown on top.

PREPARATION TIME: *5 to 6 minutes, add 10 minutes if cooking meat*
TOTAL TIME: *50 to 60 minutes*

Anything-Goes Crescent Rolls

One of the most versatile items in the grocery store is a can of refrigerator crescent rolls. You can create just about any bread by adding a favorite spice, meat, or herb. The ones that follow run the gamut from sweet to salty and can be served at a variety of meals.

Tomato Basil Crescents

SERVES 8 (OR MORE AS APPETIZERS)

1 (8-ounce) can refrigerator crescent rolls

1 (3-ounce) jar pesto sauce (with olive oil base)

1 (5-ounce) jar sun-dried tomato tapenade

Cookware needed: baking sheet

Unroll the triangles of dough and, onto each one, spread 1 scant teaspoon of pesto sauce and 1 heaping teaspoon of sun-dried tomato tapenade. Re-roll the crescents and place them on a baking sheet.

Bake according to package directions. Wrap in aluminum foil to reheat.

PREPARATION TIME: *5 minutes*
TOTAL TIME: *17 to 25 minutes*

The
Finishing Touch

For appetizers, or smaller appetites, the rolls can be cut in half before baking—they rise into a lovely knot. This applies to all the refrigerator crescent recipes.

Cinnamon Crescents

SERVES 8

1 (8-ounce) can refrigerator crescent rolls

8 tablespoons superfine granulated sugar

Cinnamon

3 tablespoons melted butter (optional)

Cookware needed: baking sheet

Unroll the triangles of dough and, onto each, sprinkle 1 teaspoon of sugar. Dust them all generously with cinnamon and re-roll the crescents.

Bake them on a baking sheet according to package directions. Wrap in aluminum foil to reheat.

Add a yummy touch to this sweet bread by brushing the crescents with the melted butter just before removing them from the oven.

PREPARATION TIME: *5 minutes*
TOTAL TIME: *17 to 25 minutes*

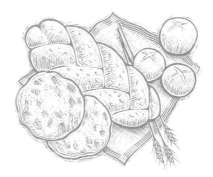

Ham Biscuits in a Flash

SERVES 8

¼ pound sliced ham (if you want to be authentic, use Smithfield or Virginia Country Ham)

2 tablespoons olive oil

or

½ (8-ounce) jar deviled Smithfield ham

1 (8-ounce) can refrigerator crescent rolls

Cookware needed: mixing bowl, baking sheet

If using sliced ham, combine it with the olive oil and mince it in a blender or food processor.

Unroll the triangles of dough and spread about 1 tablespoon of the ham mixture onto the upper third of each one.

Re-roll the triangles and put them on a baking sheet. Bake according to package directions. Wrap in aluminum foil to reheat.

PREPARATION TIME: *5 minutes (plus 5 more if grinding the ham)*
TOTAL TIME: *17 to 30 minute*

"It is not mere chance or legend which gives
the Smithfield ham honorable acclaim throughout the
world. The rich, pervading flavor of the slices is quite
unlike anything else in the way of pork.
Something more than a hundred years ago, Queen Victoria
of England ordered for Buckingham Palace a shipment
of six hams a week from Smithfield, Virginia. The order
has never been canceled. The shipments have never been
interrupted, even in times of war."

—MORRIS MARKEY, "THE TASTY PIG," 1949

Easy Sausage Swirls

YIELDS 40 SWIRLS

2 (8-ounce) cans refrigerator
crescent rolls

2 tablespoons hot mustard

1 pound bulk hot pork sausage

Cookware needed: baking sheet

Separate the rolls into four rectangles and spread each one with mustard.

Spread each rectangle with a thin layer of sausage.

Re-roll and chill the crescents until ready to bake.

Thinly slice each roll (10 swirls to a roll) and place the rounds on an ungreased baking sheet.

Bake according to package directions.

PREPARATION TIME: *5 minutes*
TOTAL TIME: *17 to 25 minutes*

Seeded Bread Sticks

SERVES 8 OR MORE

1 (8-ounce) can refrigerator
crescent rolls

Vegetable oil cooking spray

Poppy seeds

Sesame seeds

Sea salt

Dried onion (optional)

Cookware needed: baking sheet
or large pizza stone

Unroll and lay the crescent roll dough out in one single layer on a baking sheet, or shape to fit a large pizza stone, pressing all the perforated edges together to seal them.

Spray the surface of the dough with vegetable oil spray.

Sprinkle both kinds of seeds over the entire surface of the dough. Then sprinkle with salt and onion, less generously than with the seeds.

Bake according to package directions.

Remove from the oven and cut into sticks about 1 inch wide and 3 inches long.

PREPARATION TIME: *5 minutes*
TOTAL TIME: *17 to 25 minutes*

Sage Advice

A pizza cutting wheel comes in handy when cutting the bread sticks.

Fabulous Finales

THOSE TRAYS the waiters bring around at the end of a meal with a slice of triple chocolate mousse topped with raspberry sauce; a crimped lemon galette prepared with zest of lemon; a plum tart with swirls of dried apricots and toasted almonds; and a mocha torte with toffee drizzled over the top are, well...*over* the top.

Never underestimate the appeal of a sweet to round out the perfect meal, but a good dessert need not require a double boiler, a candy thermometer, and a pastry tube to be delicious. Take my experience last Thanksgiving.

While looking through the pile of cookbooks that are always by my side of the bed, I came upon a dessert recipe for "Sin." How could I resist?

This is what I read, "Mix [chocolate wafer] crumbs and melted butter. Press into bottom of 13 x 8-inch pan. Chill until firm."

Hhmmmm, I thought. I can cut out that step. I'll just use a storebought Oreo Cookie crust.

For the filling, I was supposed to "Crush chilled [toffee] candy bars and mix together with [vanilla] ice cream."

Now let's see. After doing all that, I'm going to end up with butter brickle ice cream. Why not just buy a quart, I concluded.

Finally, whip

"Or, just buy an aerosol can of whipped cream," I said out loud.

So that's what I did. I bought an Oreo Cookie crust; filled it with butter brickle ice cream, and squirted a fancy border of whipped cream around the edge—Sinful Butter Brickle Ice Cream Pie (page 257).

Thanksgiving dinner came and went and it was dessert time. I brought out slices of homemade (for real) brownies, Old-Fashioned Lemon Chess Pie (it's so simple I've included it in the book, page 250), and *From Storebought to Homemade* Sinful Butter Brickle Ice Cream Pie.

"I'll have some of that ice cream pie," my daughter piped up. "Me too," "me too," "me too," everyone around the table chimed in.

No one touched a single one of those other desserts I had taken the time to prepare.

Not only was the last slice of ice cream pie gobbled up, there wasn't even a crumb of storebought Oreo Cookie crust left on a single plate.

The moral of the story is this: Simple, easy desserts work just fine.

Fruit Platter

EVERY TIME you walk into a well-lighted, cheerful grocery store, I'll wager that you stroll by the fruit display just to enjoy the beautiful array of pears, apples, grapes, and berries. It's a feast for the eyes...and for the palate as well.

Somehow, in these days of layered cakes and fancy tortes, we seem to have forgotten how succulent and satisfying a simple arrangement of fresh fruits can be at the end of a meal. Next time you're having guests over, make a pretty centerpiece of nothing but fruit on a platter. Then, when dessert time comes around, pass a fruit plate, followed by a bowl of flavored cream. You'll be amazed how much everyone will enjoy this traditional, but seldom served dessert.

Sage Advice

For an even simpler fruit tray, arrange small grape clusters and apple wedges (sprinkled with lemon juice as described) on a plate. On a separate plate, put ½-inch slices of French bread and wedges of Brie, blue, and Camembert cheese. Garnish the bread and cheese tray with two or three flower blossoms or a few plump blueberries and mint leaves for color.

**SERVINGS VARY WITH FRUITS USED
(QUANTITY GIVEN FOR APPROXIMATELY 8 PEOPLE)**

2 red and 2 green apples

Juice of 1 lemon

4 large seedless oranges
(or tangerines, a can of
mandarin oranges, or a jar
of orange sections)

A combination (your choice) of
1-pint containers of blueberries, blackberries, raspberries

1 quart strawberries

½ pound seedless grapes

2 or 3 kiwi

Almonds, toasted

Flavored Whipped Cream
(recipe follows)

Caramel and/or chocolate sauce
(optional)

Cookware needed: medium bowl,
platter

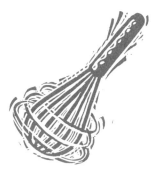

Wash and core the apples. Slice them into wedges and put them in a bowl. Or use the one-step apple corer/slicer that can be found in most grocery stores.

Squeeze lemon juice, or, if using bottled lemon juice, dribble the juice over the apples to keep them from discoloring. Refrigerate.

Peel and section the oranges or tangerines, or drain if using fruit from a can or jar.

Wash and pat dry the grapes. Snip small clusters from one bunch to be used to decorate the platter.

Rinse the berries and allow them to dry in a strainer or on paper towels.

Peel the kiwi, and slice them into rings.

To arrange the platter, put one or two large clusters of grapes in the center of a round platter. Surround them with a circle of apple wedges, kiwi slices, smaller grape clusters, and orange or tangerine sections.

These can be arranged in like groups—placing together all the red apples, all the kiwi circles, etc. or interspersed—apple slice, orange section, kiwi slice, grape cluster, apple slice, orange section, and so forth.

Sprinkle berries and almonds on top.

Pass the platter with a serving spoon and fork and follow it with a dish of Flavored Whipped Cream and, depending on how decadent you feel, bowls of hot caramel and chocolate sauce.

■ ■ ■ ■ ■ ■ ■ ■

PREPARATION TIME: *approximately 20 minutes,*
depending on the amount of fruit
TOTAL TIME: *same*

The
Finishing Touch

Any time you
are serving fruits for
dessert, it is nice to have
a small bowl or dish of
storebought chocolates
on hand for the serious
chocoholic. Chocolate
covered raspberry or
orange sticks, chocolate
covered nuts, or even
chocolate covered
miniature pretzels
will do nicely.

"Strawberries, and
only strawberries,
could now be thought
or spoken of."

—JANE AUSTEN

Flavored Whipped Cream

YIELDS APPROXIMATELY 3 CUPS

1 pint whipping cream

3 tablespoons confectioners' sugar

one of the following flavorings: a vanilla or almond extract, or a liqueur such as crème de menthe or crème de cocoa

Cookware needed: stainless steel or copper mixing bowl

Pour the carton of whipping cream into a prechilled stainless steel or copper mixing bowl. Begin to beat on high with an electric mixer. Add the confectioners' sugar slowly and continue to beat until soft peaks form (be careful that you don't beat too long, or the cream will yellow and turn to butter!). Stir in the flavoring (begin with 1 tablespoon and add more to taste).

PREPARATION TIME: *10 minutes*
TOTAL TIME: *10 minutes*

Flan

IF, when you read "flan," you're expecting to have to pull out the dreaded double boiler, think again.

Instead, next time you're at the grocery store, pick up as many packages of Kozy Shack or other ready-to-serve flans as you need and try this trick.

SERVINGS VARY ACCORDING TO NUMBER OF GUESTS

Ready-to-serve flan

1 jar whole berry preserves

Cool Whip or whipped cream

Mint leaves or fresh fruit for a garnish

Cookware needed: individual dessert plates or ramekins

Turn the flans out onto individual dessert plates or suitable ramekins.

Top them with a spoonful of your favorite whole berry preserves and a dollop of Cool Whip or whipped cream. Garnish them with mint leaves or fresh fruit to complement the preserves (strawberries, blueberries, blackberries, whatever).

PREPARATION TIME: *5 minutes*
TOTAL TIME: *5 minutes*

Pots de Crème

JUST as easy to assemble is this *From Storebought to Homemade* version of Pots de Crème, which is a fancy way of saying cream in a pot (small, individual, and very fancy pots though they be).

SERVES 4

1 box instant vanilla pudding mix, or 4 ready-to-serve individual cups of pudding

A nice liqueur such as Cointreau or Grand Marnier, Amaretto, or Framboise

Cookware needed: mixing bowl

If using instant pudding mix, prepare the pudding according to package directions. Stir ¼ cup of liqueur into the pudding and then put it into individual dessert dishes (demitasse cups or small bowls work very well for this).

Garnish each serving with a complementary fruit—mandarin oranges for Cointreau or Grand Marnier, roasted almonds for Amaretto, and raspberries or strawberries for Framboise.

PREPARATION TIME: *5 minutes*
TOTAL TIME: *5 minutes*

Baked Tipsy Apples

SERVINGS VARY

Stouffer's Escalloped Apples, frozen (as needed)

toasted, sliced almonds for a garnish

½ cup brandy

1 (12-once) jar caramel sauce

Cookware needed: baking dish or casserole, mixing bowl

Before baking the apples according to package directions, sprinkle with ¼ cup of brandy.

While the apples are baking, combine a jar of caramel sauce with another ¼ cup of brandy.

To serve, heat the brandy sauce in the microwave, or on the stovetop. Either put some of the sauce on the plate, place the apples on top, and garnish with toasted sliced almonds, or, put the apples on the plate, garnish it with the almonds, and drizzle the sauce over the top of the apple.

Serve with whipped cream.

PREPARATION TIME: *10 minutes*
TOTAL TIME: *50 minutes*

Frozen Oranges

I'VE NEVER seen frozen oranges served in a restaurant, and I've had them only a couple of times at dinner parties. Don't ask me why. They are the best and the absolutely perfect way to end a summertime dinner.

SERVINGS VARY, 1 ORANGE PER GUEST

Seedless oranges—as many as you need.

Cookware needed: a knife— that's the joy of this recipe!

Wash and dry the oranges. Slice off the top third and replace it.

Put the oranges in the freezer for the day or overnight. Just before serving dinner, take them out, remove the tops, and they'll be ready to eat (with a spoon) when it's time for dessert.

PREPARATION TIME: *5 minutes, unless you add a Finishing Touch*
TOTAL TIME: *same*

Sage Advice

When selecting the oranges, choose those with a flattened base so they'll sit up well on the plate. If available, blood oranges are best because of their vibrant color.

The Finishing Touch

Garnish each orange with a swirl of whipped cream, a sprig of fresh mint, or a few fresh raspberries. Serve them with your favorite cookies (my choice would be Milanos, orange-flavored thins, Pirouettes, or even a chocolate-covered orange candy) or splurge and get a really rich chocolate cake or torte from a local bakery or the bakery department of your grocery store.

Here's a great opportunity to pull out the squirt bottle, fill it with chocolate sauce, and make a design on the plate before placing the orange. Or, if, in one of your "I'm-going-to-fix-a-fancy-dish" moments you bought a kitchen torch, now's the chance to use it. Sprinkle the orange with granulated sugar and caramelize it.

The Basic Poached Pear

NEED an unusual, even elegant, dessert to dress up an ordinary meal? Try pears.

I've yet to figure out why pears are seldom served, when they are so delicious and so easy to prepare in such a wide variety of ways. Oh yes, did I mention that they are also good for you?

Begin with either fresh or canned pears. (If you choose fresh pears, you will want to poach them, but that's a simple task.) Combine with a flavored juice, garnish with an already made or fresh topping, and you're through.

Read through these options and see which ones tickle your taste buds. Then try one or two. I'll wager that pears will begin appearing more often around your house.

Sage Advice

Whether using fresh or canned pears, add either mint leaves, or 2 or 3 cloves and a cinnamon stick, or even a little flavored complementary fruit liqueur to the liquid. For example, to orange juice, add 1 to 2 tablespoons of Grand Marnier, or to Welch's wild raspberry blend, add Kirsch.

SERVES 4

Pears—if fresh, select firm (not quite ripe) Bosc or other pears that are in season, or canned

Some suggested flavored juices are:

cranapple juice

orange juice

juice drained from any canned cocktail fruits

your favorite mixed or blended fruit drink that you have on hand (see page 18)

If using canned pears:

Cookware needed: large bowl or baking dish or casserole

Drain the pears and place them in a bowl. Pour enough liquid (your choice) over them to cover. (Though it's not necessary, if you quickly heat the liquid in the microwave before pouring it over the pears, the pears will absorb the flavor more readily.)

Refrigerate for at least 2 hours. Serve with some of the liquid on individual dessert plates.

PREPARATION TIME USING CANNED PEARS: *5 to 10 minutes*
TOTAL TIME: *10 minutes, plus 2 hours to chill*

If using fresh pears:

Cookware needed: large bowl or saucepan or baking dish or casserole

Peel 4 whole pears. If you wish to leave them whole with the stem on, do so. Otherwise, halve the pears and remove the core.

Pears can be poached on top of the stove (in a saucepan), in a microwave, or in the oven (in a baking dish). The result is just about the same, so do what is most convenient for you. To poach on the stovetop, bring the liquid (see below) to the boiling point and then add the pears. But if microwaving or baking, place the pears in the dish, and then add the liquid.

Use approximately 2 cups of one of the suggested juices for every 4 whole pears or 8 halves.

If poaching on the stovetop, simmer the pears for approximately 15 minutes, or until they begin to soften. Microwaving takes about 10 to 15 minutes.

If baking, cook them at 350 degrees for approximately 30 minutes, basting occasionally for a richer taste.

Once the pears have cooked, chill them, juice and all, for about 4 hours. Serve with some of the cooking liquid on individual dessert plates.

■■■■■■■■■

PREPARATION TIME USING FRESH PEARS: *15 to 20 minutes*
TOTAL TIME: *varies with cooking method from 15 to 30 minutes, plus 4 hours to chill*

The
Finishing Touch

Add a few small berries—raspberries, blueberries, or sliced strawberries—to each dish for color and flavor. Mint leaves are another pretty addition. A dollop of rich vanilla ice cream is a delicious accompaniment, as is a liberal dousing of ready-to-serve boiled custard from the dairy section. And if you're feeling really indulgent, top it all off with a little chocolate—shaved, a prepared topping, or even a piece or two served on the side.

Cheesy Chocolate Pears

HERE is yet another way to serve up a quick pear dessert. It combines three delicious flavors—pear, cheese, and chocolate. Since it is "assembled" on the dessert plates themselves, there isn't even a bowl to clean up.

SERVES 4

8 well-shaped canned, pear halves, drained

Lemon juice

4 ounces cream cheese, softened—a fruit flavor, if you wish, or a more sophisticated creamy cheese such as chèvre

Chocolate sauce, your favorite commercial brand

½ cup nuts (pecans, chopped walnuts, or slivered almonds)

Cookware needed: just the serving utensils

Place 2 pear halves on each dessert plate.

Squeeze a little lemon juice on the pears for flavor.

Spoon some cream cheese into the cavity of each pear. Drizzle chocolate sauce over and around the pears and sprinkle the nuts around them.

PREPARATION TIME: *10 minutes*
TOTAL TIME: *10 minutes*

The
Finishing Touch

Thawed frozen berries, or even a gourmet preserve that is filled with large pieces of fruit, can be substituted for the chocolate sauce.

Fruit Pizza

SPEAKING of easy fruit desserts, this fruit pizza is one that daughter Joslin brought back from a trip to visit her Pennsylvania in-laws. Kelly Seiler, Mike's stepsister and a busy young mother herself, made it by gathering the fruits from a salad bar. I suggest that you do too, but as a guide the following list of ingredients includes canned or jarred fruits.

SERVES 6 TO 8

For the pizza:

1 (16-ounce) roll slice-and-bake sugar cookies

1 (8-ounce) package cream cheese, softened

1 (8-ounce) can pineapple chunks, drained

1 (11-ounce) can mandarin orange slices, drained

1 (8-ounce) can apricot halves, drained, juice reserved

2 cups halved green grapes

1 (6-ounce) jar maraschino cherries, drained

For the glaze:

½ cup reserved apricot juice

1 tablespoon cornstarch

¼ teaspoon cinnamon

Cookware needed: 14-inch pizza pan

Sage Advice

Have fun with this dessert pizza! Try substituting slice-and-bake chocolate chip cookie dough and/or a flavored cream cheese. You can also use an apricot jam (heated in the microwave for 30 seconds) instead of the glaze.

Preheat the oven to 350 degrees.

Pat sugar cookie dough into a 14-inch pizza pan.

Bake for 7 to 10 minutes or until golden brown.

Cool completely.

Spread the cream cheese over the crust.

Layer the fruits over the cream cheese in the order they are listed.

Combine all the glaze ingredients in a small saucepan and cook over medium heat until syrupy. Cool thoroughly.

Spoon the glaze over the fruit.

Chill the pizza and serve cold.

The Finishing Touch

This pizza can be topped with Cool Whip or whipped cream before serving.

PREPARATION TIME: *15 minutes*
TOTAL TIME: *approximately 20 minutes to bake and cool the cookie crust, plus a few hours to chill thoroughly*

Let Them Eat Pie!

Thank goodness my daughter has a wonderful mother-in-law who loves to bake. My poor child has been cake-deprived ever since her first birthday in 1971.

Trying to be a good mother, I had invited several friends with infants and toddlers over for a proper birthday celebration. But when the big day arrived, Joslin refused to take a morning nap and her brother, three year-old Langdon, dragged Kirk and Rodney, the little boys from next door, in to play—in the middle of the kitchen floor, of course.

Did I get aggravated? No. I simply put the eggs back in the fridge and the flour sifter back in the cabinet. For on that fateful day I took the path of no aggravation—I bought Joslin a birthday cake from the nearest grocery store. It was a great party and a family tradition was born. In our house, birthday cakes are storebought. Even today.

Unfortunately, though, my easy way out backfired the year Langdon was eight or nine and he went to his friend David Moore's birthday party. As he was leaving, Langdon made a point (I'd threatened him with no cartoons for a week if he forgot) of thanking Mrs. Moore for the nice party.

"That was great cake," he chirped, adding, "Did you buy it at the A&P?"

"Langdon!" his hostess replied, "aren't you ashamed! That was a homemade cake."

"I meant it as a compliment," Langdon replied. "Mother has tried them all. Kroger. Food Lion. Winn Dixie. A&P makes the best birthday cakes of all!"

These days, when I scoot up to Richmond, Virginia, to see Joslin and Mike and the two grandsons, I can always tell if Nancy Sweger, Mike's mom, has been there. The remains of a fabulous, home-baked cake are the telltale signs.

Me? I prefer pies. You don't have to worry about them rising (or falling) or trying to get the icing to just the right consistency.

It is sinfully easy to buy a ready-to-fill pie shell right off the grocer's shelf and then spend a minimum amount of time making a delicious filling for it. That's enough to take care of my creative dessert urges when Nancy's not around to bake cakes for everyone to enjoy!

Lemonade Pie

ONE of my earliest cooking memories is of making this frozen lemon dessert in our un-air-conditioned kitchen. There were no ready-made graham cracker pie shells, or food processors then, so my job was to crush the graham crackers. Thank goodness that's all changed!

SERVES 12 OR MORE

1 (14-ounce) can condensed milk

1 (16-ounce) container Cool Whip

1 (6-ounce) can frozen lemonade

2 graham cracker pie crusts

Cookware needed: mixing bowl

Chill the can of milk for an hour or so. Then combine it with the Cool Whip and lemonade and beat with an electric mixer until frothy.

Pour or spoon the mixture into the pie shells.

Refrigerate the pies for several hours or until well set before cutting.

PREPARATION TIME: *15 minutes*
TOTAL TIME: *several hours for the chilling*

*The
Finishing Touch*

In those pre-ready-to-fill graham cracker crust days, we made the crust by combining the crumbled graham crackers with a little melted butter and a sprinkle of sugar. We would save some of this concoction to use as a topping for the pie. It was awfully good. So, if you have the time, make up a little of this topping and everyone will think you even made the crusts!

Old-Fashioned Lemon Chess Pie

EARLY ON, in the Appetizers and Hors d'oeuvres chapter, I mentioned how compiling these recipes has taken me on a sentimental journey through my family's lives. And I've mentioned all sorts of relatives, blood kin and step-kin.

Funny, but whenever I think of Lemon Chess Pie, I remember my former sister-in-law's now former husband (how's that for a distant relation!) and how much Buddy loved this pie. He always asked me to fix it for family dinners, and I did, although not without mentioning that it would be a lot of trouble, but I'd do it "just for him."

In truth, if you can read a recipe and hold an electric mixer, you can make this pie that is guaranteed to please!

SERVES 6 TO 8 PEOPLE

1 teaspoon flour

1 ½ cups sugar

2 lemons

3 large eggs, well beaten

1 teaspoon butter, melted

1 cup milk

1 unbaked, prepared pie shell

Cookware needed: mixing bowl, small bowl

Preheat the oven to 350 degrees.

Combine the flour and sugar.

Squeeze the lemons into a small bowl, making sure to get all the juice and remove the seeds—which is why it is wise to do this separately.

Grate as much of the lemon rind as possible into the flour and sugar mixture and then add the lemon juice, the eggs, and the butter, stirring well.

Gradually add the milk and continue to mix well.

Pour the filling into the pie shell and bake for 45 minutes or until firm, lightly browned, and thoroughly set in the middle.

PREPARATION TIME: *15 to 20 minutes*
TOTAL TIME: *approximately 1 hour*

Chocolate Chess Pie

ANOTHER old-fashioned favorite, and as easy as the previous one (maybe even easier because you don't have to squeeze the lemons or grate them) is this Chocolate Chess Pie.

SERVES 6 TO 8 PEOPLE

2 large eggs
1 stick butter, softened (not melted)
2 cups sugar
2 tablespoons flour
4 tablespoons cocoa

Pinch of salt
1 (5-ounce) can evaporated milk
2 teaspoons vanilla extract
1 unbaked, prepared pie shell
Cookware needed: mixing bowl

Preheat the oven to 350 degrees.

Beat together the eggs, butter, sugar, flour, cocoa, and salt, until well blended.

Add the evaporated milk and vanilla, and, when thoroughly combined, pour the mixture into the pie shell.

Bake for 40 minutes or until firm and thoroughly set in the middle.

PREPARATION TIME: *10 minutes*
TOTAL TIME: *approximately 45 minutes*

The
Finishing Touch

To "gild the lily," so to speak, garnish the pie with Cool Whip or whipped cream, and ½ cup pecan pieces or some grated chocolate.

Brownie Pie

CHOCOLATE AND NUTS. Reminds me of brownies... which is exactly what this next pie is...Brownie Pie. It was a favorite dessert in North Carolina in the late 1970s, but like so many delicious foods, it doesn't seem to have been around lately. With all the chocoholics there are these days, it's time to resurrect it!

SERVES 6 TO 8 PEOPLE

1 cup sugar

½ cup flour

2 large eggs, beaten

½ cup butter

1 cup chopped or broken pecans

1 cup chocolate chips

1 teaspoon vanilla extract

1 unbaked, prepared pie shell

Cookware needed: 1 mixing bowl, small bowl or saucepan to melt the butter

Preheat the oven to 350 degrees.

Combine the sugar and the flour and add the eggs.

Melt the butter and allow it to cool slightly, then stir it into the egg mixture, followed by the pecans, chocolate chips, and vanilla.

Pour the filling into the pie shell and bake for 45 minutes.

PREPARATION TIME: *10 minutes*
TOTAL TIME: *approximately 1 hour*

Coconut Fruit Pie

IT'S HARD to beat a chocolate pie, but this fruit and nut pie, and Millionaire's Pie (page 254), are awfully good, and so ridiculously easy to prepare that you can make them at the drop of a hat. This one needs to be baked, the other chilled, which may help you decide which one to try first.

SERVES 6 TO 8 PEOPLE

1 stick butter
2 large eggs, lightly beaten
1 cup sugar
½ cup flaked coconut
½ cup pecans

½ cup raisins (I like the golden ones, or a mixture)
1 teaspoon distilled white vinegar
1 unbaked, prepared pie shell
Cookware needed: mixing bowl

Preheat the oven to 350 degrees.

Melt the butter, allow it to cool, and then, one at a time so they will be well blended, stir in the eggs, then the sugar, coconut, pecans, raisins, and vinegar.

Pour the filling into the pie shell and bake for 35 to 40 minutes.

PREPARATION TIME: *15 minutes*
TOTAL TIME: *1 hour*

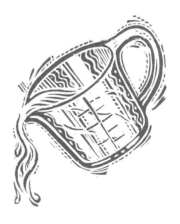

Millionaire's Pie

THIS LUSCIOUS, silky pie calls for a baked pie shell, and the flaky contrast with the gooey filling is really good. But if you're running short on time, you can substitute a graham cracker crust to eliminate that step. Do remember to chill the pineapple, though. Simply put the can in the refrigerator as soon as you bring it home from the grocery store.

SERVES 6 TO 8 PEOPLE

1 fully baked pie shell, or graham cracker crust

1 (8-ounce) package cream cheese, softened

2 cups confectioners' sugar

1 cup chilled crushed pineapple, drained

1 (12-ounce) container Cool Whip, softened, at room temperature

½ cup chopped pecans (optional)

Cookware needed: mixing bowl

If using a traditional pastry shell, bake it according to package directions.

Combine the cream cheese, sugar, pineapple, and Cool Whip and blend well.

Transfer the filling to the pie shell and, if you wish, sprinkle the top with chopped pecans.

Cover and chill for several hours.

PREPARATION TIME: *10 minutes*
TOTAL TIME: *4 to 5 hours for chilling*

Brown Sugar Pie

IF YOU LOVE pecan pie, and who doesn't, this is an excellent, ever-so-slightly different version of that Southern favorite. This recipe comes in really handy if you don't happen to have the Karo syrup that you need to make true pecan pie.

SERVES 6 TO 8 PEOPLE

1 cup brown sugar
½ cup granulated sugar
1 egg
½ eggshell milk

1 unbaked, prepared pie shell
½ to 1 cup pecans, halved or broken (optional)
Cookware needed: mixing bowl, electric mixer

Preheat the oven to 325 degrees.

Combine the sugars, the egg, and the milk, and pour the mixture into the pie shell.

If you cover the top with nuts, most people will think they're eating a pecan pie—and they are, almost.

Bake for 50 to 55 minutes, or until completely set in the middle.

PREPARATION TIME: *10 minutes*
TOTAL TIME: *approximately 1 hour*

"Eggs can be kept for some time by smearing the shells with butter or lard, then packed in plenty of bran or sawdust, the eggs not allow to touch one another; or coat the eggs with melted paraffin."

—*THE WHITE HOUSE COOK BOOK* BY HUGO ZIEMANN AND MRS. F. L. GILLETTE, 1926

Sage Advice

Did the measurement of "½ eggshell milk" catch your eye? I almost translated this into its "1 tablespoon" equivalent, as is typically done in today's cookbooks, but then you would miss the fun surprise of finding yourself measuring milk using this natural cup. And why dirty the plastic or metal variety if you don't have to?

The Finishing Touch

Not only do I recommend adding the pecans, I suggest that you top the pie with whipped cream or hard sauce and sprinkle cinnamon or chocolate shavings over it. Let's face it. If you're going to be eating this much pure sugar, a little more indulgence won't kill you.

Almost Sugar-Free Pie

BACK to that old question, "You don't eat like this all the time, do you?" The answer, "No, of course not!" hasn't changed, either.

One reason I don't indulge in these wonderful rich desserts at every meal is that my husband, Bob, has diabetes, just like almost everyone else in his father's family. It is inherited. So I watch his diet like a hawk.

Ironically, one of my father's relatives was Dr. Elliott Joslin, founder of the famed Joslin Diabetic Clinic in Boston, but I know of no diabetes in our family, so I've had to learn all about this far-reaching problem.

One thing I've learned is that more and more people, diabetic or not, are watching their sugar intake seriously. That makes this very good pie a great alternative to sugar-filled ones. I try to have it when offering more than one dessert, but oftentimes I serve it to everyone and no one suspects it is almost "sugar free," with only a few grams of sugar in the pie crust and natural sugars in the fruit (if you add no-sugar-added fruits to the mix).

Read through the recipe and decide what fruit flavor you're in the mood for—strawberry, cherry, lemon, raspberry, whatever, then buy complementary Jell-O and yogurt.

SERVES 6 TO 8 PEOPLE

1 (3-ounce) box sugar-free Jell-O (your favorite flavor)

1 cup hot water

½ cup cold water

1 (8-ounce) container sugar-free yogurt (a flavor to complement the Jell-O)

1 (8-ounce) container Cool Whip, softened, at room temperature

½ cup canned fruit in natural juices, drained and/or chopped nuts of your choice (optional)

1 graham cracker pie crust

Cookware needed: mixing bowl

Prepare the Jell-O using the hot water and the cold water. Allow it to partially jell in the refrigerator—about 30 minutes.

Stir in the yogurt and Cool Whip and, if you wish, fruit and/or nuts.

Pour the filling into the graham cracker crust and chill, or freeze.

PREPARATION TIME: *10 minutes*
TOTAL TIME: *allow for jelling and then chilling or thawing time, approximately 3 to 4 hours*

Sinful Butter Brickle Ice Cream Pie

"**TELL ME** again exactly how you made that butter brickle ice cream pie," the eager young bride asked when I told her the story (included in the introduction to this chapter) of how I converted the complicated recipe for "Sin" into a 3-step sinfully easy new recipe. Just for the record, it goes like this.

SERVES 6 TO 8 PEOPLE

1 pint butter brickle ice cream or Coffee HEATH® Bar crunch ice cream

1 Oreo cookie pie crust
1 can whipped topping
Cookware needed: None

Soften the ice cream just enough to spread it in the pie shell. Cover the pie with plastic wrap or aluminum foil and put it in the freezer. Just before serving, add a frilly border of whipped topping.

PREPARATION TIME: *10 minutes*
TOTAL TIME: *1 to 2 hours to chill*

Easy Enough Crème de Menthe Pie

EASY ENOUGH? Once you've practiced on the "sinfully" easy pie above, you'll be ready to move up to this equally easy Crème de Menthe Pie, which is wonderful in the summertime.

SERVES 6 TO 8 PEOPLE

1 pint whipping cream
1 (7-ounce) jar marshmallow cream

¼ cup Crème de Menthe
1 Oreo cookie pie crust
Cookware needed: 2 mixing bowls

Whip the cream and set aside.

Whip the marshmallow cream and Crème de Menthe together and fold the mixture into the whipped cream.

Pour the filling into the pie shell, cover the pie with plastic wrap, and freeze for at least 3 hours.

PREPARATION TIME: *15 minutes*
TOTAL TIME: *3 hours minimum freezing time*

Angels to the Rescue

I still remember the day my mother tried to make an angel food cake. What I don't remember is *why* she tried to do it. We'd bought angel food cakes many times from the grocery store and the bakery.

Knowing Mother, she probably did it for the same reason some people climb mountains—just to prove she could. But she couldn't. The cake was a disaster, and she was still talking about "all those egg whites" for days on end.

I've never even tried to make an angel food cake, but many times a store-bought angel food cake has saved the day. That's why I've called these various angel food cake desserts "Angels to the Rescue"—they involve all the complexity of purchasing an angel food cake and selecting the finishing flavor that will best complement your meal.

Hawaiian Angel

SERVES 8 TO 12

1 (8-ounce) container Cool Whip, softened, at room temperature

3 tablespoons sugar

½ teaspoon vanilla extract

¼ cup maraschino cherries, quartered

1 (8-ounce) can crushed pineapple, well drained

1 cup minimarshmallows

1 (2-ounce) package chopped walnuts

1 angel food loaf cake

Cookware needed: mixing bowl, serrated knife

Empty the Cool Whip into a mixing bowl and fold in the remaining filling ingredients, then chill the mixture for about 20 minutes.

Using a serrated-edge knife, cut a 1-inch horizontal slice from the top of the cake, then cut out a ring 2 inches wide and 2 inches deep from the inside, leaving a hollow.

Fill the cake with the chilled filling. Replace the top slice.

Frost the top and sides of the cake with additional Cool Whip or whipped cream and chill.

Slice to serve.

PREPARATION TIME: *15 to 20 minutes*
TOTAL TIME: *at least 1 hour to chill*

Angel Creams

MAKES APPROXIMATELY 16 CREAMS

1 angel food loaf cake

1 (16-ounce) container sour cream

8 tablespoons light brown sugar

Food coloring (optional)

Cookware needed: cookie sheet, serrated knife

Using a serrated-edge knife, cut the cake in half horizontally, then crosswise into bars or squares. Separate the individual cakes, laying them out on a cookie sheet or a plate.

Combine the sour cream and brown sugar. If desired, divide the mixture into 2 or 3 portions and tint each one with a different food coloring.

Ice the top of each cake, and place the cakes in the refrigerator to chill until serving time.

PREPARATION TIME: *15 to 20 minutes*
TOTAL TIME: *about 40 minutes to chill*

Strawberry Angel Short Cake

FOR this delicious summer dessert, buy a cake, slice it, and top with sweetened fresh sliced strawberries and a dollop of Cool Whip or whipped cream. Or, try this variation on the theme:

SERVES 8 TO 12

1 (10-ounce) package frozen strawberries in heavy syrup

1 angel food tube cake

1 package strawberry Jell-O

¾ cup hot water

1 (12-ounce) container Cool Whip, softened, at room temperature

Cookware needed: saucepan, mixing bowl

Set out the strawberries to thaw while you slice the cake into three horizontal layers.

Once the strawberries have thawed, pour the syrup into a measuring cup and add enough water to equal ¾ cup.

Dissolve the strawberry Jell-O in the hot water and add the ¾ cup syrup mixture.

Chill about 30 minutes, or until partially set.

Fold ½ of the Cool Whip and the strawberries into the partially set Jell-O. If necessary, chill a little longer until the mixture is a good consistency to spread.

Spread the strawberry mixture between the layers of cake, then frost it with the remaining plain Cool Whip.

Refrigerate until ready to serve, then slice.

PREPARATION TIME: *15 to 20 minutes*
TOTAL TIME: *at least 1 hour to chill*

Chocolate-Glazed
Angel Food Cake

SERVES 8 TO 12

3 cups sifted confectioners' sugar

¼ cup unsweetened cocoa

¼ cup plus 1 ½ tablespoons hot
water

1 angel food cake

Cookware needed: mixing bowl

In a bowl, combine the first three ingredients and stir until smooth.

Drizzle the glaze over the angel food cake and serve as is, or with ice cream or an accompaniment of raspberry or strawberry sherbet.

PREPARATION TIME: *10 minutes*
TOTAL TIME: *10 minutes*

Sugar-Topped Angel Food Cake

SERVES 8 TO 12

1 ½ cups sifted confectioners'
sugar

2 tablespoons milk

½ teaspoon vanilla extract

1 angel food cake

Cookware needed: mixing bowl

In a bowl, combine the first three ingredients. Drizzle the topping over the angel food cake and serve.

PREPARATION TIME: *10 minutes*
TOTAL TIME: *10 minutes*

Lemon Delight

SERVES 8 TO 12

1 angel food cake

1 jar lemon curd sauce

1 (16-ounce) container Cool Whip, softened, at room temperature

Cookware needed: 3 knives—one to cut, one to spread, one to frost

The
Finishing Touch

Garnish the cake with yellow pansies or lemon curls, if you wish.

Using a serrated edge knife, cut the angel food cake into three horizontal layers and spread the lemon curd sauce on each layer, reassembling the cake as you go.

Frost with the Cool Whip, and chill until ready to serve.

PREPARATION TIME: *10 minutes*

TOTAL TIME: *about 40 minutes to chill*

Ice Cream Cake

THIS is a fun cake because you can do anything with it—as Kathryn Wyatt did in the 1950s. Try different ice cream flavors and pick a complementary sauce. Include nuts, candies, or sauce in the cake, or not. If you're having a special party at Christmas, St. Patrick's Day, or the Fourth of July, for example, you can carry your party theme through to the end by using an appropriate mold and tinting the icing to match the occasion.

For an unusual dessert, use pistachio and peppermint ice cream. But experiment...try chocolate and pistachio with hot fudge in the middle, vanilla ice cream and orange sherbet in the summer, or vanilla and strawberry with strawberry sauce on top. The possibilities are endless.

SERVES 8 TO 12

- 1 angel food tube cake
- 2 flavors (½ gallon containers) ice cream of your choice
- 1 (16-ounce) container Cool Whip, softened, at room temperature
- Nuts of your choice
- Sauces of your choice
- **Cookware needed:** nonstick mold (ring or another shape), or a bundt pan

Break up the angel food cake into chunks about the size of a half-dollar.

Cover the bottom of the mold with a layer of cake, then add scoops of one ice cream flavor, another layer of cake, and the other ice cream flavor, alternating until you have filled the pan. Or fill it any way you like, mixing cake and ice cream together or adding sauce or nuts to the layers.

Freeze the cake for about 2 hours, then remove it from the pan by running a knife around the edge and turning it out onto a plate.

Return the cake to the freezer to harden, then ice it with Cool Whip.

Serve the cake with a bowl of hot fudge or a fruit sauce.

PREPARATION TIME: *15 minutes to assemble, 5 minutes to ice*
TOTAL TIME: *add about 2 hours to freeze*

Sage Advice

This is a good do-ahead dessert. You can assemble the cake in the mold a day or two before your party and cover it with plastic wrap. Unmold it the morning of the party, return it to the freezer, then quickly ice the cake at serving time.

The
Finishing Touch

Decorate your cake with live flowers in the summer, or with traditional ice cream toppings such as chocolate syrup or caramel sauce, M&Ms, crushed cookies, candy bars, nuts, or a dusting of colored sugar.

Allison's Vanilla Crisps

ALLISON MOORE started baking these cookies when she was about six years old. She's now all of twelve and on her way to becoming a great cook (a talent she has inherited from her father, Jeff, according to her mother, Cyndee).

Allison found the recipe in one of her grandmother's old cookbooks (printed in 1947). Together, they made some modifications (used self-rising flour instead of all-purpose flour, cut back on the vanilla, etc.), which resulted in this updated recipe.

This revised old-fashioned treat is such a simple recipe that from the start Allison was able to make the batter herself, although Grandma helped with the oven. Now Allison makes them any time the family is in the mood for something sweet.

By the way, her family considers them the most delicious cookies in the world. What better recommendation could you ask for?

MAKES ABOUT 5 DOZEN ABSOLUTELY DELICIOUS COOKIES—AND THAT'S A QUOTE

1 stick butter

1 cup sugar

2 eggs, beaten

1 teaspoon vanilla extract

1 ⅓ cups self-rising flour

Cookware needed: mixing bowl, cookie sheet

Preheat the oven to 400 degrees.

Soften the butter and blend in the sugar. Add the eggs and beat the mixture until fluffy.

Stir in the vanilla and the flour.

Drop the cookies from a tablespoon onto a nonstick cookie sheet.

Bake for 8 minutes, or until slightly brown around the edges.

PREPARATION TIME: *15 minutes*

TOTAL TIME: *approximately 45 minutes*

Chinese Chews

I HADN'T made Chinese Chews since I was home for Christmas vacation when I was in college. In truth, I had forgotten all about them. Then Gaenell Stegall reminded me of them.

Immediately, I began plotting how my grandchildren, Benjamin and Matthew, could help me make these delectable treats for Christmas in just a year or so. But wait. That's a couple of years down the road. I can't wait that long, and neither should you.

MAKES 2 TO 3 DOZEN CHEWS

1 (12-ounce) package
    butterscotch morsels

½ cup peanut butter

1 (8-ounce) can salted peanuts

1 (5-ounce) can chow mein
    noodles

Cookware needed: saucepan

Stir the butterscotch morsels and the peanut butter together in a saucepan over medium heat, until the butterscotch is melted. Or melt the mixture in a microwave.

Add the peanuts and the chow mein noodles and stir until well blended.

Drop the mixture by spoonfuls onto wax paper and set the chews aside to cool.

Variation:

Use 1 (6-ounce) package butterscotch morsels and 1 (6-ounce) package chocolate chips.

PREPARATION TIME: *15 minutes*
TOTAL TIME: *about 1 hour to cool*

English Trifle

JUST the name alone is enticing—English Trifle. Actually, I've been told it should be Scottish Trifle, but on this side of the Atlantic, I wouldn't think the exact origin mattered much.

What *does* matter is that this time-proven favorite, which used to take hours to prepare, can now be turned out in a matter of minutes. No longer must the pudding be made in a double-boiler and the cake made from scratch. Thank goodness!

Something else that does matter is the inclusion of spirits—in this case, usually sherry. This is the sort of dessert into which, in olden days, even a teetotaler would manage to slip a little "spirit" for that once-a-year holiday treat. It absolutely brings all the flavors to life.

SERVES 10 TO 12

½ cup (or more) sherry

1 ½ cups prepared vanilla pudding or boiled custard

1-pound Sara Lee or other frozen, pound cake

½ (12-ounce) jar strawberry or raspberry preserves

Slivered almonds (toasted are best)

2 cups whipped cream

Cookware needed: mixing bowl

Add the sherry to the vanilla pudding and stir well.

Slice the pound cake while still slightly frozen.

Spread each slice with the strawberry preserves.

Lay a bottom layer of cake in a pretty crystal bowl. Sprinkle the cake with almonds. Top with the sherry and pudding mixture and a layer of whipped cream. Repeat until all the ingredients have been used. (Save a few almonds to sprinkle on the top.)

PREPARATION TIME: *10 to 15 minutes*
TOTAL TIME: *20 to 30 minutes (if you toast the almonds at the time)*

Lazy Woman Peach Cobbler

GAENELL STEGALL, who reminded me of Chinese Chews (page 265), cooks like I do. She uses every shortcut and convenience food available to turn out excellent *From Storebought to Homemade* dishes while expending a minimum of time and effort. This Lazy Woman Peach Cobbler is a good example. It also fills the house with wonderful "baking" aromas while you assemble the rest of the meal from already prepared items.

SERVES ABOUT 8

1 stick butter
1 cup all-purpose flour
1 cup milk

1 (15-ounce) can (or more) peaches, lightly drained
Cookware needed: baking dish or casserole

Preheat the oven to 350 degrees.

Melt the butter in the baking dish you are going to use.

Combine the flour and the milk, and pour the mixture over the butter.

Add the peaches and some juice and bake for 30 minutes.

PREPARATION TIME: *10 minutes or less*
TOTAL TIME: *approximately 40 minutes*

Sage Advice

You may substitute half-and-half for the milk for a much richer cobbler. Adding a little more of the peach juices will add additional flavor. Remember, too, these days canned peaches aren't just canned peaches... there are variations, like cinnamon-flavored peaches or harvest peaches that have spices already included. Try using some of these more richly flavored varieties in this easy dish, or doctor up the basic recipe by adding your own sprinkle of cinnamon or a dab or two of brown sugar. Also, remember to experiment. Try blueberries or cherries or blackberries, for example. There are many ways to make a "fruit" cobbler.

Serendipity Pumpkin Cake

WANT TO START a conversation? Read a cookbook in public.

That's what happened the day in the Houston airport that I was reading *Lagniappe,* the cookbook published by the Beaumont, Texas, Junior League.

"What are you cooking?" the attractive young woman who sat down beside me asked, as she peeped over my shoulder.

"Just checking out a recipe I was told is wonderful—and easy," I answered.

That was all she needed to hear.

"Let me tell you about the best recipe I've ever cooked," she offered. "Everyone always raves about it. And it's so easy!"

In no time, this friendly stranger was rattling off the recipe, finishing it up just as the final boarding announcement for her flight was being called. In the rush, I barely got her name, Laurie Harlow ("like the actress," she said). But I got the recipe!

Laurie was right. This recipe *is* something to rave about, and a perfect dessert to have around the holidays when time is at a premium. I've decided to call it Serendipity Pumpkin Cake in honor of our fleeting meeting.

SERVES APPROXIMATELY 12

For the cake:

1 (30-ounce) can pumpkin pie filling

1 box yellow cake mix

1 (2.5-ounce) package slivered almonds, toasted

1 stick butter, melted

For the frosting:

2 tablespoons confectioners' sugar

1 teaspoon vanilla extract

1 (8-ounce) package cream cheese, softened

1 (12-ounce) container Cool Whip, softened, at room temperature

Cookware needed: mixing bowl, 9 x 13-inch baking dish or casserole

Preheat the oven to 375 degrees.

Line a 9 x 13-inch baking dish with wax paper.

Prepare the pumpkin pie filling as directed on the can, or use one that is already flavored and ready to go into the pie crust, and spread it evenly on the wax paper.

Distribute the yellow cake mix (your choice—Pillsbury, Duncan Hines, a store brand, whatever, Laurie said) over the pumpkin mixture.

Sprinkle the almonds over the cake mix and drizzle the butter over all.

Bake for 30 minutes, or until set.

Remove the pan from the oven, allow the cake to cool, then turn the pan upside down, and pull off the wax paper.

To make the frosting, combine the confectioners' sugar, the vanilla, and the cream cheese. Mix this into the Cool Whip, and frost the cake.

■ ▪ ▪ ▪ ▪ ▪ ▪ ▪ ■

PREPARATION TIME: *30 minutes*
TOTAL TIME: *1 hour and 10 to 15 minutes*

Sage Advice
Laurie said she first made this cake when she was living in Huwull, and used crushed Macadamia nuts instead of the almonds. Almonds, walnuts, Macadamia nuts—the choice is yours.

John Josselyn, an ancient ancestor of mine on my father's side, wrote about what he found in New England when he arrived there in 1663. Included in his book, *New England Rarities Discovered* (London, 1672), is this instruction on how the housewives cook pumpkins. Once "stewed," they would then add butter, vinegar, and spice "as Ginger, &c" to make it "tart like an Apple," and serve with fish or meat.

"...When ripe, and cut them [pumpkins]
into dice, and so fill a pot with them of two or
three Gallons, and stew them upon a gentle fire a
whole day, and as they sink,...fill again with
fresh Pompions [pumpkins], not putting any
liquor [water or broth] to them; and when it is
stew'd enough, it will look like bak'd Apples...."

Bread Pudding

"**OLD FASHIONED** bread pudding, that's what I miss these days," a friend of mine said with a sigh, as he turned away the dessert menu in a fancy California restaurant.

So I was thrilled, many years later, when the nice young waitress at the very elegant Thomasville, Georgia, antiques show's Patrons' Dinner asked our table, "And would you like some bread pudding?" A unanimous YES resounded!

"Bread pudding has to be the world's oldest dessert," my host, John Breison, remarked.

Which reminds me of yet another comment a friend of mine made about bread pudding last Christmas.

Tony Muncey, a fabulous chef and CIA (Culinary Institute of America) graduate, joked that if there had been really *good* bread pudding in New Orleans the British would never have allowed themselves to be defeated there.

With bread pudding apparently on so many people's minds, I decided to include a basic recipe you can throw together in just a few minutes, with a *Finishing Touch* idea to dress it up a little if you choose.

The thing to remember about bread pudding is that it truly is delicious and very filling. It makes the perfect ending to any meal—formal or casual, company or family, seated or buffet. And, best of all, if you end a meal of rotisserie chicken, deli-mashed potatoes, and cello-bag lettuce salad with this long-favored "homemade" dessert—everyone will think you made the whole meal from scratch!

SERVES 8

4 cups French bread, preferably day-old, cubed

1 cup sugar

3 cups milk

2 eggs, beaten

2 cups raisins or currants

2 cup chopped pecans (optional)

1 tablespoon lemon zest, or even Cointreau

3 tablespoons vanilla extract

½ teaspoon cinnamon

1 recipe Hard Sauce (recipe follows), or 1 recipe Whiskey Sauce (page 272)

Cookware needed: 2-quart baking dish or casserole

Preheat the oven to 350 degrees.

Place the bread in a 2-quart baking dish.

Combine the sugar, the milk, and the eggs.

Add the raisins, pecans, lemon zest or Cointreau, vanilla, and cinnamon.

Pour the mixture over the bread.

Bake the pudding for 1 hour 15 minutes.

Serve hot with Hard Sauce or warm with Whiskey Sauce, if you wish.

PREPARATION TIME: *15 minutes*
(plus more if you make the Hard or Whiskey Sauce)
TOTAL TIME: *1 hour and 30 minutes*

The
Finishing Touch

For a special occasion, turn bread pudding into a Queen of Puddings. Do this by spreading your favorite jelly (black cherry is good) over the pudding after it is baked and still warm. Then make a meringue from scratch (see page 273) — supper was a whiz, so you have time to do this — or use Sauer's Egg White Magic. Apply the meringue in peaks to the pudding. Return it to the oven, set at 400 degrees, until the jelly is warmed and the meringue is nicely "tanned" and set, about 15 minutes.

"Food,
glorious food!"

—FROM *OLIVER*

Hard Sauce

MAKES ABOUT 1 ½ CUPS

Sage Advice

Many recipes call for whiskey in Hard Sauce, but since the Whiskey Sauce is given next, I've stuck with the vanilla here. Because Hard Sauce is hard and cold, serve it on a piping hot dessert—like bread pudding. It's like putting butter or sour cream on a baked potato.

5 tablespoons butter, softened

1 cup confectioners' sugar, sifted

Pinch of salt

1 tablespoon vanilla extract

½ cup half-and-half or heavy cream

Cookware needed: mixing bowl

To the butter (soft, not melted) gradually add the sugar, beating until well blended.

Add the pinch of salt and the vanilla, blending well.

Add the cream and beat continuously until the sauce is smooth, then refrigerate until it becomes "hard."

PREPARATION TIME: *5 to 6 minutes*
TOTAL TIME: *10 minutes plus the hardening time*

Whiskey Sauce

MAKES ABOUT 1 ⅓ CUPS

Sage Advice

You can prepare the Whiskey Sauce before dinner, up to adding the egg yolk. Cover the saucepan to keep it warm. When you are ready to serve, return the saucepan to very low heat and finish the sauce.

1 cup confectioners' sugar

½ stick butter

3 tablespoons half-and-half or heavy cream

1 egg yolk, lightly beaten

¼ cup whiskey (bourbon), the better the quality, the better the taste

Cookware needed: saucepan, mixing bowl

Combine the sugar, butter, and cream in a saucepan.

Cook over low heat until the sugar dissolves, stirring often with a wooden spoon.

Remove from the heat.

Put about ¼ of the hot sauce in a mixing bowl, and add the egg yolk, beating with a whisk until it is well blended.

Add this to the remaining sauce in the saucepan and whisk well.

Cool slightly (4 to 5 minutes), then stir in the bourbon. Serve over the warm pudding.

PREPARATION TIME: *10 minutes*
TOTAL TIME: *10 minutes*

Homemade Meringue

Whip 2 egg whites till frothy. Add ¼ teaspoon cream of tartar and continue to whip until curvy peaks form. You do not want to beat the egg whites until they are so dry that they are overly stiff. Add 4 tablespoons of confectioners' sugar, ½ to 1 teaspoon at a time. Finally add ½ teaspoon vanilla extract and beat just long enough to blend, and it's ready to use.

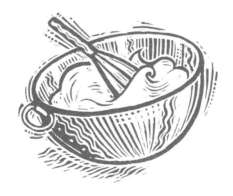

What's-in-It Ice Cream Dessert

MY LIFELONG FRIEND Anne Geyer should have written this book. I've told her so, but she's busy doing other things—like having casual dinner parties that are always relaxing and enjoyable. Why?

We should all learn from Anne's secret. She puts her emphasis on her guests and serves them delicious, but easily prepared dishes, like this wonderful ice cream dessert that I always hope will be on her menu when we're on her guest list. Thing is, I couldn't quite figure out exactly what the ingredients were.

Naturally, I asked Anne for her recipe. But rather than taking credit for it herself, Anne 'fessed up and said she must give credit where credit is due.

Anne got the recipe from her eldest daughter, Elizabeth—a busy wife, mother of two, and businesswoman in Athens, Georgia. In the Southern tradition, Elizabeth enjoys taking this dessert to friends who've had new babies, an illness or sadness in the family—or for just no reason at all.

When Elizabeth shared the recipe with her mother a few years ago, Anne admits, "I took it and ran!"

You will too—right to the grocery store to grab up the ingredients.

SERVES 12 OR MORE

12 to 16 ice cream sandwiches

1 (18-ounce) container Cool Whip, softened, at room temperature

1 pint vanilla ice cream

Chocolate sauce in a squeezable container

1 cup slivered almonds, toasted

2 ounces Kahlua

Cookware needed: large crystal bowl

"Ice" the interior of a crystal bowl large enough to hold the ingredients by putting it in the freezer till frost crystals appear, for a well-dressed appearance.

Cut the ice cream sandwiches in thirds for a good fit.

Now, begin to layer as follows: ice cream sandwich, Cool Whip, ice cream.

Spoon the Cool Whip and ice cream evenly over the sandwiches—the amount of each is up to you.

Drizzle chocolate sauce over the first layer, followed by almonds and Kahlua.

Start the layering over with more sandwiches and build several layers until you've reached the top, ending with lots of chocolate, almonds, and Kahlua on top.

Cover with plastic wrap and freeze for at least 8 hours, or for several days.

PREPARATION TIME: *15 minutes*

TOTAL TIME: *15 minutes, plus at least 8 hours "freezing" time*

You'll-Never-Guess-It's-Made-with-Cookies Icebox Dessert

AS FATE would have it, no sooner had Anne Geyer given me the recipe for What's-in-It Ice Cream Dessert, than my daughter said she'd just learned of an "icebox dessert," adding, "and you'd never guess it's made with cookies."

What's great about this dessert is that you can use whatever cookies you already have on hand, even though most of us would go with the chocolate variety.

It's as easy to make as Anne's dessert, and since it doesn't have the Kahlua, it's more of a family treat.

SERVES 8 OR MORE

1 cup milk

1 (21-ounce) package Keebler chocolate chip cookies (or another of your choosing)

1 (8-ounce) container Cool Whip, softened, at room temperature

¾ cup mini chocolate chips

¾ cup chopped pecans

Cookware needed. mixing bowl, deep casserole dish

Sage Advice

This is a wonderful recipe to prepare with the help of children. But be ready to fish an occasional cookie out of the milk, and to lose at least one or two cookies to the eager helpers themselves.

Pour the milk into a wide-mouthed measuring cup or bowl.

Dip approximately 10 cookies, one by one, into the milk for 5 to 6 seconds and then place them in the casserole. (At the end, you may need to break a cookie to fill in the corners.)

Cover this bottom layer with ⅓ of the Cool Whip, followed by ⅓ of the chocolate chips and ⅓ of the pecans.

Dip another 10 cookies and repeat this process another time.

Spread the third and final cookie and Cool Whip layer. At this point, crumble 4 or 5 additional cookies (dry—not dipped in milk) over it, then add the final ⅓ chocolate chips and pecans.

Cover the dessert with plastic wrap and chill for at least 8 hours.

PREPARATION TIME: *10 to 15 minutes*
TOTAL TIME: *15 minutes, plus 8 hours for chilling*

Cake Mix Cookies

MOST writers will tell you their most often-asked question is, "What made you write your book?"

Scores of people have asked me that very question about *From Storebought to Homemade*. When my son, Langdon, is around, he interjects, "Not *what*. Who? It was Barney. Remember those cookies he made. I've never seen you so mad in all your life, Mom."

Let me explain.

My former husband was a college president, and we used the school's catering service for many large events. Once, we were having the freshman class over for a picnic. For dessert I suggested to Barney (not his real name) that we might have really good homemade cookies—a special treat, I figured.

We got cookies all right. Cookies that the kids found worked better as Frisbees. They were the biggest and the worst cookies I've ever tasted. And ugly to boot.

"Next time," I vowed, "I'll make them myself."

And I did...but by the old time-consuming method of creaming the butter, adding the flour, vanilla, and sugar. You know the routine.

I had always looked for quick-and-easy recipes, but as the college president's wife, with so much entertaining to do—and never knowing exactly what I'd get from the catering service—I learned lots of ways to turn storebought items into "homemade" specialties.

If only I'd had Nancy Sweger's recipe for Cake Mix Cookies back then!

One thing is for sure—these days, when I come to the end of the Cake Mix Cookie dough, I always roll one extra-large cookie, about the size of a Frisbee, and mutter, "Barney, this one's for you!"

MAKES APPROXIMATELY 2 ½ DOZEN COOKIES

1 box cake mix of your choice
(see *Sage Advice*)

2 eggs, beaten

1 (8-ounce) container Cool Whip,
softened, at room temperature

1 cup confectioners' sugar

Cookware needed: mixing bowl,
cookie sheet

Sage Advice

The hardest part of this recipe is trying to decide what flavor cake mix to use—Lemon Supreme, Chocolate, White, or another one of your favorites.

Preheat the oven to 350 degrees.

Mix the cake mix, the eggs, and the Cool Whip together with a fork.

Roll the dough into balls the size of a nickel, and roll them in the confectioners' sugar.

Place the cookies on a cookie sheet, allowing room for them to spread.

Bake for 10 minutes.

Let the cookies sit for 1 minute, then remove them to an airtight container.

PREPARATION TIME: *30 minutes*
TOTAL TIME: *40 to 60 minutes*

Brunch for the Bunch

IF FONDUE has made a comeback, then brunches can't be far behind.

I've always liked brunches—both as a hostess and a guest.

One reason I particularly enjoy having a brunch is that you can serve almost any food you can think of—from egg and cheese dishes to tenderloin.

When I began thinking about which of my favorite dishes I usually prepare for this late-morning or noontime gathering, I realized that I serve a wide variety of selections—from Crab Imperial (page 99, usually an entrée but served on toast, rather than rice, for a brunch) to Cheese Garlic Grits (page 192), which appears in the Salads, Vegetables, Potatoes and Rice chapter.

So I decided to include the more traditional brunch dishes here, but also to provide a short list of recipes that appear in other chapters that work equally well for a brunch. That list appears on page 300.

Brunch provides the host or hostess with a perfect opportunity to serve a wide variety of jellies and condiments. Most farmers' markets and quaint stores have all kinds of berry jellies and preserves, and grocery store shelves are filled with vast numbers of pickles and relishes that I'm always dying to try.

If you're worried about what to serve these goodies in, don't be. You can buy unmatched saucers, that long ago lost their cups, for only a few cents at most flea markets and yard sales. Gather up a collection and have them on hand for your next brunch or buffet. The array of the condiments and colorful saucers will add charm and interest to your table.

"Condiments are like old friends—highly thought of, but often taken for granted."

MARILYN KAYTOR,
LOOK, JANUARY 29, 1963

Not-Just-for-Brunch Casserole

IF YOU haven't fixed this casserole, you must be the *only* person who hasn't!

Of all the recipes shared with me when I mentioned *From Storebought to Homemade*, this was the one I received most frequently. Interestingly, unlike many casseroles that have been around for some time (I first made it when the kids were about 8 and 10, so that was some 23 years ago now), this is one that has never been forgotten. To this day I make it for our Christmas breakfast.

But it isn't just a party or special-occasion recipe. Should you be a busy mother worried about feeding your children a good hot breakfast—or dinner for that matter—try preparing this for them. The leftovers reheat well too.

SERVES 10 TO 12

10 slices bread, cubed (crusts removed if you wish—I don't)

1 pound bulk sausage (hot or mild), cooked and crumbled, or for a quicker version, 1 (8-ounce) package cooked, diced ham

1 (8-ounce) package Cheddar cheese, grated (or a cheese mixture)

8 eggs, beaten

4 cups milk

Salt and pepper, to taste

Cookware needed: skillet, mixing bowl, deep baking dish or casserole

Put the bread cubes in a greased deep baking dish.

Add the sausage (or the ham if you're using that) and the cheese to the baking dish.

Combine the eggs, milk, and salt and pepper and pour the mixture over all, making sure it doesn't overflow.

Cover and refrigerate the casserole overnight, or for at least 8 hours, so the custard is absorbed.

When ready to bake, preheat the oven to 350 degrees. Bake the casserole for 45 to 50 minutes

PREPARATION TIME: *10 minutes (plus 10 more minutes if you use the sausage)*
TOTAL TIME: *a little more than 1 hour, plus at least 8 hours to chill*

A Side of Beans

WILL CHILDREN be at the brunch? This ready-in-no-time dish will satisfy them if they turn up their noses to your other offerings—if the grownups leave any, that is.

SERVES 4 TO 6 (OR MORE CHILDREN)

1 (13-ounce) can B&M baked beans

1 tablespoon apple cider vinegar

2 tablespoons water

1 (16-ounce) package cocktail franks

⅓ cup Cheddar cheese, grated

Cookware needed: baking dish or casserole

Preheat the oven to 350 degrees.

Combine all the ingredients, or reserve the grated cheese to sprinkle on top, and pour the mixture into a lightly greased baking dish.

Bake for 20 to 30 minutes, or until bubbly.

PREPARATION TIME: *5 minutes*
TOTAL TIME: *approximately 35 minutes*

The
Finishing Touch

This is a dish that benefits from the crunch of some crumbled potato chips sprinkled on top with the cheese.

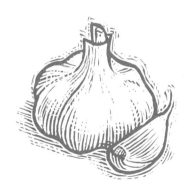

Eggnog Pancakes

EARLY ONE December morning, when the season and the weather screamed for pancakes, I discovered I had used my last egg the day before. It was then I remembered the trick for making Ice Cream Muffins (page 221). Ice cream would work here too I reasoned. But, while reaching into the refrigerator for some bacon, I saw a carton of Southern Comfort eggnog, a uniquely flavored nog, but without the spirits.

That morning we had the richest, fluffiest pancakes ever. They were so good, in fact, there was no reason to pass the syrup, just the butter.

SERVES 4 TO 6

2 cups pancake mix

1¾ to 2 cups eggnog, preferably
   Southern Comfort

Cookware needed: mixing bowl,
skillet

Sage Advice

If using all eggnog is too rich for your taste, or your cholesterol, use half eggnog and half milk. These eggnog pancakes will be very fluffy, so be forewarned if you like thin, flat pancakes.

Stir the pancake mix and eggnog together and drop the batter by spoonfuls onto a hot nonstick griddle or skillet.

PREPARATION TIME: *3 minutes*
TOTAL TIME: *10 to 15 minutes*

Baked Egg, Shrimp, and Cheese Delight

ONCE, when I served this casserole, a guest asked me what was in it. I began answering, "shrimp, Worcestershire sauce, cheese, garlic sauce...."

"Well!" she interrupted me. "Anything would be good with shrimp, Worcestershire sauce, cheese, and garlic in it!"

I have to agree.

SERVES 4 TO 6

1 cup Ragú Roasted Garlic Parmesan sauce

Cayenne pepper

Worcestershire sauce

2 cups medium, cleaned and cooked shrimp (either from the fresh seafood counter or from the frozen food section)

1 cup Cheddar cheese, grated

6 hard-boiled eggs, chopped

Cookware needed: baking dish or casserole

Sage Advice

If you have the Egg Wave™ gadget to hard boil the eggs, you avoid the tedious task of shelling them after they are cooked. But if you don't have a microwave oven, or the Egg Wave™, you can buy already hard-boiled eggs from the salad bar the same way you buy sliced celery.

Preheat the oven to 375 degrees.

Season the sauce generously with the cayenne and Worcestershire. (You can do this right in the measuring cup.)

Combine the sauce with the shrimp, cheese, and eggs in a buttered baking dish.

Bake until piping hot, about 35 minutes.

PREPARATION TIME: *15 minutes*
TOTAL TIME: *approximately 50 minutes*

Your Mother's Basic Quiche Recipe

Quiche has suffered a bad rap since your mother or grandmother used to make it. You know, the "real men don't eat..." tag line.

But as I said, if fondue can have a comeback, then brunches can't be far behind. And how can you have a brunch without quiche?

When quiche was all the rage, several "instant" varieties were available in the milk or freezer bins at the grocery store. Those can be hard to find these days. But, actually, it takes no more time to stir up the egg and milk base to make a quiche than it does to open a carton of "instant" quiche mix to pour into your frozen pie shell. Your mother will tell you (or you may remember yourself) that the time-consuming part of making a quiche was grating the cheese—but already grated cheese packs have taken care of that.

So try making a "homemade" quiche using the following formula. (It might even satisfy your "closet chef" yearnings for a while.)

The basic quiche recipe is as simple as remembering *1 to ¼—one large egg per quarter cup of milk.*

This translates into 2 large eggs and ½ cup of milk per pie shell (9-inch, not deep dish) for most quiches. But if you want to make several different quiches to put out, just the way you might make several different pies for a dessert buffet, or if you prefer to use a deep-dish pie shell, mix the eggs and milk to make the "custard" in one large batch, and pour the desired amount over whatever fillings you use.

The Proof Is in the Pie Crust

Nancy Sweger, my daughter's mother-in-law, is the only person I know who always makes her own pie crusts. The rest of us use frozen pie shells or the refrigerated pie doughs. Whichever you use—from scratch to ready-to-cook—while preparing the custard and ingredients, prepare the pie crust as follows:

- Preheat the oven to 350 degrees.
- Separate the white of one of the eggs to be used in the custard and beat it lightly. Pour the leftover egg white(s) into the quiche mixture.
- Brush a pie shell with a little of this egg white, using a pastry brush.
- Prick the bottom and sides of the pie shell with a fork.
- Bake the crust for 5 minutes (just about the amount of time it will take you to prepare the quiche for baking).

(Incidentally, you do not have to defrost a frozen pie shell.)

Sausage Quiche

THE SIMPLE QUICHE that combines those three breakfast favorites, eggs, sausage, and cheese, is a good recipe to start with.

SERVES 6

1 9-inch pie shell

3 large eggs, beaten

¾ cup milk

Salt and pepper, to taste

Cayenne pepper, to taste

1 pound cooked (hot or mild) bulk sausage

1 ½ cups Cheddar cheese, grated—*sharp* is best

Cookware needed: skillet, mixing bowl

Prepare the pie shell according to the directions above.

Do not turn off the oven.

Combine eggs, milk, and seasonings and beat lightly until well blended.

Stir in the sausage and pour the mixture into the prepared pie shell.

Distribute the cheese on top and bake for 40 to 45 minutes.

PREPARATION TIME: *15 minutes*

TOTAL TIME: *approximately 60 minutes*

Broccoli and Ham Quiche

MANY a mother has persuaded her children (even the boys) to eat their broccoli by preparing this broccoli and ham quiche. It works just as well as a brunch dish for grown-ups.

SERVES 6

■ ■ ■ ■ ■ ■ ■ ■

1 9-inch pie shell
6 large eggs, beaten
1 cup milk
½ cup sour cream
Salt and pepper, to taste
¾ cup broccoli florets, frozen or fresh

¼ to ½ cup small diced ham bits (these are available in vacuum sealed packages, as well as at the salad bar)
½ cup Cheddar cheese, grated
Cookware needed: mixing bowl

Prepare the pie shell according to the directions on page 285.

Do not turn off the oven.

Combine the eggs, milk, sour cream, and seasonings and beat lightly until well blended.

Stir in the broccoli, ham, and cheese, and pour the mixture into the prepared pie shell.

Bake for 40 to 45 minutes.

■ ■ ■ ■ ■ ■ ■ ■

PREPARATION TIME: *5 minutes*
TOTAL TIME: *approximately 50 minutes*

Fancy Crabmeat Quiche

THIS SOPHISTICATED and rich quiche uses whipped cream in place of milk (which makes for a different egg to liquid proportion), Swiss rather than Cheddar cheese, and fills a deep-dish pie shell. The recipe does call for sautéing the bacon, but the taste makes it worth it.

SERVES 6 TO 8

1 deep-dish pie shell

4 strips bacon

½ cup frozen, diced onion

1 (8-ounce) package Swiss cheese, grated

1 (6-ounce) can crabmeat

4 large eggs, beaten

1 ½ cups whipped cream

2 tablespoons dry sherry

¼ teaspoon nutmeg

Salt and pepper, to taste

Cookware needed: skillet, mixing bowl

Prepare the pie shell according to the directions on page 285. For this larger size, bake 8 to 10 minutes.

Sauté the bacon, remove it to a paper towel to drain, and reserve the drippings in the pan.

Sauté the onion in the bacon drippings. Crumble the drained bacon.

Sprinkle 1 cup of the grated Swiss cheese in the bottom of the pie shell.

Layer the crabmeat over the cheese, followed by the crumbled bacon and the onion.

Combine the eggs, cream, sherry, and seasonings, and pour the mixture into the shell.

Top with the remaining Swiss cheese.

Bake for about 40 to 45 minutes.

PREPARATION TIME: *20 minutes*
TOTAL TIME: *approximately 1 hour and 10 minutes*

No-Pie-Shell Quiche

SHOULD you not have a pie crust handy, or if you happen to have extra "custard," try this version of quiche that makes its own crust.

SERVES 8

3 eggs

1 stick butter

1 ½ cups milk

½ cup Bisquick

¼ teaspoon salt

Dash pepper

1 cup Cheddar or Swiss cheese, grated (or a combination to your liking)

½ cup chopped ham (or use bacon or sausage)

1 (10-ounce) bag frozen, chopped broccoli, defrosted

1 (4-ounce) can sliced mushrooms, drained

Cookware needed: blender; pie pan, baking dish or casserole

Preheat the oven to 350 degrees.

Put the eggs, butter, milk, Bisquick, salt, and pepper in a blender.

Blend well, stir in the cheese, and pour half the mixture into a greased pie pan.

Press the broccoli, mushrooms, and ham into the cheese and custard mixture.

Top this layer with the remaining cheese and custard mixture.

Bake for 45 minutes.

Turn off the oven and allow the quiche to set for 10 minutes.

PREPARATION TIME: *10 minutes*
TOTAL TIME: *a little more than 1 hour*

Sage Advice

Once again, the ingredients you choose to put into this quiche can be determined by your personal preference. Frozen asparagus pieces might be substituted for the broccoli, for example, or you can leave out the mushrooms but toss in some toasted almonds.

Legendary Cheese Pie

MY FRIEND ANNE GEYER and I belong to some of the same civic groups and clubs, and invariably we are called on to "bring a dish" to a luncheon meeting or reception. While I'm fretting over what to take, Anne is at home whipping together her Legendary Cheese Pie. And when she doesn't bring it, I'm always disappointed.

Like many cheese-and-egg–based dishes, this one is very versatile and can be served at a brunch, for a formal luncheon, or, cut into small pieces, as an appetizer at a cocktail party.

SERVES 8 (OR 24 AS AN APPETIZER)

10 large eggs

½ cup flour

1 teaspoon salt

1 stick butter, melted

1 (8-ounce) package Monterey Jack cheese, grated

1 (8-ounce) package sharp Cheddar cheese, grated

1 (16-ounce) container small curd cottage cheese

1 (4-ounce) can chopped green chili peppers, drained

Cookware needed: mixing bowl, 9 x 13-inch baking dish or casserole

Preheat the oven to 350 degrees.

Beat the eggs until light in color.

Add the flour, salt, butter, cheeses, and chili peppers, and stir to blend.

Pour mixture into a lightly greased 9 x 13-inch baking dish.

Bake for 35 to 40 minutes.

Cool slightly before cutting.

PREPARATION TIME: *10 minutes*
TOTAL TIME: *approximately 45 minutes*

Quick Breakfast Ring

THIS LONG-TIME favorite is sweet, and probably one that you may be familiar with. Read through the basic recipe given below, but before making it, check out some of the possible variations in *Sage Advice.* You may prefer one of those.

SERVES 16 TO 20

¼ cup brown sugar, packed

6 tablespoons butter or margarine, melted

2 tablespoons pecan halves

6 maraschino cherries, cut in half

½ cup granulated sugar

2 teaspoons cinnamon

2 (8-ounce) cans refrigerator biscuits

Cookware needed: 10-inch ring mold

Preheat the oven to 425 degrees.

Mix the brown sugar with 2 tablespoons of the butter. Spread the butter and sugar into the bottom of a 10-inch ring mold.

Arrange the nuts and cherries, cut side up, on the brown sugar.

Combine the granulated sugar and the cinnamon.

Dip each biscuit into the remaining melted butter. Then roll it in the sugar-cinnamon mixture.

Arrange the biscuits in the mold so that they are slightly overlapping.

Bake for 12 to 15 minutes.

Unmold onto serving plate immediately. The butter usually prevents the mold from sticking, but if it does stick, loosen with a knife or spatula.

PREPARATION TIME: *15 minutes*
TOTAL TIME: *30 minutes*

Sage Advice

For some variety, try these combinations for the topping: substitute 1 cup walnuts, or almonds for the pecans (without the cherries, this variation is similar to the well-known favorite, "Monkey Bread"); use a granola mixture instead of the pecans and cherries; instead of cherries, use grated orange peel.

Ham-Stuffed Apples

YOU MAY HAVE read in the Introduction my suggestion for using a fruit or vegetable as an individual serving dish. These ham-stuffed apples do just that, and they don't take very long to prepare, especially if you're having only a few guests. But I wouldn't undertake making a dozen or so of these.

SERVES 6

6 large, red unpeeled apples

8 ounces ready-to-serve cooked ham cubes or bits

2 tablespoons butter, melted

⅓ cup raisins, brown or golden

⅓ cup chopped pecans

3 tablespoons brown sugar

½ to 1 cup apple juice

Cookware needed: mixing bowl, baking dish or casserole

Cut the tops off the apples and scoop out the core with some of the fruit, but be sure to leave a thick shell to hold the stuffing.

Preheat the oven to 350 degrees.

Put approximately 1 cup of the removed apple fruit in a mixing bowl and combine it with the ham, butter, raisins, pecans, and brown sugar, mixing the ingredients well.

Spoon this mixture into the cored apples and place them in a baking dish.

Pour the juice over the apples and bake for 35 to 40 minutes, basting occasionally with the juice.

PREPARATION TIME: *30 to 40 minutes*
TOTAL TIME: *approximately 1 hour and 15 minutes*

Sausage-Apple Ring

THIS MAKE-AHEAD Sausage-Apple Ring is good any time of the year, but my Raleigh, North Carolina, friend, Judy Root, says it is particularly good to have during the Christmas season. So good, in fact, that her daughter, Susan Jordan, who lives in Paris, even dares to serve it there.

Incidentally, because you don't have to cook the sausage first, this dish is easily and quickly assembled.

SERVES 6 TO 8

Pam, or other vegetable cooking spray

2 pounds bulk sausage, hot or mild, or a combination of the two

1 cello-pack saltines (approximately 42), crushed

½ cup milk

1 cup peeled and diced apples

3 eggs, lightly beaten

Cookware needed: mixing bowl, ring mold, or if you have one, a bundt pan

Preheat the oven to 350 degrees.

Spray, or grease, a ring mold well, even if it is nonstick.

Combine the ingredients and spread the mixture evenly in the pan.

Bake for 1 hour.

Turn the pan upside down to drain on a plate covered with paper towels. (Obviously you don't want the grease draining on your countertop.)

Use a spatula to loosen the edges of the ring and unmold it onto a serving plate (or, if planning to reheat, onto an ovenproof or microwaveable plate) and serve at once, or refrigerate it until you are ready to reheat it.

PREPARATION TIME: *10 minutes*
TOTAL TIME: *1 hour and 15 minutes*

Parmesan Asparagus

IN THE LIST of additional recipes suitable for brunches (page 300), you will find several fruit or vegetable dishes from the Salads, Vegetables, Potatoes and Rice chapter (page 128). But this simple Parmesan Asparagus makes such a nice presentation on a buffet table that I have included it here.

SERVES 4 TO 6

2 (10-ounce) boxes frozen asparagus

2 tablespoons butter, melted

¼ cup dry white wine

¼ teaspoon freshly ground pepper

½ to ¾ cup Parmesan cheese, grated, or more, to taste

Cookware needed: baking dish or casserole

Preheat the oven to 400 degrees.

Cook the asparagus according to package directions, being sure not to overcook them.

Drain and place them in a shallow baking dish.

Drizzle the butter and wine over the asparagus and sprinkle them with the freshly ground pepper.

Cover all with the Parmesan cheese, adding more if you wish.

Bake for about 10 minutes, or until the cheese melts.

PREPARATION TIME: *15 minutes*
TOTAL TIME: *25 to 30 minutes*

The
Finishing Touch

For a variation, arrange slices of large, ripe tomatoes in the baking dish and top each one with 3 or 4 asparagus spears. Follow with the rest of the ingredients to make individual servings of this nice vegetable dish.

Queenly Chicken Salad

WHEN QUEEN ELIZABETH II visited the University of Virginia, my alma mater, she was served a chicken salad fit for royalty, complete with green grapes and slivered almonds. But it's the curry powder and soy sauce, plus the pineapple, that make this a special delicacy indeed.

Ever since then, this very unusual, and definitely delicious Queenly Chicken Salad has been a favorite for brunches and special luncheons.

SERVES 5

2 cups Time Trimmer, or other ready-to-serve chicken pieces, unflavored

¾ cup mayonnaise

2 teaspoons lemon juice

1 teaspoon curry powder (optional)

2 teaspoons soy sauce

1 (5-ounce) can sliced water chestnuts, drained

½ pound seedless grapes, halved

½ cup chopped celery

½ cup toasted slivered almonds

1 (8-ounce) can pineapple chunks, drained

Cookware needed: mixing bowl

The
Finishing Touch

Treat your friends and family like royalty and serve this on a pretty leaf of lettuce topped with extra slivered almonds or a swirl of lemon peel. Garnish the plate with a small bunch of grapes. And always remember to wear your very best jewelry.

Set the chicken pieces out to thaw, if necessary.

Combine the mayonnaise with the lemon juice and other seasonings.

Toss thoroughly with the chicken and remaining ingredients.

Chill in the refrigerator for 2 to 3 hours.

PREPARATION TIME: *15 minutes*
TOTAL TIME: *approximately 3 hours*

Coke-Cooked Dogs

LOOKING FOR SOMETHING you can do at the last minute for a casual brunch or backyard picnic? Many's the time I've surveyed a table set with storebought fried chicken, a big bowl of homemade Pickled Cole Slaw (page 131), a casserole of delicious Jalapeño Corn Bread (page 230), and panicked.

That's when it's time for Larry Aaron's Coke-Cooked Hot Dogs, a recipe he learned from his mom, Evelyn Groff Aaron. They're a little like my favorite, Everyone's Favorite... Meatballs (page 65) appetizer. They're cooked in a secret ingredient (in this instance the Coke) that adds an unidentifiable zing and keeps everyone guessing, "What makes them so good?"

The
Finishing Touch

Just serve in a warm bowl or on a platter, with a basket of buns and small dishes of the usual condiments nearby, or cut into small pieces and spear with toothpicks.

SERVES 0 TO 10 (OR MORE IF USED AS AN APPETIZER)

1 (12-ounce) can or bottle
  Coca-Cola
1 tablespoon ketchup or
  barbeque sauce

1 pound hot dogs
Cookware needed: skillet

Combine the Coke and ketchup or barbeque sauce in a skillet.

Prick the hot dogs with a fork.

Simmer the hot dogs in the liquid for about 5 minutes or until thoroughly hot.

PREPARATION TIME: *5 minutes*
TOTAL TIME: *10 minutes*

Open House Shrimp, Virginia-Style

TRUST ME! Don't let the long list of ingredients or the instructions frighten you off. This is a wonderful recipe that will make a hit at your next large party. Furthermore, as I suggest, you can kill two birds with one stone by preparing this recipe—food for your party and Christmas remembrances for your friends. Read on!

Kaye Anne Davis Aikins has eaten or served her mother's pickled shrimp every Christmas Eve since she was tall enough to reach the dining-room table. "No matter where we were living, Mother always cooked what she called her Virginia pickled shrimp," Kaye Anne fondly remembers. "And now I'm fixing it for my grandchildren." That makes this a four-generation Davis-Aikins family favorite.

It is so much a tradition, in fact, that it was served to the 400-plus guests at her family's Sea Island, Georgia, home when Kaye Anne's father, Bill Davis, celebrated his 95th birthday.

Of course, when Kaye Anne's mother, Alice Davis, was fixing her Virginia pickled shrimp, it took hours and hours to shell those succulent sea creatures we all love so much.

Thank goodness we can now buy the packages of frozen, shelled, and deveined raw shrimp (with tails left on) that make this family recipe a real cinch.

This is an easy recipe, but you will need a large jar to hold the ingredients. And, as I suggested at the outset, because it yields more shrimp than you can possibly use at one party, and because it can be made 4 or 5 days in advance, it's a great way to make neighborhood Christmas gifts *and* party food with a minimum of effort.

Sage Advice

Do not use already cooked shrimp as a shortcut. The shrimp need to be freshly cooked and still hot to absorb the flavor of the pickling sauce while they are cooling.

SERVES A HOUSE FULL OF SHRIMP-LOVING GUESTS!

For the Pickling Juices:

7 teaspoons salt

3 to 4 teaspoons pepper, cracked or freshly ground

2 teaspoons confectioners' sugar

2 teaspoons dry mustard

A pinch of cayenne pepper

1 cup distilled white vinegar

2 cups olive oil

2 cups water

Juice of 2 lemons

For Shrimp preparation:

10 cups water

5 pounds frozen, uncooked, peeled and deveined, ready-to-cook shrimp

2 (12-ounce) bags frozen, diced onion, defrosted and drained on paper towels (or 10 to 15 small onions, sliced or diced)

2 ounces whole bay leaves

Cookware needed: mixing bowl, 10-gallon pot, very large jar

The Finishing Touch

Serve with Ritz crackers and fancy toothpicks nearby. There's no need to have a cocktail sauce for these spicy treats.

Thoroughly mix the first 5 ingredients with the vinegar. Combine the olive oil, water and lemon juice, then add—*very* slowly—to the vinegar mixture, stirring to blend thoroughly. Set aside.

Bring the 10 cups of water to a boil and add the shrimp.

When the water comes back to a boil (after a minute of two), pour it off immediately. Do not allow the shrimp to boil or sit in the water.

In a very large jar, assemble the following layers immediately (this must be done while the shrimp are still warm in order for all the flavors to be absorbed): (1) shrimp; (2) onions; (3) bay leaves.

Repeat the layers until all the ingredients have been used.

Stir the vinegar and oil mixture again and slowly pour it over the ingredients in the jar.

Tightly screw on the top of the jar and place it in the refrigerator.

At least 3 times a day, turn the jar over to be sure all the shrimp are being properly "pickled."

To serve, empty the contents of the jar into a bowl. With a slotted spoon, scoop up the shrimp and whatever onions cling to them, and place them in a large serving dish.

PREPARATION TIME: *30 minutes*

TOTAL TIME: *2 to 3 days minimum to become really flavorful*

Lynda Bird Johnson Robb's Hot Spinach Casserole

WHEN LYNDA ROBB was a guest in our home, my Republican daughter, Joslin, was most excited. Not because Lynda was President Johnson's daughter, or Senator Robb's wife, but because her recipe for a hot spinach casserole had long been one of Joslin's favorite company dishes. You see, Lynda has long lived in Virginia, where her husband was a senator, and her recipe is a favorite among Virginians.

Lynda says that even people, who don't like spinach ask for seconds of this spicy dish.

Your guests will too...whatever state they live in.

Sage Advice

Have no fear, this casserole is a favorite of Democrats and Republicans alike.

SERVES 6 TO 8

2 (10-ounce) packages frozen, chopped spinach

2 to 3 tablespoons frozen, chopped onion

4 tablespoons butter

2 tablespoons all-purpose flour

1 (5-ounce) can evaporated milk

Freshly ground black pepper, to taste

¾ teaspoon celery salt

¾ teaspoon crushed garlic

1 teaspoon Worcestershire sauce

Small dash cayenne pepper

1 (6-ounce) roll jalapeño cheese, cut into small pieces

Croutons

Cookware needed: medium saucepan, skillet, baking dish or casserole

Preheat the oven to 350 degrees.

Cook the spinach according to package directions. Drain well, reserving ½ cup of the cooking liquid.

Sauté the onion in the butter. Add the flour and mix well.

Stir in the evaporated milk and the reserved spinach liquid (a whisk is a good tool for this).

Season the mixture with the pepper, celery salt, garlic, Worcestershire sauce, and cayenne pepper. Add the jalapeño cheese and stir until the cheese is melted.

Add the cooked spinach and blend well.

Pour the mixture into a baking dish and top it with the croutons.

Bake for 30 minutes or until bubbly.

PREPARATION TIME: *20 minutes*

TOTAL TIME: *50 minutes*

Oranges Vermouth

BY NOW you know that many of these *From Storebought to Homemade* recipes were given to me by friends and acquaintances, but the other day someone asked me *why* people give away their favorite recipes.

Her question brought back memories of the occasional time when I've asked someone for a recipe—a compliment because the dish was so delicious—only to have my request refused. Or worse, to be given the recipe, but with an essential ingredient omitted. Either way, those few experiences have left a bad taste in my mouth, so to speak.

Her question also brought to mind the wonderful comment made by my friend Mina Wood when I told her about this cookbook. She said, "Oh, I'd like to share a couple of my recipes in your cookbook so my daughters-in-law, who are wives, mothers, and career women, and other young girls like them, can have them."

I can't imagine a more generous thought. To me it exemplifies sharing the best you have with those you love in order to enhance their lives.

So, for Alex, Lalla, and Anne Wood, and for others like them, here's a wonderful dessert recipe that makes a light and delicious finale for a fancy dinner party, a family gathering, or a brunch.

The
Finishing Touch

Serve the orange sections in pretty crystal dishes and garnish each serving with raspberries, strawberries, or a few seedless green grapes for complementary taste and color. Orange or raspberry chocolate candies, or orange-flavored Milano cookies, are also nice accompaniments.

SERVES 4

⅓ cup sugar

½ cup vermouth

2 whole cloves

4 large seedless oranges, or a jar of orange sections

Cookware needed: mixing bowl

Combine the sugar, vermouth, and whole cloves in a covered bowl.

Carefully peel the oranges and separate the sections, if using fresh. Place the oranges in the bowl, cover, and refrigerate overnight. Remove the cloves and serve.

PREPARATION TIME: *10 minutes, less if using bottled orange sections*
TOTAL TIME: *overnight for chilling*

Among the many other dishes in this book suitable for brunches are the following:

- Almost any recipe in Appetizers, especially Dressed Up English Muffins (page 53) and Curried Chicken Bits (page 63)
- Individual cups or mugs filled with a chilled or hot soup, including Love Apple Fromage (page 77), Chilled Strawberry (page 81), or Virginia Cream of Peanut Soup (page 80)
- Either beef or pork tenderloin, served cold and thinly sliced, or the Wild Rice and Sausage entrée (page 119), or Crab Imperial recipe (page 99), all in Easy Entrées
- A colorful jelled salad, such as Avocado or Tomato Aspic (page 143 or page 148) or the Mango Soufflé (page 146) is always a good choice
- And for the accompaniments, try a grits dish (pages 192-193), Scalloped Corn (page160), or a Baked Fruit dish (pages 176-177)

■ ■ ■ ■ ■ ■ ■

I'VE BEEN GIVEN this recipe many times, and by many names—Life's a Cake, the Happiness Cake, and the Cake of Human Kindness, for starters. But the first time it was shared with me was when I was giving a talk in Bartlesville, Oklahoma, many years ago. No matter what its name, it rings as true now as it did when it was first written:

1 cup good thoughts	2 cups sacrifice
1 cup kind deeds	2 cups well-beaten faults
1 cup consideration for others	3 cups forgiveness

Mix thoroughly. Add tears of Joy, Sorrow and Sympathy.

Flour with Love and Kindly service.

Fold in Prayer and Faith.

Pour all into your daily life. Bake with the heat of Human Kindness. Serve with a Smile. Serves all the Starved Souls who hunger.

Index